Atlas of Nail Disorders Across All Skin Colors

Shari R. Lipner

Atlas of Nail Disorders Across All Skin Colors

A Comprehensive Guide to Navigating Nails

Springer

Shari R. Lipner
Department of Dermatology
Weill Cornell Medicine
New York, NY, USA

ISBN 978-3-031-74271-2 ISBN 978-3-031-74272-9 (eBook)
https://doi.org/10.1007/978-3-031-74272-9

This Springer imprint is published by the registered company Springer Nature Switzerland AG
The registered company address is: Gewerbestrasse 11, 6330 Cham, Switzerland

To my husband, Igor, for his love, support, and inspiration.

To my beautiful children, Justin, Emily, and Evan, who bring me joy every day.

To my parents, Ferne and Henry, for their love, patience, support, and encouragement.

To my sisters and brother, Alyson, Lindsi, and Steven, for always being there for me.

In memory of my grandparents, Idee and Jack, for their love and devotion and whom I miss every day.

Preface

While there are many dermatology and nail disorder atlases that are available, none thus far include images from a wide range of skin colors. The impetus for writing this atlas was based on our prior studies showing that there is a scarcity of images of nail disorders in darker-skinned individuals in dermatology textbooks, nail disorder textbooks, journal articles, and Web-based dermatology curriculums for medical students, residents, and attendings. We also found a strikingly similar paucity of images of nail disorders in public education print- and Web-based materials geared to laypeople and patients. We know that this dearth of images in darker-skinned individuals likely has a real impact, because we also found that darker-skinned individuals have longer time to diagnosis of certain nail conditions compared to light-skinned patients. Therefore, we aim to fill this knowledge gap in the diagnosis of nail disorders with this atlas of nail conditions that has equal numbers of images of light-, medium-, and dark-skinned patients. We hope that our work improves diagnosis and outcomes for patients with both common and uncommon nail disorders.

New York, NY, USA　　　　Shari R. Lipner

Acknowledgments

The writing of an atlas covering the broad scope of nail unit disorders across the skin spectrums is dependent on a group effort, which is possible only with the support and enthusiasm of many individuals. We are extremely grateful to Dr. Jane Bellet, Dr. Nilton Gioia Di Chiacchio, Holly Evans, Dr. Chander Grover, Dr. Eckart Haneke, Dr. Thomas Knackstedt, Dr. Bertrand Richert, Janice Schwartz, Dr. Antonella Tosti, and the Pachyonychia Congenita Project for all their image contributions.

I would like to thank Dr. Richard Scher, my mentor, my friend, my supporter, and my teacher, without whom none of this would have been possible.

I am extremely grateful to Rachel Hill, who was my right hand in organizing and coordinating the writing of the atlas. She diligently made changes to our outline and formatting as ideas for improvement arose and handled all the coordination with the co-authors and with the publisher. I appreciate all the time and effort that she dedicated to this project to pull this off seamlessly.

I am also very thankful to Rachel Hill, Kaya Curtis, and Eden Axler, who wrote the bulk of chapters in this atlas and really took this on completely as part of their 1-year nail disorder research fellowship.

I would like to thank each and every one of the medical students and resident authors for writing and working with me on numerous drafts and for collecting the broad range of images that make this atlas so useful and special.

Finally, I would like to thank the entire staff at Springer, particularly Michelle Tam and Lee Klein, who were extremely supportive from the first idea of this atlas to its completion.

Contents

Contributors

Eden Axler, BS Albert Einstein College of Medicine, Bronx, NY, USA

Zi-Ning Choo, BS Weill Cornell Medical College, New York, NY, USA

Kaya L. Curtis, BA Weill Cornell Medical College, New York, NY, USA

Noelle Desir, BA Weill Cornell Medical College, New York, NY, USA

Rachel C. Hill, BS Weill Cornell Medical College, New York, NY, USA

Verena Isak, MD Department of Dermatology, Weill Cornell Medicine, New York, NY, USA

Apostolos Katsiaunis, BS Tufts University School of Medicine, Boston, MA, USA

Shari R. Lipner, MD, PhD Department of Dermatology, Weill Cornell Medicine, New York, NY, USA

Yuna Oh, MD Department of Dermatology, Weill Cornell Medicine, New York, NY, USA

Brianna Olamiju, MD Department of Dermatology, Weill Cornell Medicine, New York, NY, USA

Michael Ong, BS Weill Cornell Medicine, New York, NY, USA

Rachel E. Reingold, MD Department of Dermatology, Weill Cornell Medicine, New York, NY, USA

Jose W. Ricardo, MD Department of Dermatology, Weill Cornell Medicine, New York, NY, USA

Part I

Infectious Nail Disorders

Acute Paronychia

1

Apostolos Katsiaunis and Shari R. Lipner

1.1 Description of Disease

Acute paronychia (AP) is the most common hand infection and is characterized by erythema, edema, and pain involving the nail folds that resolves within six weeks [1, 2]. AP develops from disruption and bacterial invasion of the nail fold.

1.2 Epidemiology

1.2.1 Sex

AP affects both sexes equally. In a retrospective analysis by Desai et al. out of 2512 emergency department paronychia cases (both acute and chronic), 54.5% of patients were male [3]. Manicuring and needle-associated paronychia more commonly affected women (58.9% and 55.5%, respectively, $P < 0.0001$). Injuries with sports equipment and knives more commonly affected men (63.0%, and 61.5%, respectively (both $P < 0.0001$) [3].

1.2.2 Age

In the study of 2512 paronychia patients by Desai et al., the mean age was 27.6 ± 20.6 years [3]. Overall, 74.2% of patients reporting manicuring or beauty tools, 73.6% reporting needles or nails, and 79.5% reporting knives as the paronychia cause, were ages 21 years and over. In contrast, 68.8% of patients reporting doors or drawers, and 87.4% reporting sports equipment as the paronychia cause were under the age of 21 years [3].

S. R. Lipner, *Atlas of Nail Disorders Across All Skin Colors*,
https://doi.org/10.1007/978-3-031-74272-9_1

1.2.3 Race

AP studies lack substantial racial demographic data. The retrospective study of 2512 paronychia patients by Desai et al. reported similar proportions of White (25.6%) and Black (28.6%) patients [3]. Paronychia causes varied by race. Overall, 25.9% of patients reporting manicuring equipment, 27.3% reporting footwear, and 30.8% reporting knives as the cause of paronychia were White, while 40.2% reporting doors/drawers, 33.6% reporting needles/nails, and 51.6% reporting sports equipment, as the cause of paronychia were Black ($P < 0.0001$) [3].

1.3 Risk Factors

Trauma to the nail unit is the most common risk factor [4]. Manual labor, penetrating trauma, and nail care practices, including aggressive manicures and artificial nails, are risk factors. Biting, picking, and sucking the nails or fingers are also risk factors. Onychocryptosis [5], pemphigus vulgaris, pustular psoriasis, and reactive arthritis may predispose individuals to AP [6–8]. Medications, including epidermal growth factor receptor inhibitors, cytotoxic chemotherapy agents, systemic retinoids, and antiretroviral drugs are also associated with AP [9–11].

1.4 Etiology

AP is typically caused by the introduction of skin flora organisms including *Staphylococcus aureus* and *Streptococcus pyogenes* into the nail folds [1]. Other aerobic bacteria, such as gamma-hemolytic streptococci and *Klebsiella pneumoniae,* and anaerobic organisms are each responsible for 25% of cases. Exposure to oral secretions may increase infection risk from aerobic bacteria, including *Eikenella corrodens,* and anaerobic bacteria, such as *Fusobacterium*, *Peptostreptococcus*, *Prevotella*, and *Porphyromonas* spp. [1]. Contact with livestock may lead to infection by *Pasteurella multocida* [6]. Isolates of *Pseudomonas aeruginosa*, Coliforms, and *Proteus vulgaris* have also been reported [6]. Nonbacterial pathogens including *Candida albicans* and herpes simplex virus are less common causes [6].

1.5 Clinical Features

Patients typically present 2–5 days after the inciting cause with acute onset of redness, pain, swelling, and sensitivity in the nail folds of one digit [8, 12]. Applying pressure to the nail fold may express pus. The presence of pallor and fluctuance necessitate incision and drainage [13].

1.6 Clinical Features in Skin of Color

Clinical features of AP in patients with skin of color have not been described in the literature; however, longitudinal melanonychia is common in this population.

1.7 Requirements for Diagnosis

To diagnose AP, a detailed patient history and thorough physical examination are important. Wound culture from the affected digit is recommended given the increasing frequency of methicillin-resistant *Staphylococcus aureus* infections [14]. In a retrospective study of 758 patients who underwent incision and drainage for paronychia, 4% had positive cultures [15]. The digital pressure test, pressing thumb and index finger together to check for skin blanching, may help in uncovering abscesses [16]. Imaging, including ultrasonography and radiographs, may be useful if deeper infections, including osteomyelitis or atypical clinical presentations, are suspected [17].

1.8 Cases

Figures 1.1, 1.2, 1.3, 1.4, 1.5, 1.6, and 1.7 demonstrate the presentation of AP in a clinical setting.

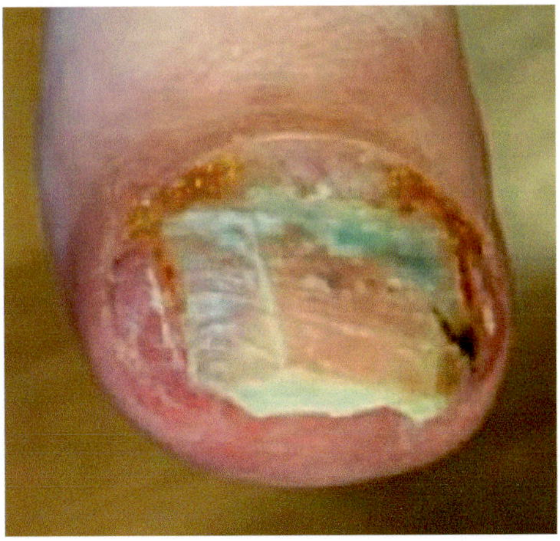

Fig. 1.1 31-Year-old female, Fitzpatrick type I, acute paronychia, with erythema of the lateral nail folds and honey-colored crust involving the great toenail

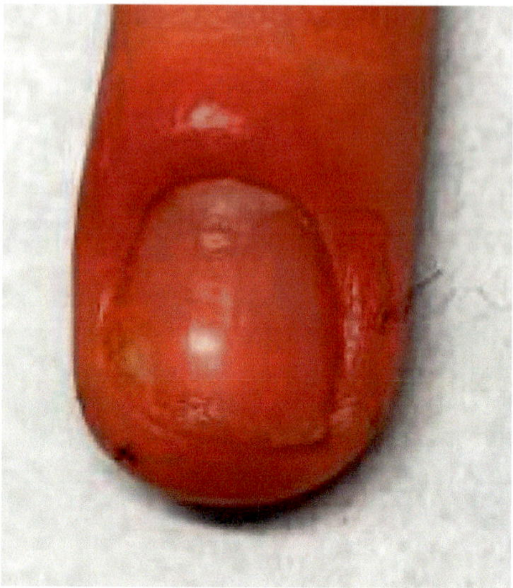

Fig. 1.2 35-Year-old female, Fitzpatrick type II, acute paronychia, with erythema and tenderness involving the proximal and lateral nail folds of the fingernail. The cuticle is missing

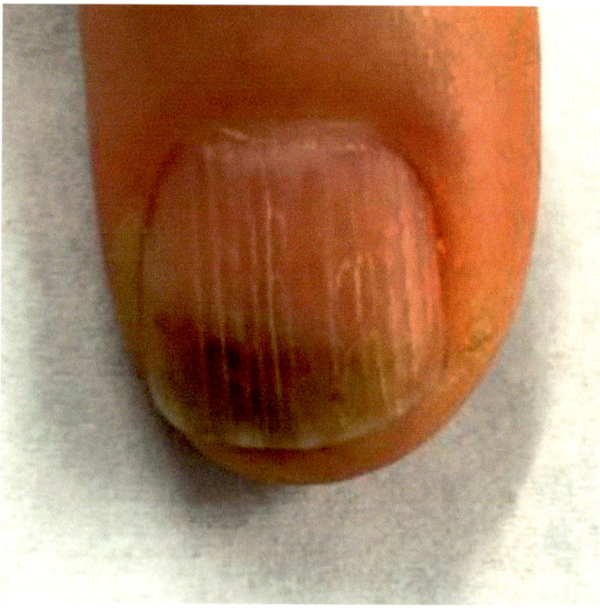

Fig. 1.3 62-Year-old female, Fitzpatrick type II, acute paronychia, with a collection of pus within the right lateral nail fold of the fingernail and distal onycholysis

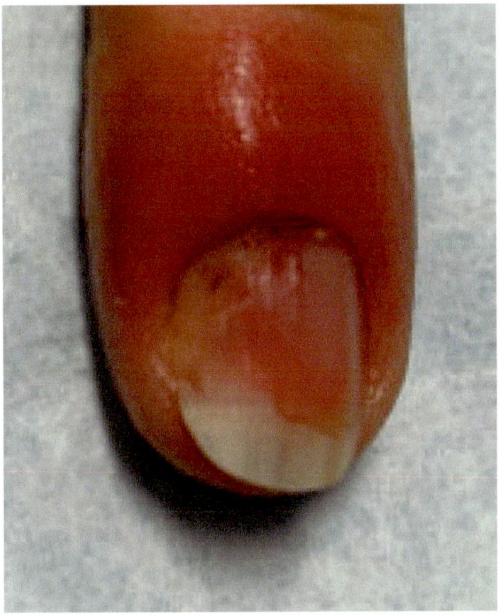

Fig. 1.4 44-Year-old female, Fitzpatrick type III, acute paronychia, with erythema and tenderness involving the lateral and proximal nail folds of the fingernail and distal onycholysis

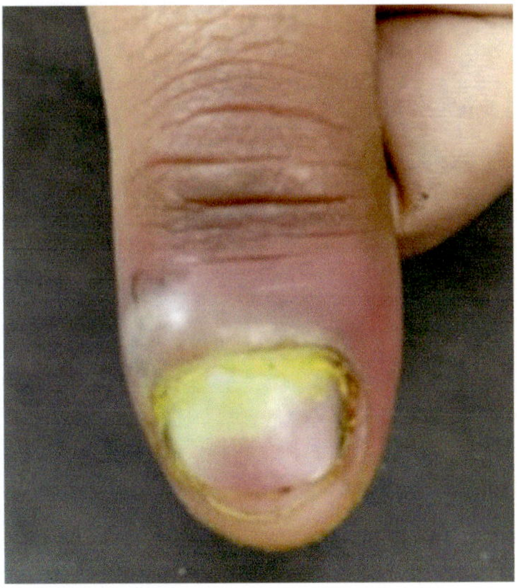

Fig. 1.5 Patient, Fitzpatrick type IV, acute paronychia, presenting with abscess formation along the lateral and proximal thumbnail fold [5] (*from* Bansal and Relhan V [5]; *with permission*)

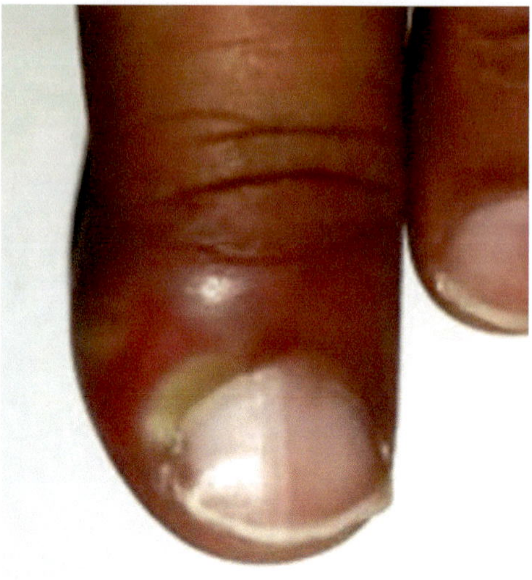

Fig. 1.6 Patient, Fitzpatrick type V, acute paronychia, presenting with erythema, swelling, and pus discharge along the lateral and proximal nail fold of the third digit [5] (*from* Bansal and Relhan V [5]; *with permission*)

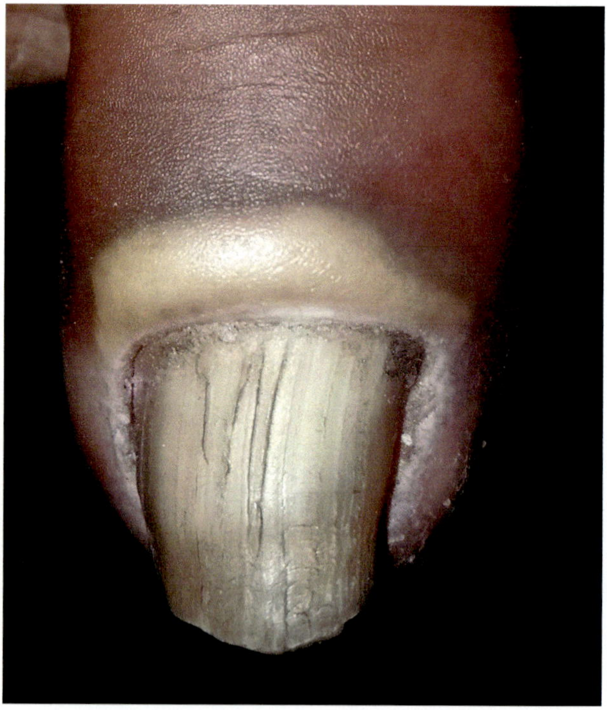

Fig. 1.7 Patient, Fitzpatrick type VI, acute paronychia, presenting with erythema, swelling, and abscess formation along the proximal nail fold [17] (*from* Oakley and Gomez [18]; *with permission*)

References

1. Rigopoulos D, Larios G, Gregoriou S, Alevizos A. Acute and chronic paronychia. Am Fam Physician. 2008;77(3):339–46.
2. Flevas DA, Syngouna S, Fandridis E, Tsiodras S, Mavrogenis AF. Infections of the hand: an overview. EFORT Open Rev. 2019;4(5):183–93. https://doi.org/10.1302/2058-5241.4.180082.
3. Desai AD, Wang Y, Nadarajah CC, Lipner SR. Cross-sectional analysis of paronychias in the National Electronic Injury Surveillance System 1999–2018. Skin Appendage Disord. 2022;8(6):454–61. https://doi.org/10.1159/000525032.
4. Leggit JC. Acute and chronic paronychia. Am Fam Physician. 2017;96(1):44–51.
5. Relhan V, Bansal A. Acute and chronic paronychia revisited: a narrative review. J Cutan Aesthet Surg. 2022;15(1):1–16. https://doi.org/10.4103/JCAS.JCAS_30_21.
6. Shafritz AB, Coppage JM. Acute and chronic paronychia of the hand. J Am Acad Orthop Surg. 2014;22(3):165–74. https://doi.org/10.5435/JAAOS-22-03-165.
7. Lee HE, Wong WR, Lee MC, Hong HS. Acute paronychia heralding the exacerbation of pemphigus vulgaris. Int J Clin Pract. 2004;58(12):1174–6. https://doi.org/10.1111/j.1742-1241.2004.00111.x.
8. Baran R, Barth JDR. Nail disorders: common presenting signs, differential diagnosis, and treatment. Churchill Livingstone; 1991. https://doi.org/10.1001/archderm.1992.01680110146031.
9. Robert C, Sibaud V, Mateus C, et al. Nail toxicities induced by systemic anticancer treatments. Lancet Oncol. 2015;16(4):e181–9. https://doi.org/10.1016/S1470-2045(14)71133-7.
10. Garden BC, Wu S, Lacouture ME. The risk of nail changes with epidermal growth factor receptor inhibitors: a systematic review of the literature and meta-analysis. J Am Acad Dermatol. 2012;67(3):400–8. https://doi.org/10.1016/j.jaad.2011.10.009.
11. Figueiras DA, Ramos TB, Marinho AKOF, Bezerra MSM, Cauas RC. Paronychia and granulation tissue formation during treatment with isotretinoin. An Bras Dermatol. 2016;91(2):223–5. https://doi.org/10.1590/abd1806-4841.20163817.
12. Jebson PJ. Infections of the fingertip. Paronychias and felons. Hand Clin. 1998;14(4):547–55. viii
13. Tosti A, Piraccini BM, Ghetti E, Colombo MD. Topical steroids versus systemic antifungals in the treatment of chronic paronychia: an open, randomized double-blind and double dummy study. J Am Acad Dermatol. 2002;47(1):73–6. https://doi.org/10.1067/mjd.2002.122191.
14. Goldstein BG, Goldstein AO, Tosti A. Paronychia. UpToDate.
15. Fowler JR, Ilyas AM. Epidemiology of adult acute hand infections at an urban medical center. J Hand Surg Am. 2013;38(6):1189–93. https://doi.org/10.1016/J.JHSA.2013.03.013.
16. Turkmen A, Warner RM, Page RE. Digital pressure test for paronychia. Br J Plast Surg. 2004;57(1):93–4. https://doi.org/10.1016/j.bjps.2003.10.014.
17. Aluja Jaramillo F, Quiasúa Mejía DC, Martínez Ordúz HM, González Ardila C. Nail unit ultrasound: a complete guide of the nail diseases. J Ultrasound. 2017;20(3):181–92. https://doi.org/10.1007/s40477-017-0253-6.
18. Oakley A, Gomez J. Paronychia. DermNet. 2017. https://dermnetnz.org/topics/paronychia. Accessed 21 Feb 2024.

Green Nail Syndrome

2

Apostolos Katsiaunis and Shari R. Lipner

2.1 Description of Disease

Green nail syndrome (GNS), also known as chloronychia, was first described in 1944 and presents as green nail plate discoloration. It is due to colonization by *Pseudomonas aeruginosa* [1], an aerobic, coccobacillus, gram-negative bacterium found in moist environments [2]. The bacterium produces the blue-green pigments, pyoverdin and pyocyanin, which account for the characteristic green discoloration [3, 4].

2.2 Epidemiology

2.2.1 Sex

GNS may disproportionately affect women. In a retrospective analysis of 23 GNS patients by Ohn et al. (2020), there were 17 (73.9%) female and 6 (26.1%) male patients [5]. In another retrospective study by Ohn et al. (2021) including 32 GNS patients, 19 (59.4%) were female and 13 (40.6%) were male [6]. In a case series of 26 patients with GNS by Geizhals et al., 21 (80.7%) were female, and 5 (19.2%) were male [2].

2.2.2 Age

GNS may be associated with older age. In the retrospective analysis of 23 patients by Ohn et al. (2020), the average age was 53.8 ± 12.2 years (range: 32–81) [5]. In their case series of 26 patients, Geizhals et al. reported an average age of 59 years (range: 24–81) [2]. Ohn et al. (2021) reported an average age of 54.5 ± 15.1 in their retrospective study of 32 patients [6]. The absence of patients younger than 24 suggests that GNS might be uncommon among young adults and children.

S. R. Lipner, *Atlas of Nail Disorders Across All Skin Colors*,
https://doi.org/10.1007/978-3-031-74272-9_2

2.3 Risk Factors

A moist environment increases the risk for GNS. Dry skin is less likely to be colonized or infected by *P. aeruginosa* [3, 4]. Chronic exposure to water, soaps, detergents, onychotillomania, and trauma are risk factors [7]. Occupations and activities involving repeated immersion in water, such as those of homemakers, dishwashers, cooks, gardeners, janitors, plumbers, nail salon workers, bakers, barbers, swimmers, and healthcare personnel, predispose to GNS [7–11]. Wearing tight-fitting shoes for extended periods, especially in military recruits and soccer players, and exercise are associated with GNS [3, 4]. The use of artificial nails and nail polishes might increase the risk of GNS infection, though the evidence is limited [8]. Chronic paronychia, onychotillomania, nail psoriasis, and onychomycosis are also predisposing factors for GNS [8–11]. In the retrospective analysis of 23 patients by Ohn et al. (2020), 13 (56.5%) patients reported a previous history of nail diseases, including 12 (52.2%) patients with a history of onychomycosis and one (4.3%) with nail psoriasis [5]. The retrospective study of 32 patients by Ohn et al. (2021) reported that 22 (68.8%) patients had a history of onychomycosis [6]. In the case series of 26 patients by Geizhals et al., a history of nail trauma was reported in 11.5% of patients [2].

2.4 Clinical Features

GNS presents with nail plate discoloration, ranging from green to green-black, blue-grey, green-brown, and green-yellow, brown, or black [2, 3]. In the case series of 26 patients by Geizhals et al., green and green-brown discolorations were most common [2]. Ohn et al. (2021) reported that dermoscopy showed structureless green patterns in all patients, and the average number of colors was 2.6 ± 0.9 per patient [6].

GNS usually affects one or two nails and may occur in both fingernails and toenails [12]. GNS may affect one nail at a time, particularly the first digit, and the patient's dominant hand [2, 5, 6]. The retrospective study of 32 patients by Ohn et al. (2021) noted single-digit involvement in 87.5% of patients [6]. The retrospective study of 23 patients by Ohn et al. (2020) noted the great toenail or thumbnail was involved in 22 (95.7%) patients [5]. The case series of 26 patients by Geizhals et al. noted involvement of the great toenail or thumbnail in 47.6% and 80% of patients, respectively. In this study, there was right-hand predominance (80.8%), and 76.9% of patients presented with onycholysis [2].

The nail itself is typically not painful. However, the nail folds may be inflamed, presenting with edema, erythema, and pain [12]. The condition is not self-limiting. In their retrospective studies, Ohn et al. reported mean disease durations of 11.9 months in 23 patients (2020) and 10.7 months in 32 patients (2021) [5, 6]. Geizhals et al. noted a mean time to presentation of 4 months, with all 26 patients showing resolution after three months of nightly treatment with gentamicin 0.3% topical solution, with three recurrences that resolved after the second round of treatment [2].

2.5 Clinical Features in Skin of Color

No current literature specifically describes GNS in patients of color. Melanonychia may be present, which may obscure the green discoloration, making the diagnosis more challenging.

2.6 Requirements for Diagnosis

Diagnosis of GNS may be made based on distinct clinical and dermoscopic observations. In more challenging cases, a nail plate clipping with histopathology and gram stain and/or a wound culture from the affected area may be performed [1].

2.7 Cases

Figures 2.1, 2.2, 2.3, 2.4, 2.5, and 2.6 demonstrate the presentation of GNS in a clinical setting.

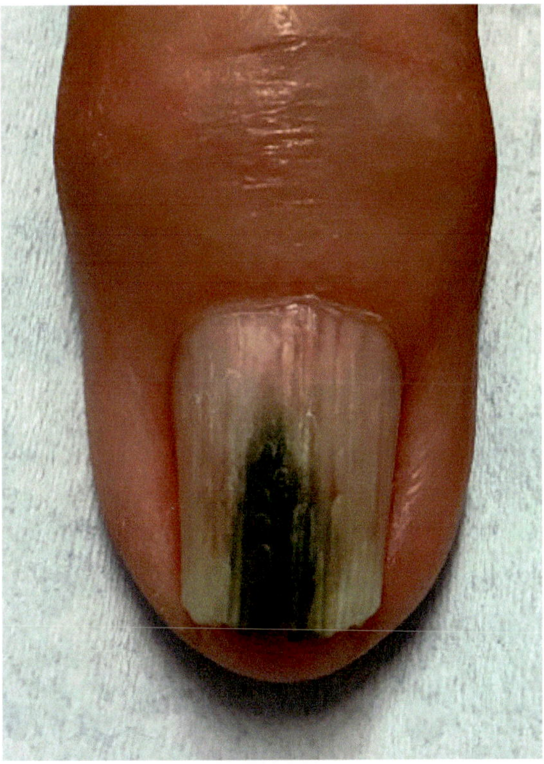

Fig. 2.1 84-Year-old female, Fitzpatrick type I, green nail syndrome, with green nail plate discoloration involving the fingernail

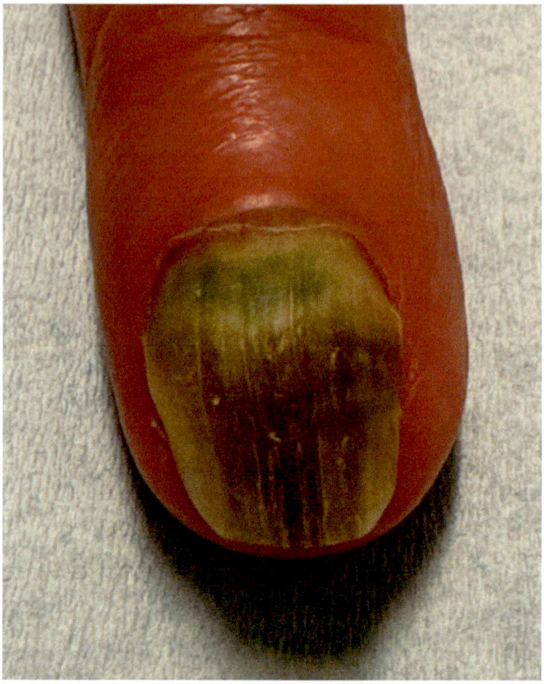

Fig. 2.2 81-Year-old female, Fitzpatrick type II, green nail syndrome, with green nail plate discoloration involving the fingernail

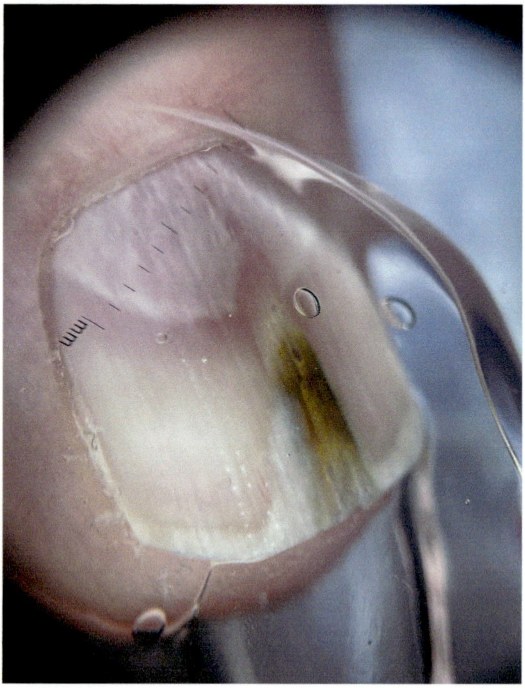

Fig. 2.3 58-Year-old male, Fitzpatrick type II, green nail syndrome, dermoscopy showing structureless green areas on right thumbnail nail plate

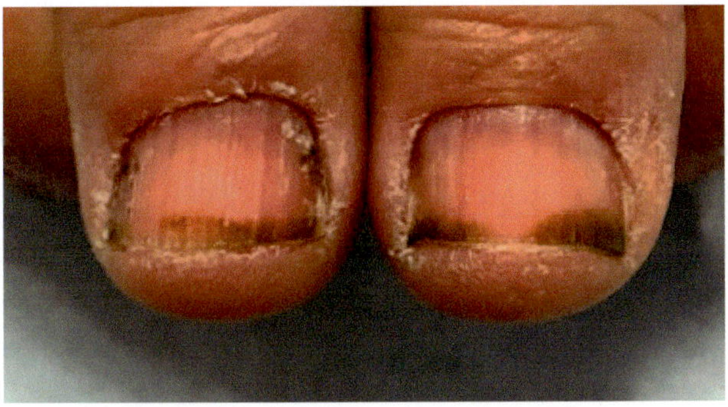

Fig. 2.4 57-Year-old male, Fitzpatrick type III, green nail syndrome, with a history of chronic paronychia and green nail plate discoloration involving the thumbnails

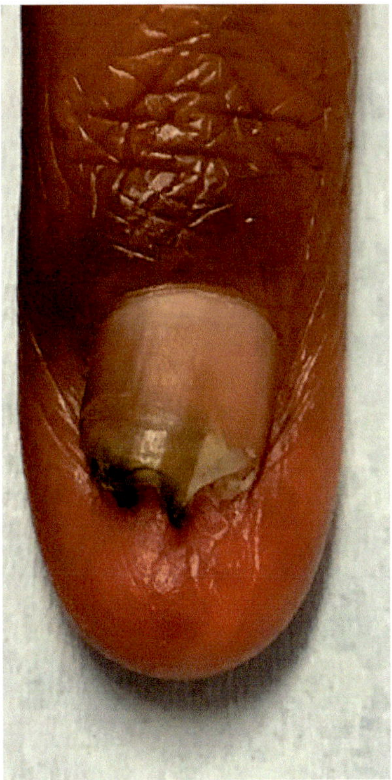

Fig. 2.5 37-Year-old female, Fitzpatrick type IV, green nail syndrome, with a pincer nail and green nail plate discoloration involving the fingernail

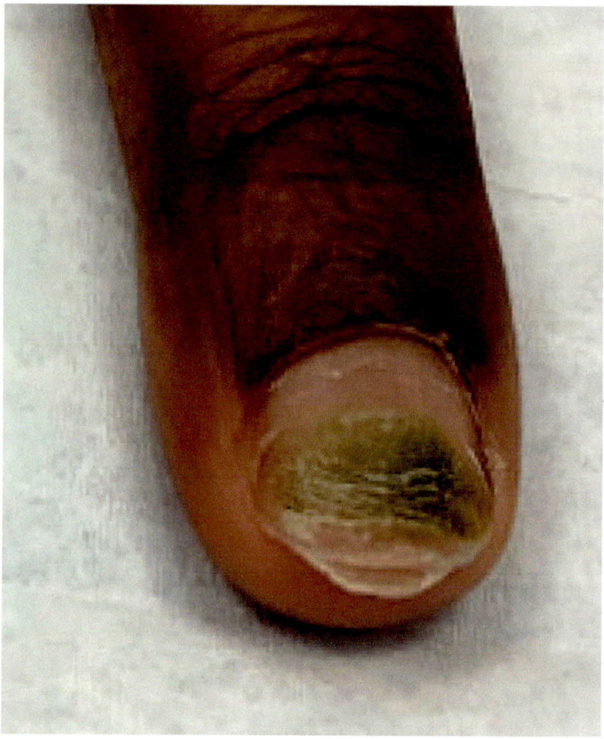

Fig. 2.6 40-Year-old female, Fitzpatrick type V, green nail syndrome, with green nail plate discoloration involving the fingernail

References

1. Goldman L. Greenish pigmentation of nail plates from bacillus pyocyaneus infection. Arch Dermatol Syphilol. 1944;49(2):136. https://doi.org/10.1001/archderm.1944.01510080048014.
2. Geizhals S, Lipner SR. Retrospective case series on risk factors, diagnosis and treatment of Pseudomonas aeruginosa nail infections. Am J Clin Dermatol. 2020;21(2):297–302. https://doi.org/10.1007/s40257-019-00476-0.
3. Chiriac A, Brzezinski P, Foia L, Marincu I. Chloronychia: green nail syndrome caused by Pseudomonas aeruginosa in elderly persons. Clin Interv Aging. 2015;10:265–7. https://doi.org/10.2147/CIA.S75525.
4. Gish D, Romero BJ. Green fingernail. J Fam Pract. 2017;66(5):E7–9.
5. Ohn J, Yu DA, Park H, Cho S, Mun JH. Green nail syndrome: analysis of the association with onychomycosis. J Am Acad Dermatol. 2020;83(3):940–2. https://doi.org/10.1016/j.jaad.2020.01.040.
6. Ohn J, Hur K, Park H, Cho S, Mun JH. Dermoscopic patterns of green nail syndrome. J Eur Acad Dermatol Venereol. 2021;35(7):e464–6. https://doi.org/10.1111/jdv.17224.
7. Stone OJ, Mullins JF. The role of Pseudomonas aeruginosa in nail disease. J Invest Dermatol. 1963;41:25–6.
8. Rigopoulos D, Rallis E, Gregoriou S, et al. Treatment of pseudomonas nail infections with 0.1% octenidine dihydrochloride solution. Dermatology. 2009;218(1):67–8. https://doi.org/10.1159/000171816.

9. Hengge UR, Bardeli V. Images in clinical medicine. Green nails. N Engl J Med. 2009;360(11):1125. https://doi.org/10.1056/NEJMicm0706497.
10. Matheson N, Weekes M, Coggle S. Skier's toe: traumatic onycholysis complicated by Pseudomonas chloronychia. BMJ Case Rep. 2009;2009:bcr0720092074. https://doi.org/10.1136/bcr.07.2009.2074.
11. Yang YS, Ahn JJ, Shin MK, Lee MH. Fusarium solani onychomycosis of the thumbnail coinfected with Pseudomonas aeruginosa: report of two cases. Mycoses. 2011;54(2):168–71. https://doi.org/10.1111/j.1439-0507.2009.01788.x.
12. Romaszkiewicz A, Sławińska M, Sobjanek M, Nowicki RJ. Nail dermoscopy (onychoscopy) is useful in diagnosis and treatment follow-up of the nail mixed infection caused by Pseudomonas aeruginosa and Candida albicans. Postepy Dermatol Alergol. 2018;35(3):327–9. https://doi.org/10.5114/ada.2018.76232.

Onychomycosis

3

Verena Isak, Eden Axler, and Shari R. Lipner

3.1 Description of Disease

Onychomycosis is a fungal infection of the nails, most commonly caused by dermatophytes and rarely by non-dermatophyte molds (NDMs) and yeasts. It is the most frequently encountered nail disorder in clinical practice. Onychomycosis predominantly affects the toenails, most commonly the great toenail(s), and there is a strong association with tinea pedis [1–3]. There are several onychomycosis subtypes, with distal lateral subungual onychomycosis (DLSO) being the most common (87%) [4]. Other types include superficial white onychomycosis (SWO), proximal subungual onychomycosis (PSO), total dystrophic onychomycosis (TDO), and fungal melanonychia (FM) [2].

3.2 Epidemiology

While onychomycosis is prevalent worldwide, both prevalence and type of infection display geographic variations. The cited prevalence varies widely, with an average of 11.4% (range: 5–17.7% as mean lower and upper limit) and a weighted average prevalence of 5.5% worldwide [5, 6]. Geographically, South America has the highest reported mean prevalence (18.8%), followed by Asia (12.1%), North America (9%), and Europe (8.9%); prevalence data from Africa is scarce [5].

3.2.1 Sex

Most population-based studies show a predilection of onychomycosis among men. Male-to-female ratios of 1.28–2.32:1 are reported [2, 5, 7–9]. A few studies report male-to-female ratios of 0.44–0.92 [10, 11].

S. R. Lipner, *Atlas of Nail Disorders Across All Skin Colors*,
https://doi.org/10.1007/978-3-031-74272-9_3

3.2.2 Age

Prevalence and incidence of onychomycosis increase with advancing age. It is rare in children, with a reported prevalence of <1% [12, 13]. The prevalence in the adult population was four-fold higher in patients 60 years or older vs. <60 years in a cross-sectional study including 30,000 patients [4]. A survey-based study of 2,468 patients selected randomly from the Icelandic National Registry found an odds ratio of 2.74 for onychomycosis in people 50 years or older vs. those 16–49 years [14].

3.3 Etiology

Several population- and hospital-based studies implicate dermatophytes as the most common pathogens responsible for onychomycosis (65–85%); of those, *Trichophyton rubrum* is by far the most common dermatophyte, followed by *T. mentagrophytes* [1–5]. NDMs, including include *Acremonium*, *Fusarium*, *Scopulariopsis*, and *Aspergillus* spp., infrequently cause onychomycosis [15, 16]. The remaining onychomycosis cases are caused by yeasts, including *Candida albicans*, *parapsilosis*, *guilliermondii*, and *tropical.* However, clinicopathologic correlation is necessary as many are contaminants rather than pathogens [4, 15].

3.3.1 Proximal Subungual Onychomycosis

Although PSO is the rarest form of onychomycosis in the general population, it is commonly observed in patients with AIDS and may be an early clinical sign of HIV infection. A study including 62 individuals with both AIDS and onychomycosis reported that 54 of them (88.7%) had PSO [17].

3.3.2 Fungal Melanonychia

FM may be due to 21 species of dematiaceous and 8 species of non-dematiaceous fungi, which produce melanin, giving them a brown-to-black appearance when cultured [18]. Among the most common causes of FM are the dematiaceous fungus *Scytalidium dimidiatum* and the non-dematiaceous dermatophyte *T. rubrum* [18]. Less commonly, yeasts, including *Candida* and certain non-dermatophyte fungi, can cause FM [19]. The rise in global travel and migration has contributed to its spread [18].

3.4 Risk Factors

Predisposing factors for onychomycosis include a diagnosis of tinea pedis in the patient or their family members, history of nail trauma, hyperhidrosis, malignancy, peripheral vascular disease, chronic kidney disease, diabetes mellitus, immunosuppression including HIV, use of occlusive shoes, warm humid weather, and visiting pools [3, 6, 14, 16].

3.5 Clinical Features

Clinical examination findings of onychomycosis typically include yellow nail discoloration, onycholysis, brittleness, crumbling and thickening of nails, and subungual hyperkeratosis [20]. Symptoms may include pain, difficulties with fitting into shoes, and paresthesias. Secondary bacterial infections may occur in severe cases if left untreated [3, 20].

3.5.1 Dermatophytoma

An important onychomycosis subtype is dermatophytoma, a compact subungual mass containing fungal elements, specifically hyphae, and spores [6, 21]. Clinically, dermatophytomas present as dense white or yellow patches or longitudinal streaks, often accompanied by subungual hyperkeratosis beneath the onycholytic area. They can also appear as opaque yellow, orange, or white patches in the nail plate or subungual region [22].

3.5.2 Distal Lateral Subungual Onychomycosis

DLSO manifests as subungual hyperkeratosis, leading to varying degrees of nail plate onycholysis. Patients typically exhibit white or yellow discoloration of the nail plate along with subungual debris [6]. On dermoscopy, the most prevalent pattern indicative of DLSO is a fringed proximal border within the onycholytic area. Longitudinal striae, resembling an aurora borealis with vertical streaks of varying colors, are also typical [6]. In a prospective study examining dermoscopic features of 60 nails with DLSO, longitudinal striae and jagged proximal edges were present in all patients, with intermittent spiked patterns in 78.3% of nails, chromonychia in 38.3%, and distal irregular termination in 11.7% of cases [23].

3.5.3 Proximal Subungual Onychomycosis

PSO, also referred to as proximal white subungual onychomycosis, is a rare onychomycosis subtype. PSO develops when pathogens invade the nail unit through the proximal nail fold and cuticle, penetrate the newly formed nail plate, and migrate distally. Clinically, PSO is characterized by subungual hyperkeratosis, proximal onycholysis, leukonychia, and the destruction of the proximal nail plate. The infection spreads from the proximal nail fold across the lunula, progressively involving all nail plate layers [24].

3.5.4 White Superficial Onychomycosis

WSO predominantly targets the superficial layers of the nail plate, mainly affecting toenails [25]. Clinically, WSO is marked by white or yellow patches on the nail surface, termed "pseudo-leukonychia," which form a chalky-white, firm, platelike layer that adheres to the nail plate and can be easily scraped off [25]. Dermoscopic examination shows several small, white, or yellow opaque and friable patches on the nail plate [26]. Epilumination microscopy can identify these white flakes as fungal colonies. As the infection progresses, it can encompass a significant portion of the nail surface, potentially leading to erosion and eventual nail plate loss [25].

3.5.5 Total Dystrophic Onychomycosis

TDO represents the advanced stage of nail fungal infection causing complete nail plate dystrophy [27]. This severe form of onychomycosis usually begins as DLSO, but can also develop from other subtypes, particularly PSO. Clinically, TDO is characterized by nail plate crumbling, thickening, ridging of the nail bed, and accumulation of subungual debris [28]. In a prospective study analyzing dermoscopic features in 122 onychomycosis cases, 15% of TDO patients showed a spiked pattern, 40% had longitudinal striae, and all (100%) exhibited distal irregular termination and a ruined appearance [29].

3.5.6 Fungal Melanonychia

Onychomycosis may uncommonly present as melanonychia, defined as brown-to-black nail pigmentation. FM may appear clinically similar to nail unit melanoma [19, 30]. The pattern of pigmentation in FM can vary from a thin band to complete nail plate pigmentation and can affect one or multiple nails. In a prospective study including 14 patients with FM (20 nails), 10 had only one affected nail, 3 had two affected nails, and 1 had four affected nails [31]. Distinctive features of FM include irregular white to yellow pigmentation and a "jagged edge" with sharp longitudinal whitish grooves [19]. In a retrospective study evaluating dermoscopic features including 20 patients with FM and 14 patients with nail unit melanoma, a "white or yellow streak" was more common in the FM group (90%) compared to the nail unit melanoma group (0%). Additionally, a reverse triangular pattern, caused by fungal invasion from the distal nail plate, was prevalent in the FM group (50.0%), but absent in the melanoma group (0%) [19]. In a retrospective study including 42 cases of FM, 52.3% of nails presented with either white streaks or jagged edges [32]. The most common pigmentation patterns were homogeneous brown (35.7%), homogeneous black (21.4%), homogeneous grey (21.4%), clumped/granular black (16.6%), and irregular longitudinal black (9.5%) pigmentation. Pseudo-Hutchinson's sign was observed in 9.5% of the nails [32].

3.6 Clinical Features in Skin of Color

In patients with skin of color, physiologic longitudinal melanonychia, presenting as grey-brown longitudinal bands, can potentially obscure the early signs of onychomycosis. Additionally, differentiating FM from benign melanocytic activation can be more challenging in skin of color patients due to overlapping pigmentation features. These features can delay diagnosis and treatment, underscoring the need for heightened clinical awareness.

3.7 Diagnosis

Diagnosis of onychomycosis cannot be made based on clinical examination alone. Mycological confirmation is necessary. Culture on sabouraud dextrose agar can identify the fungal species and its viability, but due to the slow growth of fungi, it can take up to 4 weeks and has low sensitivity (53%). Direct microscopy with potassium hydroxide (KOH), Parker's blue-black ink, or fluorescent stain is a rapid in-office test but does not identify the causative strain, is expertise dependent, and has the lowest sensitivity (48%) compared to other techniques. Histology of nail clippings with periodic acid Schiff or Grocott's methenamine silver staining has a turnaround time of a few days and has an 82% sensitivity. Molecular tests, including polymerase chain reaction, can identify the causative organism and demonstrate both high sensitivity (85%) and high specificity (94%) [33–35].

3.8 Cases

Figures 3.1, 3.2, 3.3, 3.4, 3.5, 3.6, 3.7, 3.8, 3.9, and 3.10 show the presentation of onychomycosis in a clinical setting.

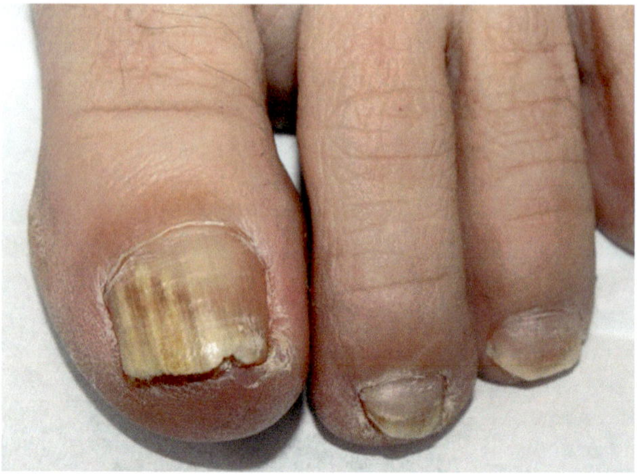

Fig. 3.1 68-Year-old female, Fitzpatrick type II, left great toenail with onychomycosis and dermatophytoma, with thickening, onycholysis, and subungual debris. There are also white/yellow streaks

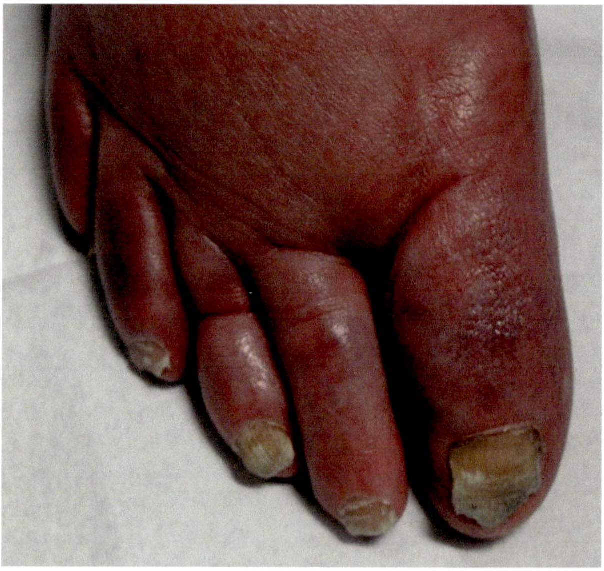

Fig. 3.2 79-Year-old female, Fitzpatrick type II, onychomycosis, with xanthonychia and thickening of right toenails

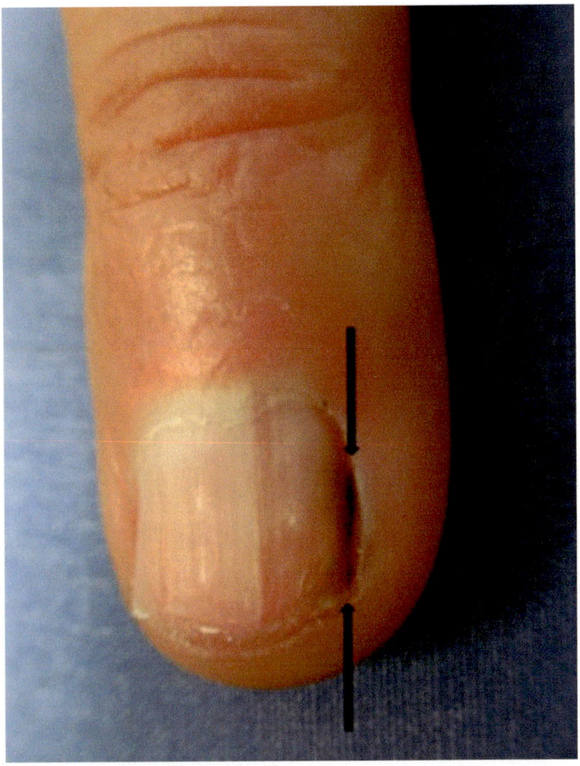

Fig. 3.3 79-Year-old male, Fitzpatrick type II, fungal melanonychia. Right fourth distal finger with a solitary black linear vertical nail plate streak (located between the tips of the black arrows). The culture of the fungal melanonychia grew *Candida parapsilosis* [30] (image reproduced under Creative Commons Attribution License. PMID: 33959438)

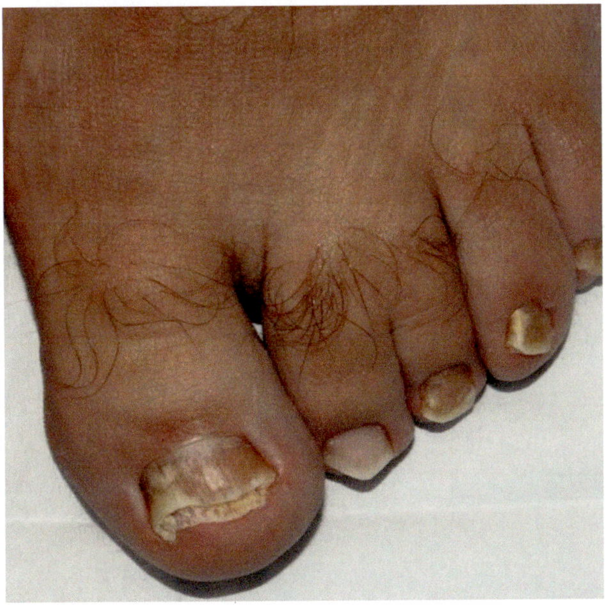

Fig. 3.4 39-Year-old male, Fitzpatrick type II, onychomycosis with dermatophytoma, with onycholysis, subungual debris, and white/yellow patches on the left toenails, sparing the left second toenail

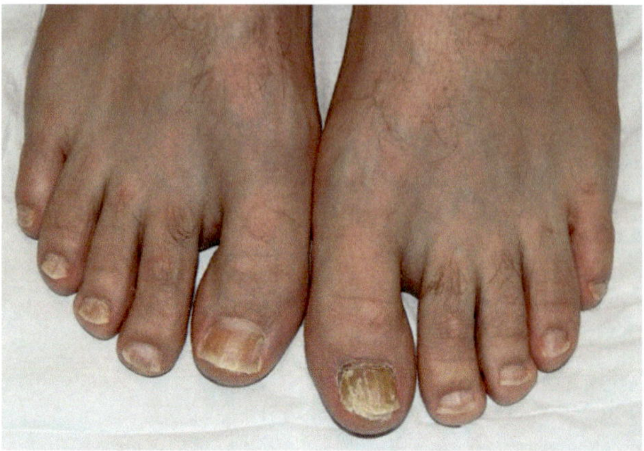

Fig. 3.5 34-Year-old male, Fitzpatrick type II, onychomycosis with thickening, xanthonychia, onycholysis, and subungual debris of the left great toenail and all of the right toenails

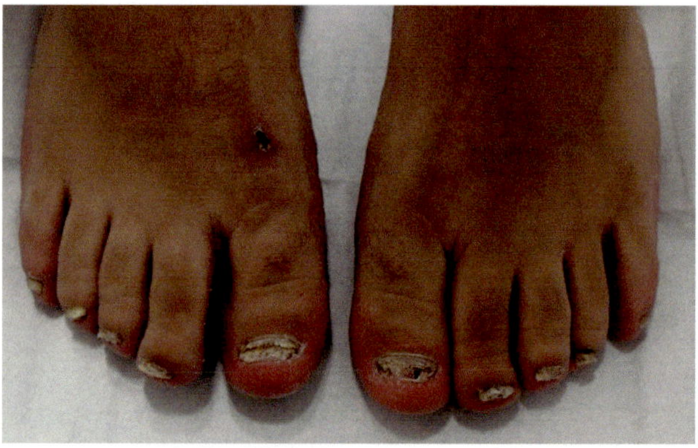

Fig. 3.6 27-Year-old male, Fitzpatrick type III, onychomycosis, with xanthonychia, thickening, onycholysis, and subungual hyperkeratosis of all toenails

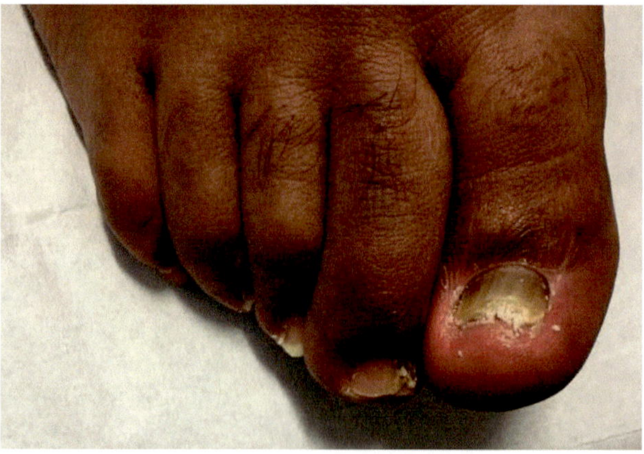

Fig. 3.7 51-Year-old male, Fitzpatrick type IV, onychomycosis, with onycholysis with subungual debris involving great toenail and second toenail medially. There is significant toe overlap

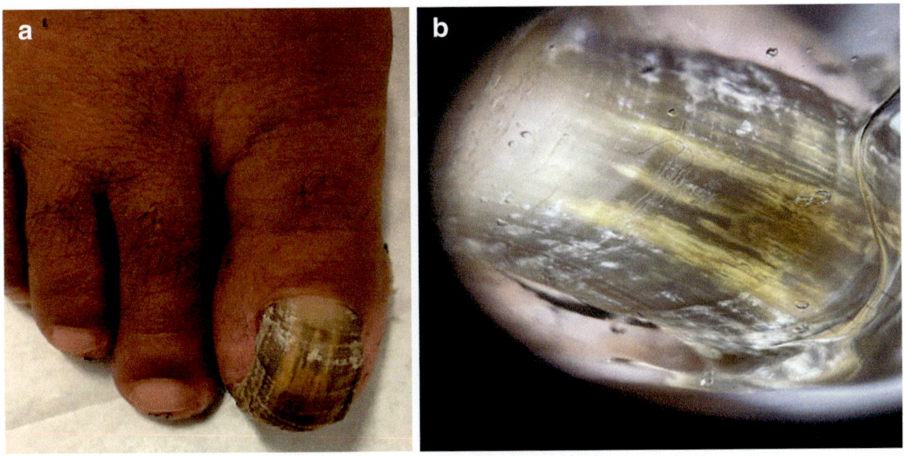

Fig. 3.8 (**a**) 47-Year-old female, Fitzpatrick type V, with thickening, melanonychia, parrot beak appearance, and yellow streaks of the right great toenail on clinical examination. (**b**) Clinical findings were enhanced with dermoscopy

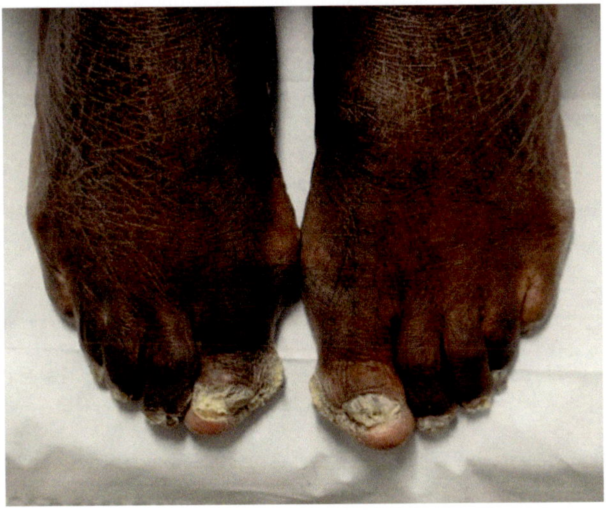

Fig. 3.9 75-Year-old man, Fitzpatrick type V, onychomycosis, with thickening and crumbling of all toenails

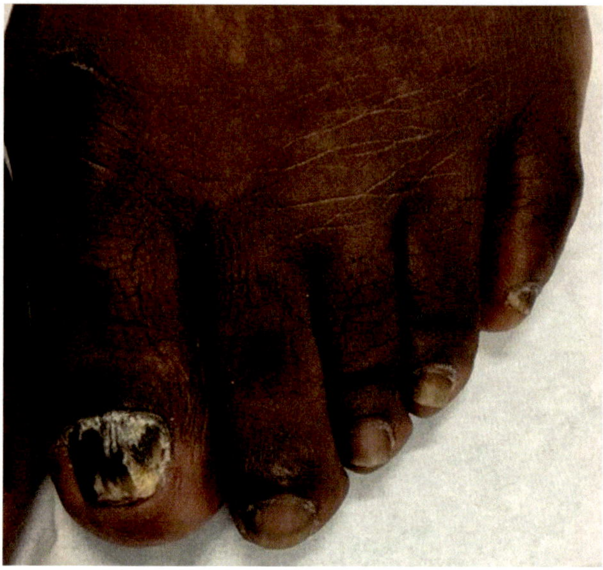

Fig. 3.10 76-Year-old female, Fitzpatrick type V, onychomycosis with thickening with diffuse brown discoloration involving the left great toenail

References

1. Vlahovic TC. Onychomycosis: evaluation, treatment options, managing recurrence, and patient outcomes. Clin Podiatr Med Surg. 2016;33(3):305–18. https://doi.org/10.1016/j.cpm.2016.02.001.
2. Asz-Sigall D, Tosti A, Arenas R. Tinea unguium: diagnosis and treatment in practice. Mycopathologia. 2017;182(1–2):95–100. https://doi.org/10.1007/s11046-016-0078-4.
3. Lipner SR, Scher RK. Onychomycosis: treatment and prevention of recurrence. J Am Acad Dermatol. 2019;80(4):853–67. https://doi.org/10.1016/j.jaad.2018.05.1260.
4. Gupta AK, Gupta G, Jain HC, et al. The prevalence of unsuspected onychomycosis and its causative organisms in a multicentre Canadian sample of 30 000 patients visiting physicians' offices. J Eur Acad Dermatol Venereol. 2016;30(9):1567–72. https://doi.org/10.1111/jdv.13677.
5. Sigurgeirsson B, Baran R. The prevalence of onychomycosis in the global population: a literature study. J Eur Acad Dermatol Venereol. 2014;28(11):1480–91. https://doi.org/10.1111/jdv.12323.
6. Lipner SR, Scher RK. Onychomycosis: clinical overview and diagnosis. J Am Acad Dermatol. 2019;80(4):835–51. https://doi.org/10.1016/j.jaad.2018.03.062.
7. Degreef H, del Palacio A, Mygind S, Ginter G, Pinto Soares A, Zuluaga de Cadena A. Randomized double-blind comparison of short-term itraconazole and terbinafine therapy for toenail onychomycosis. Acta Derm Venereol. 1999;79(3):221–3. https://doi.org/10.1080/000155599750011020.
8. Sahin I, Oksuz S, Kaya D, Sencan I, Cetinkaya R. Dermatophytes in the rural area of Duzce, Turkey. Mycoses. 2004;47(11–12):470–4. https://doi.org/10.1111/j.1439-0507.2004.01025.x.
9. Sigurgeirsson B, Steingrímsson O, Sveinsdóttir S. Prevalence of onychomycosis in Iceland: a population-based study. Acta Derm Venereol. 2002;82(6):467–9. https://doi.org/10.1080/000155502762064665.
10. Sais G, Jucglà A, Peyrí J. Prevalence of dermatophyte onychomycosis in Spain: a cross-sectional study. Br J Dermatol. 1995;132(5):758–61. https://doi.org/10.1111/j.1365-2133.1995.tb00722.x.

11. Roberts DT. Prevalence of dermatophyte onychomycosis in the United Kingdom: results of an omnibus survey. Br J Dermatol. 1992;126(Suppl 39):23–7. https://doi.org/10.1111/j.1365-2133.1992.tb00005.x.
12. Gupta AK, Sibbald RG, Lynde CW, et al. Onychomycosis in children: prevalence and treatment strategies. J Am Acad Dermatol. 1997;36(3 Pt 1):395–402. https://doi.org/10.1016/s0190-9622(97)80215-0.
13. Vestergaard-Jensen S, Mansouri A, Jensen LH, Jemec GBE, Saunte DML. Systematic review of the prevalence of onychomycosis in children. Pediatr Dermatol. 2022;39(6):855–65. https://doi.org/10.1111/pde.15100.
14. Sigurgeirsson B, Steingrímsson O. Risk factors associated with onychomycosis. J Eur Acad Dermatol Venereol. 2004;18(1):48–51. https://doi.org/10.1111/j.1468-3083.2004.00851.x.
15. Ghannoum MA, Hajjeh RA, Scher R, et al. A large-scale north American study of fungal isolates from nails: the frequency of onychomycosis, fungal distribution, and antifungal susceptibility patterns. J Am Acad Dermatol. 2000;43(4):641–8. https://doi.org/10.1067/mjd.2000.107754.
16. Svejgaard EL, Brandrup F, Kragballe K, et al. Oral terbinafine in toenail dermatophytosis. A double-blind, placebo-controlled multicenter study with 12 months' follow-up. Acta Derm Venereol. 1997;77(1):66–9. https://doi.org/10.2340/0001555555776669.
17. Dompmartin D, Dompmartin A, Deluol AM, Grosshans E, Coulaud JP. Onychomycosis and AIDS. Clinical and laboratory findings in 62 patients. Int J Dermatol. 1990;29(5):337–9. https://doi.org/10.1111/j.1365-4362.1990.tb04755.x.
18. Finch J, Arenas R, Baran R. Fungal melanonychia. J Am Acad Dermatol. 2012;66(5):830–41. https://doi.org/10.1016/j.jaad.2010.11.018.
19. Kim HJ, Kim TW, Park SM, et al. Clinical and dermoscopic features of fungal melanonychia: differentiating from subungual melanoma. Ann Dermatol. 2020;32(6):460–5. https://doi.org/10.5021/ad.2020.32.6.460.
20. Gupta AK, Stec N, Summerbell RC, et al. Onychomycosis: a review. J Eur Acad Dermatol Venereol. 2020;34(9):1972–90. https://doi.org/10.1111/jdv.16394.
21. Lipner SR, Scher RK. Evaluation of nail lines: color and shape hold clues. Cleve Clin J Med. 2016;83(5):385–91. https://doi.org/10.3949/ccjm.83a.14187.
22. Gupta AK, Wang T, Cooper EA. Dermatophytomas: clinical overview and treatment. J Fungi (Basel). 2022;8(7). https://doi.org/10.3390/jof8070742.
23. Nargis T, Pinto M, Shenoy MM, Hegde S. Dermoscopic features of distal lateral subungual onychomycosis. Indian Dermatol Online J. 2018;9(1):16–9. https://doi.org/10.4103/idoj.IDOJ_40_17.
24. Elewski BE. Onychomycosis: pathogenesis, diagnosis, and management. Clin Microbiol Rev. 1998;11(3):415–29. https://doi.org/10.1128/cmr.11.3.415.
25. Ploysangam T, Lucky AW. Childhood white superficial onychomycosis caused by Trichophyton rubrum: report of seven cases and review of the literature. J Am Acad Dermatol. 1997;36(1):29–32. https://doi.org/10.1016/s0190-9622(97)70321-9.
26. Grover C, Jakhar D, Sharma S. The grid pattern of white superficial onychomycosis. Indian J Dermatol Venereol Leprol. 2020;86(5):568–70. https://doi.org/10.4103/ijdvl.IJDVL_699_19.
27. Baran R, Hay RJ, Tosti A, Haneke E. A new classification of onychomycosis. Br J Dermatol. 1998;139(4):567–71. https://doi.org/10.1046/j.1365-2133.1998.02449.x.
28. Hay RJ, Baran R. Onychomycosis: a proposed revision of the clinical classification. J Am Acad Dermatol. 2011;65(6):1219–27. https://doi.org/10.1016/j.jaad.2010.09.730.
29. Devi Sangeetha A, Gopalakrishnan K, Ramachandran R, Narasimhan M, Ramraj B. A descriptive study of onychoscopic features in various subtypes of onychomycosis. Med J Armed Forces India. 2022;78(Suppl 1):S219–s225. https://doi.org/10.1016/j.mjafi.2021.03.019.
30. Ohn J, Choe YS, Park J, Mun JH. Dermoscopic patterns of fungal melanonychia: a comparative study with other causes of melanonychia. J Am Acad Dermatol. 2017;76(3):488–493.e2. https://doi.org/10.1016/j.jaad.2016.08.013.
31. Kilinc Karaarslan I, Acar A, Aytimur D, Akalin T, Ozdemir F. Dermoscopic features in fungal melanonychia. Clin Exp Dermatol. 2015;40(3):271–8. https://doi.org/10.1111/ced.12552.

32. Elmas ÖF, Metin MS. Dermoscopic findings of fungal melanonychia. Postepy Dermatol Alergol. 2020;37(2):180–3. https://doi.org/10.5114/ada.2020.94836.
33. Gupta AK, Baran R. Ciclopirox nail lacquer solution 8% in the 21st century. J Am Acad Dermatol. 2000;43(4 Suppl):S96–102. https://doi.org/10.1067/mjd.2000.109068.
34. Wilsmann-Theis D, Sareika F, Bieber T, Schmid-Wendtner MH, Wenzel J. New reasons for histopathological nail-clipping examination in the diagnosis of onychomycosis. J Eur Acad Dermatol Venereol. 2011;25(2):235–7. https://doi.org/10.1111/j.1468-3083.2010.03704.x.
35. Kondori N, Abrahamsson AL, Ataollahy N, Wennerås C. Comparison of a new commercial test, dermatophyte-PCR kit, with conventional methods for rapid detection and identification of Trichophyton rubrum in nail specimens. Med Mycol. 2010;48(7):1005–8. https://doi.org/10.3109/13693781003743130.

Subungual Warts

4

Zi-Ning Choo and Shari R. Lipner

4.1 Description of Disease

Cutaneous warts (verrucae) are benign epidermal tumors resulting from human papillomavirus (HPV) infection of keratinocytes. Verruca that affects the nail unit may be periungual, involving the lateral and proximal nail folds, or subungual, occurring underneath the nail plate [1]. Subungual warts comprise a relatively small fraction of all verruca; a cross-sectional analysis of 108 patients estimated that only approximately 5% of verruca are subungual [2]. Periungual and subungual warts are most commonly caused by HPV subtypes 1, 2, 4, 24, and 57. HPV subtypes 16, 18, 52, 58, and 73 are rare causes and are associated with malignant transformation to squamous cell carcinoma. Butcher's warts, which are hand warts associated with meat handling professions, are caused by HPV subtype 7 and may occasionally involve the nail unit [1].

Morphologically, subungual warts are the most often common warts (verruca vulgaris) [1]. Histopathological features include acanthosis, digitated epidermal hyperplasia, parakeratotic cells with entrapped red blood cells, hypergranulosis, and tortuous capillaries in the dermal papillae. Koilocytes, keratinocytes with nuclear enlargement, irregular nuclear membrane contours, nuclear hyperchromasia, and a perinuclear halo, are pathognomonic [3].

4.2 Epidemiology

4.2.1 Sex

Verruca are common in both sexes [4]. Prior studies have not demonstrated a sex bias in common wart frequency among either pediatric or adult patients. A survey-based study of 12,377 participants ages 18–74 years across five European countries estimated a lifetime prevalence of verruca of 27%, with an estimated prevalence of 24–26% in men and 28–30% in women [5]. A cross-sectional study of Australian

S. R. Lipner, *Atlas of Nail Disorders Across All Skin Colors*,
https://doi.org/10.1007/978-3-031-74272-9_4

school children ages 4–18 years estimated that the prevalence of verruca was 22% in both males and females [6]. While large-scale studies specifically addressing subungual wart prevalence have not been performed, a cross-sectional analysis of 108 verrucae cases in India showed a slight male predominance in subungual warts, though this finding is limited by a small sample size [2].

4.2.2 Age

The age distribution of subungual warts has not been studied. However, verruca in general may affect individuals of any age and is particularly common among children and adolescents ages 5–20 years, with peak incidence between ages 12 and 16 years and declining thereafter [6, 7].

4.2.3 Other Factors

Subungual warts are caused by infection of abraded or macerated skin with HPV. Hence, behaviors causing nail plate and nail fold damage, including nail picking, nail biting, and chronic immersion in water, increase risk [8]. Nail biting and nail picking may also cause autoinoculation and spread of lesions to the face and lips [3]. Fingernails are more often affected than toenails, perhaps because hands are more frequently exposed to sources of HPV infection. In addition, immunosuppressed patients are at higher risk of developing subungual warts, and may have numerous recurrent warts affecting multiple nails (see risk factors).

4.3 Risk Factors

Risk factors for subungual and periungual warts include occupations and behaviors that damage the integrity of the nail plate and nail folds because repetitive maceration allows human papillomaviruses to penetrate the damaged epidermis [1]. The prevalence of active butcher's warts is estimated at 33.3% among slaughterhouse workers and 34.1% among butchers [9, 10]. Cases of multiple and recurrent subungual and periungual warts in the setting of nail biting have also been reported [11, 12].

Immunosuppression and immunodeficiency are important risk factors for the development of all warts, including subungual warts. Human immunodeficiency virus infection is associated with multiple and recurrent verrucae in less common locations, including the periungual and subungual regions [13–15]. HPV is one of the most frequent infections in transplant recipients. A cross-sectional study of 189 renal transplant patients found a steady increase in the incidence of warts after transplant, reaching 65% among patients with transplants for more than five years [16, 17].

A positive association between warts and atopic dermatitis in children and adolescents has been reported. A survey of 9417 children aged up to 17 years found that a self-reported history of atopic dermatitis in the setting of another atopic disease (e.g. allergic rhinitis, asthma, food allergy) modestly increased the odds of having verruca (OR 1.83, 95% CI [1.82–1.84], $p < 0.001$) [18].

4.4 Clinical Features

Subungual warts develop weeks to years after inoculation with HPV and are most often asymptomatic. However, rarely patients may report severe pain, mimicking the pain associated with glomus tumors. Subungual warts usually affect the hyponychium at first, growing slowly toward the nail bed and then causing onycholysis. Size varies between one and ten mm in diameter with a rough keratotic surface. Morphologies include nodular lesions causing onycholysis or linear growth, and those producing a longitudinal band of onycholysis and splinter hemorrhages. Most frequently, subungual warts are located on the lateral aspect of the proximal nail fold. Warts on the proximal nail fold may present with periungual hyperkeratosis resembling a hyperkeratotic cuticle [3].

Suggestive physical examination findings include the presence of black dots upon paring of the lesion (indicating pinpoint bleeding), pain with lesion compression due to nerve endings feeding the lesion, and the presence of interrupted skin folds, known as dermatoglyphics [8]. A dermoscopy of verrucae will show numerous densely packed papilla, each containing a central red or black dot or loop representing vessels, surrounded by a white halo. The vessels may sometimes be associated with hemorrhage, which appears as irregularly distributed, small, red to black to brown tiny dots or streaks [19, 20].

In contrast to verruca in other locations, which often spontaneously resolve over months to years, subungual warts rarely resolve without treatment and are challenging to treat. They have a high recurrence rate and risk of permanent damage to the nail matrix with aggressive therapy. Complications of subungual warts include bone erosions, autoinoculation of the face and lips in nail biters, and rare malignant transformation to squamous cell carcinoma, most often in immunosuppressed individuals [3, 8].

4.5 Clinical Features in Skin of Color

In skin of color patients, verruca may be skin-colored, pink, or any shade of brown or gray. Verrucae are more likely to be hyperpigmented in darker skin. Scales may appear whitish, yellowish, or any shade of brown or gray.

4.6 Requirements for Diagnosis

The diagnosis of subungual warts can often be made clinically, but a biopsy may be needed to rule out other diagnoses, such as squamous cell carcinoma when the presumed verruca does not respond to therapy. A substantial fraction of subungual squamous cell carcinomas are verrucous carcinomas, which often present as a verrucous lesion mimicking a viral wart [21, 22]. High-risk features necessitating biopsy include a long-standing lesion in an older adult, immunocompromise, or treatment refractoriness. An X-ray of the affected digit may be necessary to rule out exostosis [3].

4.7 Cases

Figures 4.1, 4.2, 4.3, 4.4, 4.5, and 4.6 demonstrate the presentation of subungual warts in a clinical setting.

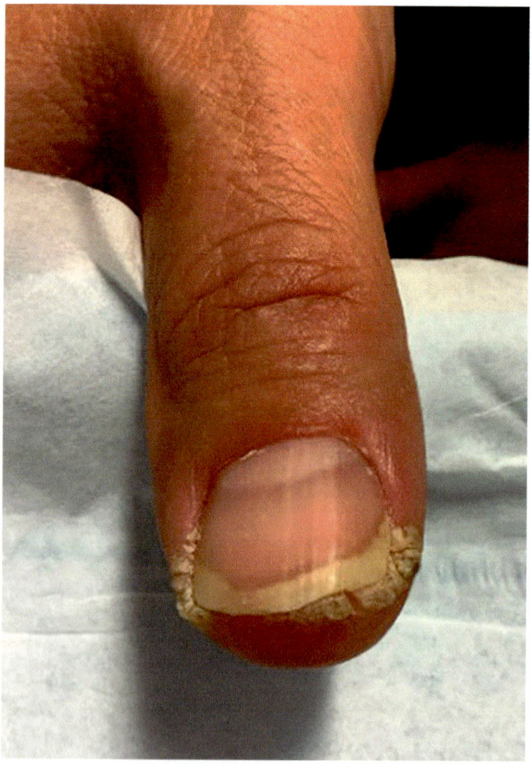

Fig. 4.1 66-Year-old male, Fitzpatrick type II, subungual and periungual verrucae, with verrucous papules involving the lateral nail folds and hyponychium of the right thumbnail

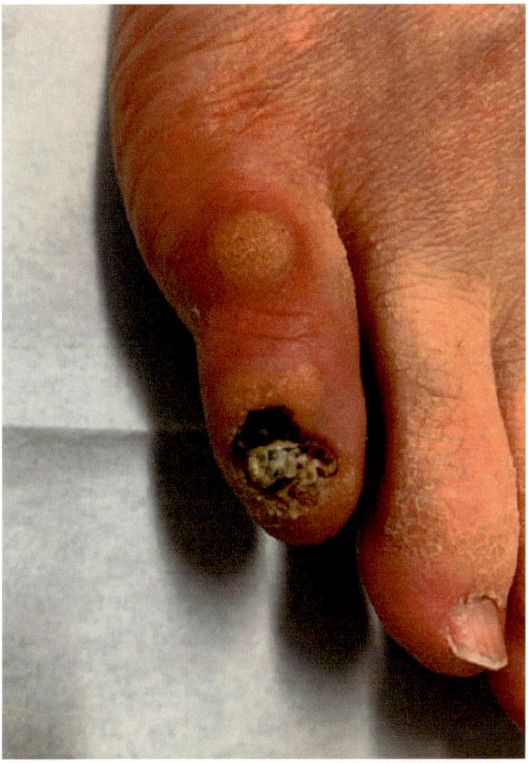

Fig. 4.2 59-Year-old male, Fitzpatrick type III, subungual verruca, with nail plate crumbling involving the right fifth toenail. The heme near the cuticle is secondary to a prior intralesional bleomycin injection

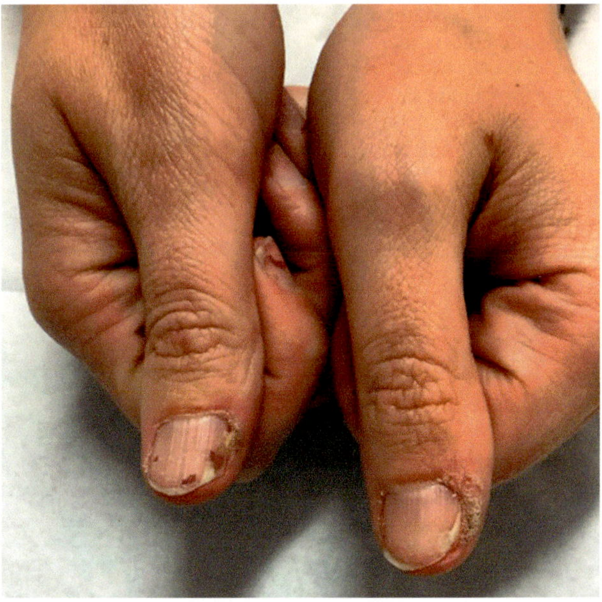

Fig. 4.3 30-Year-old female, Fitzpatrick type IV, periungual verrucae, with onycholysis involving bilateral thumbnails and verrucous plaques involving the nail folds

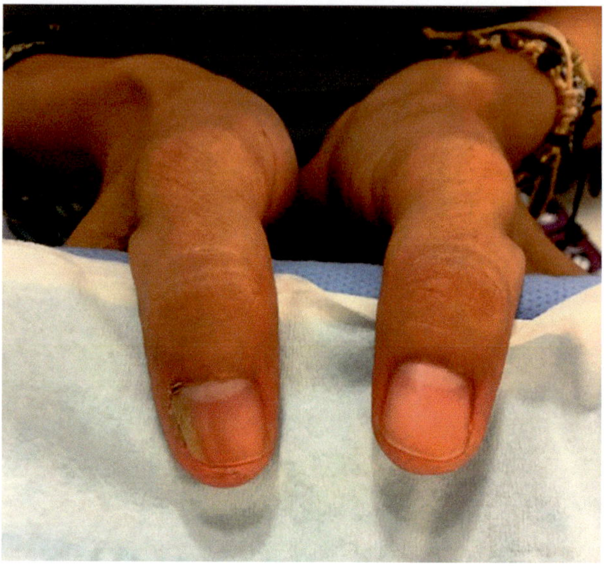

Fig. 4.4 45-Year-old female, Fitzpatrick type IV, subungual verruca, with onycholysis and subungual hyperkeratosis of the right thumbnail

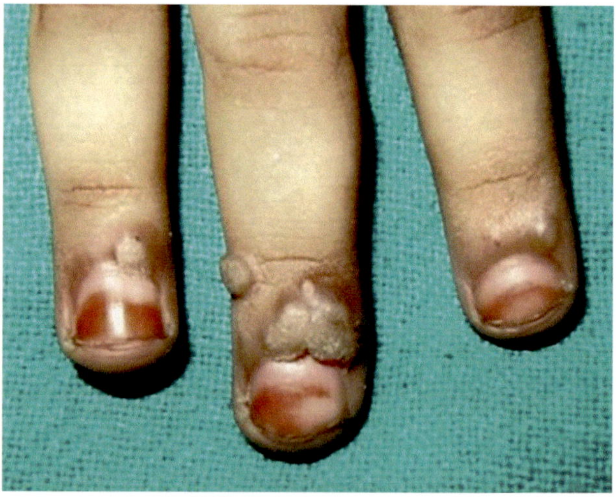

Fig. 4.5 7-Year-old female, Fitzpatrick type V, periungual verrucae involving the proximal nail folds of the second, third, and fourth digits of the right hand (reproduced with permission from Singer et al. [23])

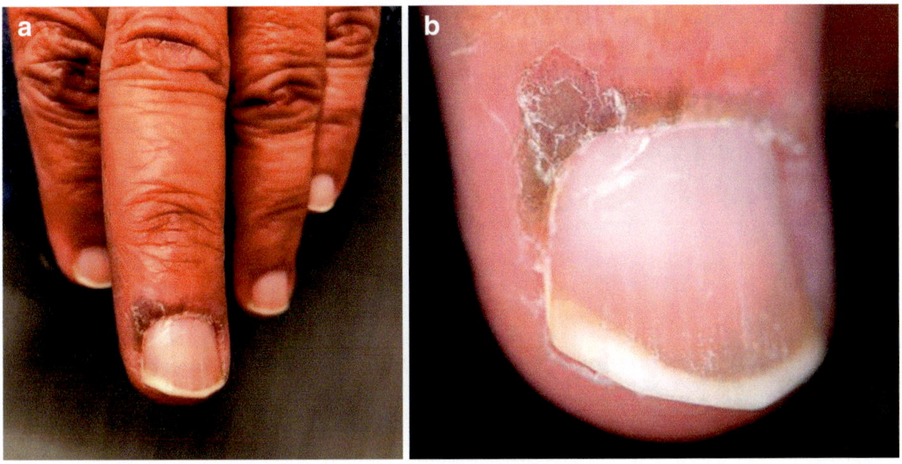

Fig. 4.6 (**a**) 69-Year-old female, Fitzpatrick type V, periungual verruca, with hyperkeratosis involving the nail fold of the right third fingernail. (**b**) Enhanced with dermoscopy

References

1. Jablonska S, Orth G, Obalek S, Croissant O. Cutaneous warts clinical, histologic, and virologic correlations. Clin Dermatol. 1985;3:71–82.
2. Ghadgepatil SS, Gupta S, Sharma YK. Clinicoepidemiological study of different types of warts. Dermatol Res Pract. 2016;2016:7989817.
3. Pasch M, Haneke E, Baran R, Thomas L, Richert B. Tumors of the nail apparatus and adjacent tissues. In: Baran & Dawber's diseases of the nails and their management. Wiley; 2019. p. 675–824. https://doi.org/10.1002/9781119323396.ch21.
4. Laurent R, Kienzier J-L. Epidemiology of HPV infections. Clin Dermatol. 1985;3:64–70.
5. Kilkenny M, Marks R. The descriptive epidemiology of warts in the community. Australas J Dermatol. 1996;37:80–6.
6. Van Haalen FM, Bruggink SC, Gussekloo J, Assendelft WJJ, Eekhof JAH. Warts in primary schoolchildren: prevalence and relation with environmental factors. Br J Dermatol. 2009;161:148–52.
7. Kilkenny M, Erlin K, Young R, Marks R. The prevalence of common skin conditions in Australian school students: 1. Common, plane and plantar viral warts. Br J Dermatol. 1998;138:840–5.
8. Tosti A, Piraccini BM. Warts of the nail unit: surgical and nonsurgical approaches. Dermatologic Surg. 2001;27:235–9.
9. KEEFE, M., et al. Cutaneous warts in butchers. Br J Dermatol. 1994;130:9–14.
10. Majewski S, Jablonska S, Favre M, Orth G. Human papillomavirus type 7 and Butcher's warts. Arch Dermatol. 2001;137:1655–6.
11. Halteh P, Scher RK, Lipner SR. Onychophagia: a nail-biting conundrum for physicians. J Dermatol Treat. 2017;28:166–72.
12. Shin J-O, et al. Onychophagia: detailed clinical characteristics. Int J Dermatol. 2022;61:331–6.
13. Porro AM, et al. Detection and typing of human papillomavirus in cutaneous warts of patients infected with human immunodeficiency virus type 1. Br J Dermatol. 2003;149:1192–9.
14. Coates SJ, Leslie KS. What's new in HIV dermatology? F1000Res. 2019;8:F1000.

15. Aftergut K, Cockerell CJ. UPDATE ON THE CUTANEOUS MANIFESTATIONS OF HIV INFECTION: clinical and pathologic features. Dermatol Clin. 1999;17:445–71.
16. Schmook T, et al. Viral warts in organ transplant recipients: new aspects in therapy. Br J Dermatol. 2003;149:20–4.
17. Dyall-Smith D, Trowell H, Dyall-Smith ML. Benign human papillomavirus infection in renal transplant recipients. Int J Dermatol. 1991;30:785–9.
18. Silverberg JI, Silverberg NB. Childhood atopic dermatitis and warts are associated with increased risk of infection: a US population-based study. J Allergy Clin Immunol. 2014;133:1041–7.
19. Chauhan P, et al. Dermoscopy of infectious dermatoses (infectiouscopy) in skin of color—a systematic review by the international dermoscopy society "imaging in skin of color" task force. Dermatol Pract Concept. 2023;13:e2023309S.
20. Errichetti E, et al. Dermoscopy in general dermatology (non-neoplastic dermatoses) of skin of colour: a comparative retrospective study by the International Dermoscopy Society. Eur J Dermatol. 2020;30:688–98.
21. Riddel C, Rashid R, Thomas V. Ungual and periungual human papillomavirus–associated squamous cell carcinoma: a review. J Am Acad Dermatol. 2011;64:1147–53.
22. Batalla A, Feal C, Rosón E, Posada C. Subungual squamous cell carcinoma: a case series. Indian J Dermatol. 2014;59:352–4.
23. Singal A, Grover C. Efficacy and safety of intralesional bleomycin in the management of ungual warts. Skin Appendage Disord. 2020;6:346–50.

Part II

Inflammatory Nail Disorders

Nail Eczema

5

Eden Axler and Shari R. Lipner

5.1 Description of Disease

Eczema is a common skin condition marked by recurring episodes of inflammation due to a disruption in the skin's protective barrier [1]. Palmoplantar eczema can trigger periungual inflammation, disrupting nail matrix function and leading to nail changes [2]. Periungual eczema may originate from atopy or finger sucking. Over time, cuticle loss can result in chronic paronychia or bacterial and *Candida* spp. superinfections [3].

5.2 Epidemiology

In a prospective study including 777 atopic dermatitis patients, nail dystrophy was present in 16% [4].

5.2.1 Children

Nail changes secondary to eczema may be more common in older vs. younger children with atopic dermatitis. In a prospective study of 235 atopic dermatitis patients ages 2–19 by Chung et al. [1], 24 (10.2%) patients had nail findings [1]. On average, children with atopic dermatitis and fingernail involvement were older than those without fingernail involvement (10.13 ± 4.36 vs. 7.21 ± 4.91, $P = 0.026$) [1].

5.2.2 Correlation with Severity

A correlation between nail dystrophy and eczema severity has been suggested. In the prospective study by Chung et al. [1], the presence of toenail dystrophy was correlated with higher eczema severity scores (OR 1.15, $P = 0.030$) [1]. In a

S. R. Lipner, *Atlas of Nail Disorders Across All Skin Colors*,
https://doi.org/10.1007/978-3-031-74272-9_5

prospective study of 100 patients with atopic dermatitis analyzed with capillaroscopy, there was a positive association between the presence of nail findings, including pitting, trachyonychia, decreased capillary density, and avascular areas, with the severity of eczema defined by the scoring atopic dermatitis score (all $P < 0.05$) [5].

5.3 Risk Factors

Risk factors for nail changes associated with eczema have not been well studied, though risk factors for atopic dermatitis involving the skin include personal and family history of eczema, asthma, seasonal allergies, stress, cigarette smoke exposure, skin irritants, farm and rural living, and outdoor and indoor pollutants [6, 7].

5.4 Clinical Features

In the prospective study by Chung et al., the most common nail finding observed in children with atopic dermatitis was nail pitting (25%), followed by koilonychia (16.7%), leukonychia (12.5%), brachyonychia (8.3%), melanonychia (8.3%), onychomadesis (8.3%), and onycholysis (8.3%) [1]. Four patients had multiple findings concurrently, with all four presenting with koilonychia, nail pitting, and onychoschizia, and three also presenting with Beau's lines [1].

5.5 Clinical Features in Skin of Color

In individuals with darker skin tones, longitudinal melanonychia often accompanies other characteristic nail findings.

5.6 Requirements for Diagnosis

The diagnosis of nail eczema is mainly based on clinical examination. Patients presenting with suspected nail eczema are asked about the history of eczema or rashes involving the hands, feet, and digits, because a rash may or may not be present at the time of diagnosis. Since the differential diagnosis includes nail psoriasis and onychomycosis, a clipping with histopathology can be used to rule out these other entities.

5.7 Cases

Figures 5.1, 5.2, 5.3, 5.4, 5.5, 5.6, and 5.7 demonstrate the manifestations of nail eczema in a clinical setting.

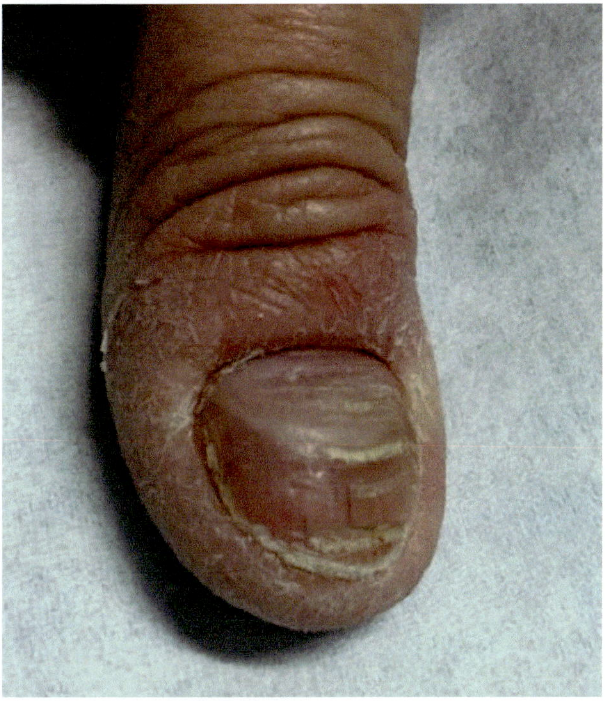

Fig. 5.1 75-Year-old female, Fitzpatrick type II, nail eczema, with xerotic patches of the right thumb. There are wide grooves in the nail plate and the cuticle is mostly absent

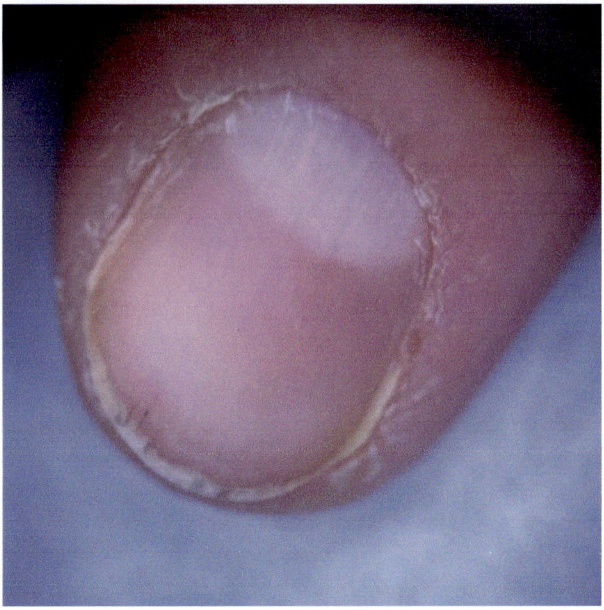

Fig. 5.2 31-Year-old female, Fitzpatrick type II, nail eczema. With contact dermoscopy, the wide grooves are obliterated with the ultrasound gel. Dermoscopy shows splinter hemorrhages

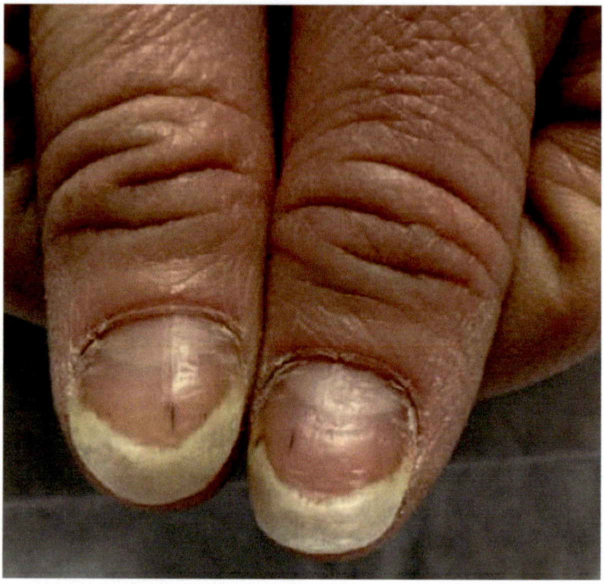

Fig. 5.3 40-Year-old female, Fitzpatrick type II, nail eczema, with bilateral thumbnails with onycholysis, wide grooves in the nail plate, splinter hemorrhages, and xerotic patches on the nail folds

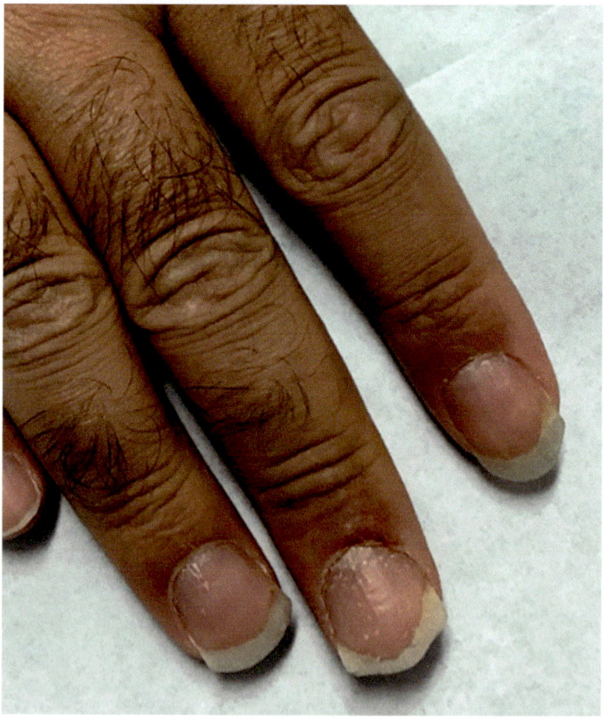

Fig. 5.4 38-Year-old male, Fitzpatrick type III, nail eczema, with onycholysis and wide grooves involving the left third fingernail

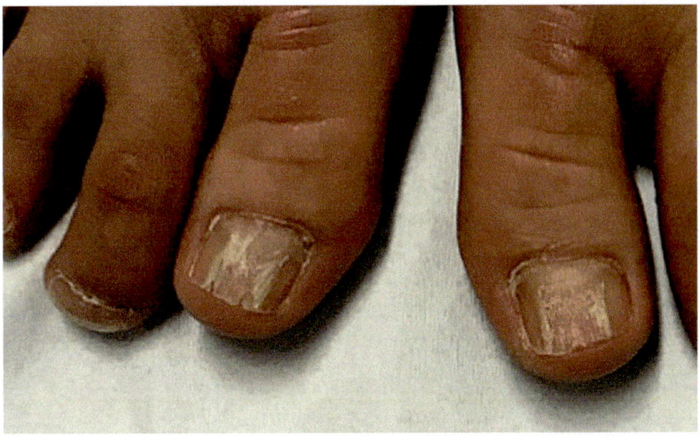

Fig. 5.5 36-Year-old female, Fitzpatrick type III, nail eczema, with onychorrhexis with sandpaper texture involving the bilateral great toenails

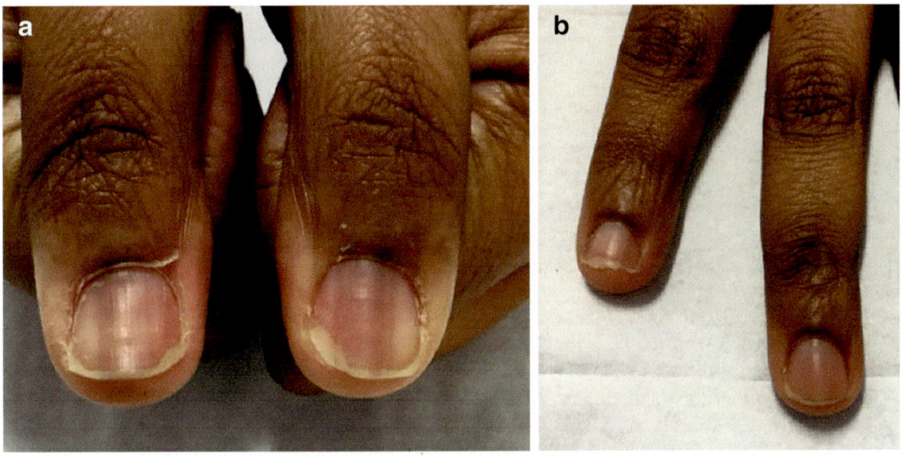

Fig. 5.6 (**a** and **b**) 38-Year-old female, Fitzpatrick type V, nail eczema, with onycholysis and wide transverse grooves involving the bilateral thumbnails and right fifth fingernail. There are also grey longitudinal bands involving the thumbnails

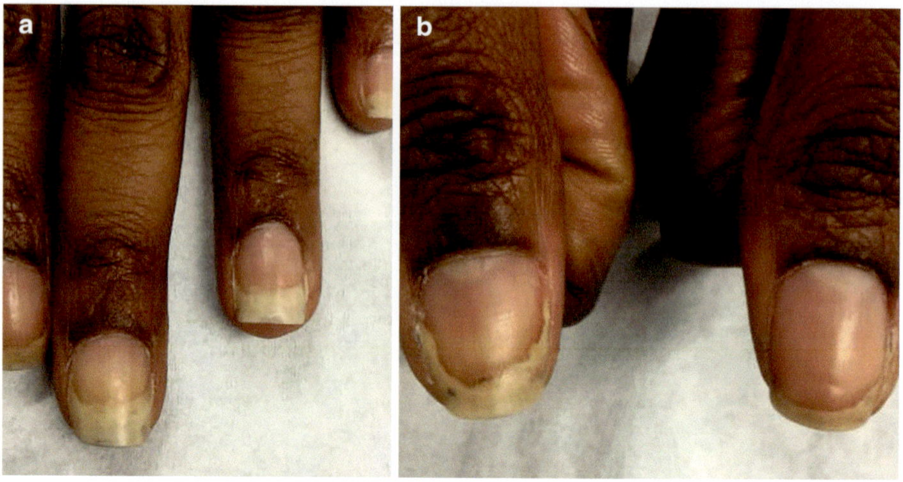

Fig. 5.7 (**a** and **b**) 44-Year-old female, Fitzpatrick type V, nail eczema, with onycholysis involving the fingernails and wide transverse grooves involving the left thumbnail, right second fingernail, and right third fingernail

References

1. Chung BY, Choi YW, Kim HO, Park CW. Nail dystrophy in patients with atopic dermatitis and its association with disease severity. Ann Dermatol. 2019;31(2):121–6. Epub 2019/04/01. https://doi.org/10.5021/ad.2019.31.2.121.
2. Milanesi N, D'Erme AM, Gola M. Nail improvement during alitretinoin treatment: three case reports and review of the literature. Clin Exp Dermatol. 2015;40(5):533–6. Epub 2015/02/17. https://doi.org/10.1111/ced.12584.
3. Richert B, André J. Nail disorders in children: diagnosis and management. Am J Clin Dermatol. 2011;12(2):101–12. https://doi.org/10.2165/11537110-000000000-00000.
4. Simpson EL, Thompson MM, Hanifin JM. Prevalence and morphology of hand eczema in patients with atopic dermatitis. Dermatitis. 2006;17(3):123–7. Epub 2006/09/08. https://doi.org/10.2310/6620.2006.06005.
5. Arslan Uku S, Demir B, Cicek D, Inan Yuksel E. Assessment of nail findings in children with atopic dermatitis. Clin Exp Dermatol. 2021;46(8):1511–7. Epub 2021/08/04. https://doi.org/10.1111/ced.14783.
6. Kantor R, Silverberg JI. Environmental risk factors and their role in the management of atopic dermatitis. Expert Rev Clin Immunol. 2017;13(1):15–26. Epub 2016/07/28. https://doi.org/10.1080/1744666x.2016.1212660.
7. Wan J, Mitra N, Hoffstad OJ, Gelfand JM, Yan AC, Margolis DJ. Variations in risk of asthma and seasonal allergies between early- and late-onset pediatric atopic dermatitis: a cohort study. J Am Acad Dermatol. 2017;77(4):634–40. Epub 2017/08/14. https://doi.org/10.1016/j.jaad.2017.06.013.

Nail Lichen Planus

6

Eden Axler and Shari R. Lipner

6.1 Description of Disease

Lichen planus (LP) is an inflammatory condition that may affect the skin, scalp, mucosa, and nails. Nail lichen planus (NLP) may cause permanent nail loss and have a negative impact on daily functioning [1–3]. Therefore, early recognition, diagnosis, and treatment are necessary. NLP is characterized by longitudinal nail plate ridging and fissuring [2]. As the disease progresses, a dorsal pterygium, or scar, may develop, resulting in permanent nail loss [4, 5]. Approximately 4–12% of individuals with NLP experience permanent damage to at least one nail [6]. Little is known about disease pathophysiology, although abnormal toll-like receptor activity is hypothesized to play a role [1].

6.2 Epidemiology

LP may involve the skin, mucosa, scalp, and nails or may be isolated to the nails [7]. In a prospective study including 75 patients with cutaneous LP, nail findings were present in 28% of patients, with a mean age of 58.1 +/– 12.6 years with female predominance (57.14%) [8]. In a retrospective study of 24 patients with isolated NLP, the average age was 47 years [9]. It is estimated that 10–15% of NLP cases are in children [1].

6.3 Clinical Features

NLP impacts fingernails more often than toenails. In a retrospective study of 67 NLP patients, 94% had fingernail involvement (average: seven fingernails), and 54% had toenail involvement (average: three toenails) [10]. Clinical features of NLP often overlap with other nail dystrophies, and therefore no single finding

S. R. Lipner, *Atlas of Nail Disorders Across All Skin Colors*,
https://doi.org/10.1007/978-3-031-74272-9_6

may be pathognomonic [5]. NLP variants include trachyonychia and bullous NLP [5]. NLP may affect the nail matrix or nail bed, and it often affects both. Nail bed disease signs include onycholysis, subungual hyperkeratosis, salmon patches or oil spots, splinter hemorrhages, and distal splitting [4, 11]. Nail matrix signs include nail pitting, leukonychia, red lunula, and crumbling [11]. In a cross-sectional study with 31 NLP patients, predominant nail findings were longitudinal ridging (74.2%), splinter hemorrhages (58.1%), trachyonychia (25.8%), nail pitting (22.45%), and transverse ridging (19.4%) [12]. More severe NLP changes include complete fissuring, deep grooves, splits exceeding 5 mm in length, onycholysis exceeding 50%, erythema of the lunula, dorsal pterygium, and anonychia [2].

6.4 Clinical Features in Skin of Color

In individuals with darker skin tones, longitudinal melanonychia often accompanies other characteristic nail findings. Clinical presentation of NLP may vary amongst individuals, regardless of skin color.

6.5 Risk Factors

Risk factors for LP include hepatitis C virus, autoimmune disease, internal malignancies, dyslipidemia, anxiety, depression, and viral infection [13, 14]. An association between NLP and metal allergy has been explored in a retrospective study with 115 LP patients. The prevalence of metal allergy in NLP patients was higher compared to oral LP patients (59% vs. 27%, $P < 0.05$) [15]. Further research is needed to clarify specific risk factors for NLP.

6.6 Requirements for Diagnosis

Clinical features may be highly suggestive of NLP. Nail biopsy, preferably using a longitudinal excision, may be necessary in challenging cases. In a cohort study of 45 patients with confirmed cutaneous LP with nail findings who underwent nail biopsy, histopathological features of NLP were sawtooth acanthosis and a widespread lichenoid infiltrate closely adhering to the dermo-epidermal junction, accompanied by basal layer liquefaction. A less common diagnostic feature of NLP is hypergranulosis of the nail bed epithelium [5].

6.7 Cases

Figures 6.1, 6.2, 6.3, 6.4, 6.5, and 6.6 demonstrate the presentation of NLP in a clinical setting.

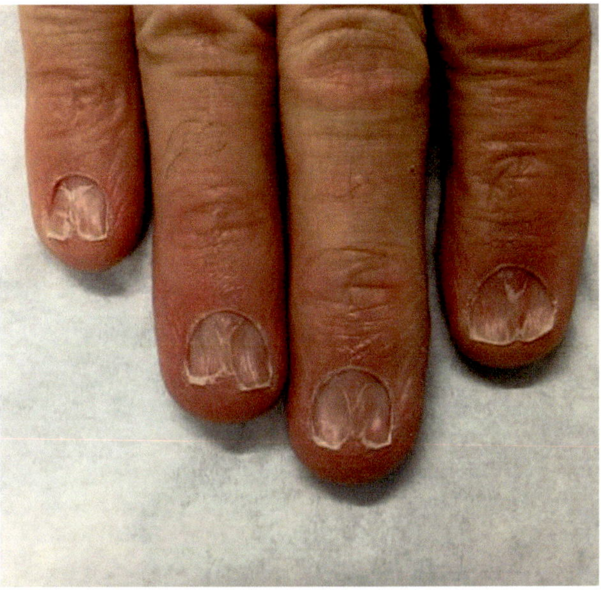

Fig. 6.1 53-Year-old male, Fitzpatrick type II, nail lichen planus, with longitudinal ridging, koilonychia, and nail splitting of the right fingernails

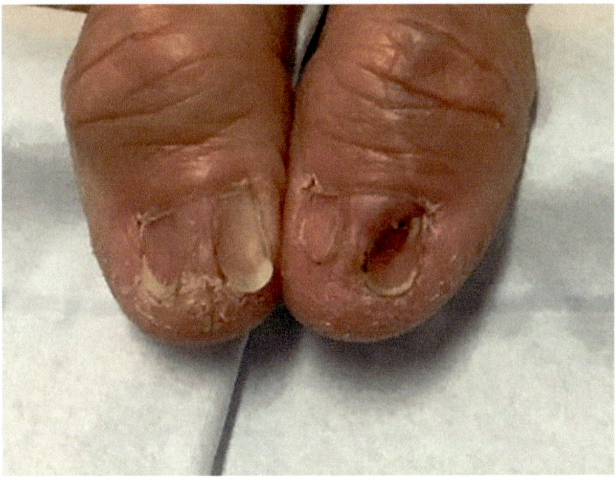

Fig. 6.2 79-Year-old female, Fitzpatrick type II, nail lichen planus, with nail plate atrophy and dorsal pterygium of the bilateral thumbnails

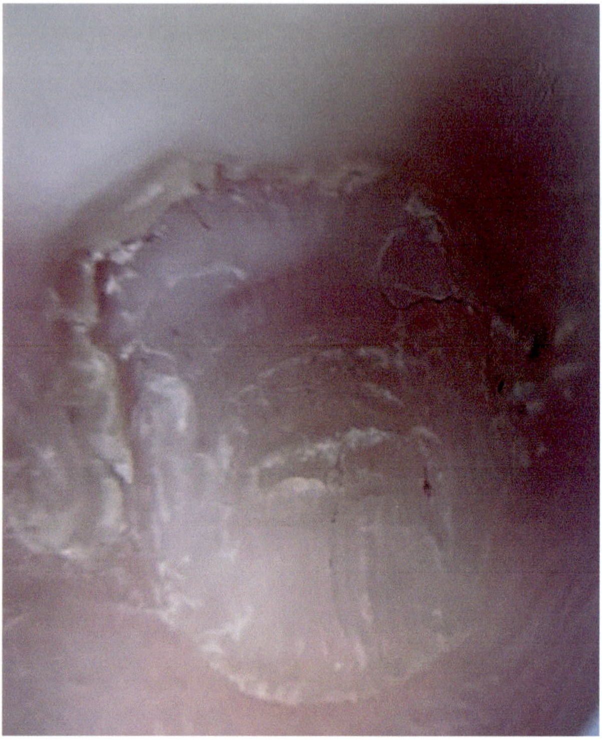

Fig. 6.3 53-Year-old female, Fitzpatrick type II, nail lichen planus. Dermoscopy shows nail plate thinning, ragged cuticles, and nail plate atrophy

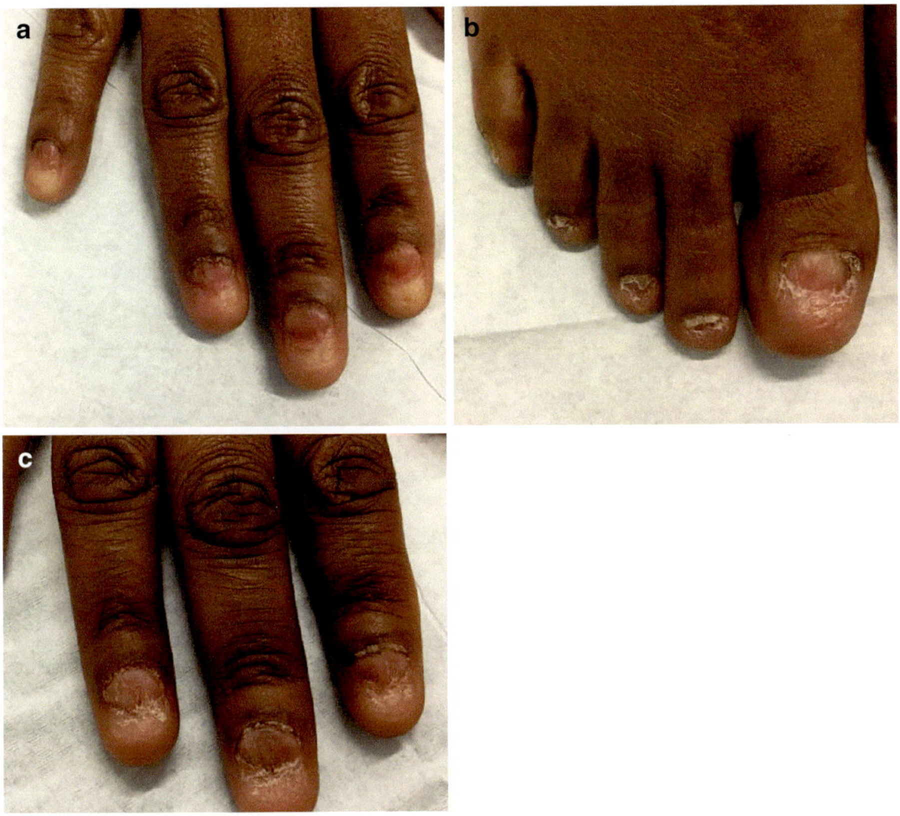

Fig. 6.4 (**a–c**) 48-Year-old female, Fitzpatrick type IV, nail lichen planus, with longitudinal melanonychia, nail plate atrophy, and nail loss

Fig. 6.5 35-Year-old female, Fitzpatrick type V, nail lichen planus, with longitudinal melanonychia, pterygium, and onycholysis of the right fingernails

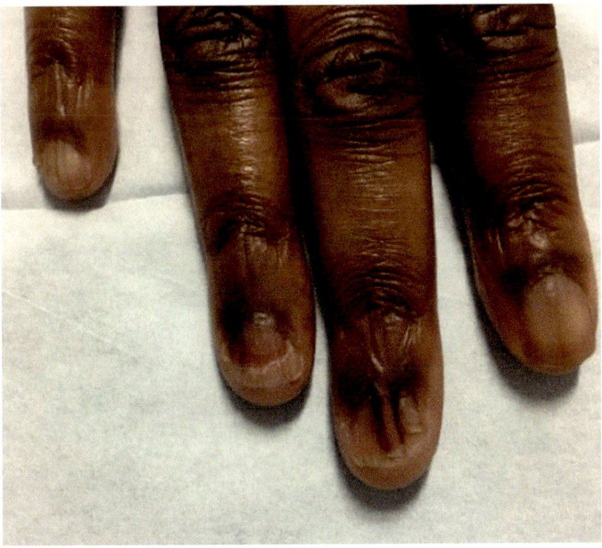

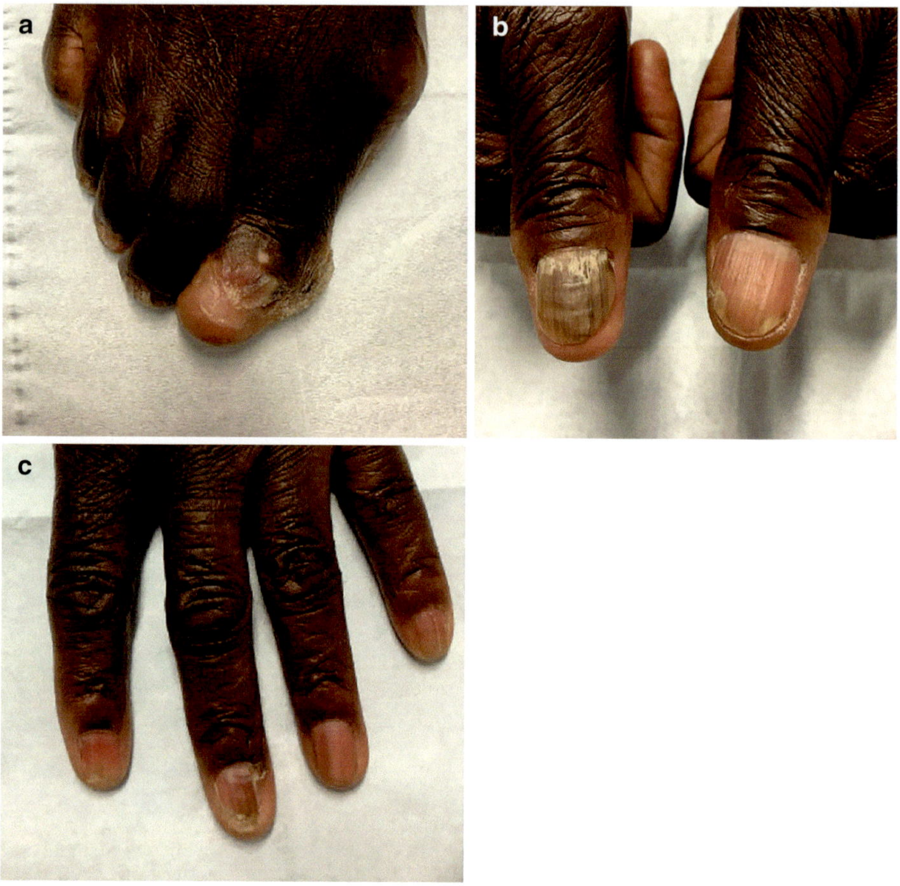

Fig. 6.6 (**a–c**) 67-Year-old male, Fitzpatrick type VI, nail lichen planus, with longitudinal melanonychia, longitudinal ridging, nail plate splitting, and nail loss

References

1. Gupta MK, Lipner SR. Review of nail lichen planus: epidemiology, pathogenesis, diagnosis, and treatment. Dermatol Clin. 2021;39(2):221–30. https://doi.org/10.1016/j.det.2020.12.002.
2. Iorizzo M, Tosti A, Starace M, et al. Isolated nail lichen planus: an expert consensus on treatment of the classical form. J Am Acad Dermatol. 2020;83(6):1717–23. https://doi.org/10.1016/j.jaad.2020.02.056.
3. Dehesa L, Tosti A. Treatment of inflammatory nail disorders. Dermatol Ther. 2012;25(6):525–34. https://doi.org/10.1111/j.1529-8019.2012.01516.x.
4. Lipner SR. Nail lichen planus: a true nail emergency. J Am Acad Dermatol. 2019;80(6):e177–8. https://doi.org/10.1016/j.jaad.2018.11.065.
5. Kharghoria G, Grover C, Bhattacharya SN, Sharma S. Histopathological evaluation of nail lichen planus: a cross-sectional study. J Cutan Pathol. 2021;48(1):11–7. https://doi.org/10.1111/cup.13783.
6. Grover C, Kharghoria G, Baran R. Nail lichen planus: a review of clinical presentation, diagnosis and therapy. Ann Dermatol Venereol. 2022;149(3):150–64. https://doi.org/10.1016/j.annder.2022.01.010.

7. Tziotzios C, Lee JYW, Brier T, et al. Lichen planus and lichenoid dermatoses: clinical overview and molecular basis. J Am Acad Dermatol. 2018;79(5):789–804. https://doi.org/10.1016/j.jaad.2018.02.010.
8. Żychowska M, Żychowska M. Nail changes in lichen planus: a single-center study. J Cutan Med Surg. 2021;25(3):281–5. https://doi.org/10.1177/1203475420982554.
9. Tosti A, Peluso AM, Fanti PA, Piraccini BM. Nail lichen planus: clinical and pathologic study of twenty-four patients. J Am Acad Dermatol. 1993;28(5 Pt 1):724–30. https://doi.org/10.1016/0190-9622(93)70100-8.
10. Goettmann S, Zaraa I, Moulonguet I. Nail lichen planus: epidemiological, clinical, pathological, therapeutic and prognosis study of 67 cases. J Eur Acad Dermatol Venereol. 2012;26(10):1304–9. https://doi.org/10.1111/j.1468-3083.2011.04288.x.
11. Hwang JK, Grover C, Iorizzo M, et al. Nail psoriasis & nail lichen planus: updates on diagnosis & management. J Am Acad Dermatol. 2023;90:585. https://doi.org/10.1016/j.jaad.2023.11.024.
12. Sharma S, Kaur J, Bassi R, Sekhon HK. Dermatoscopy of nail lichen planus: a boon for early diagnosis. J Clin Aesthet Dermatol. 2021;14(7):34–7.
13. Gorouhi F, Davari P, Fazel N. Cutaneous and mucosal lichen planus: a comprehensive review of clinical subtypes, risk factors, diagnosis, and prognosis. ScientificWorldJournal. 2014;2014:742826. https://doi.org/10.1155/2014/742826.
14. Hong S, Fan R, Cohen JM. Lichen planus is associated with depression and anxiety: a cross-sectional study in the all of us research program. Arch Dermatol Res. 2023;315(5):1417–9. https://doi.org/10.1007/s00403-022-02459-4.
15. Nishizawa A, Satoh T, Yokozeki H. Close association between metal allergy and nail lichen planus: detection of causative metals in nail lesions. J Eur Acad Dermatol Venereol. 2013;27(2):e231–4. https://doi.org/10.1111/j.1468-3083.2012.04561.x.

Nail Psoriasis

7

Eden Axler and Shari R. Lipner

7.1 Description of Disease

Psoriasis is a chronic inflammatory condition that may affect the skin, scalp, genitalia, nails, and joints, and is characterized by epidermal hyperproliferation resulting in erythematous to brown plaques with grey or silver scale [1]. Approximately 5–10% of psoriasis patients have only nail changes without skin involvement [2].

7.2 Epidemiology

7.2.1 Sex

Nail psoriasis (NP) may be more common in men. In a prospective study by Pourchot et al. [3] including 313 children with psoriasis, nail findings occurred in 43% of males vs. 22% of females ($P < 0.001$). In a cross-sectional study including 3,531 psoriasis patients, 40.9% had nail involvement, with men being affected 11.2% more frequently than women [4].

7.2.2 Adult Patients

In a prospective cohort study including 4,016 adults with skin psoriasis, 24.5% had nail involvement, with a higher prevalence observed with increasing psoriasis severity [5].

S. R. Lipner, *Atlas of Nail Disorders Across All Skin Colors*,
https://doi.org/10.1007/978-3-031-74272-9_7

7.2.3 Children

In the prospective study by Pourchot et al. [3], 32.3% of children with psoriasis had nail findings, with associations between nail involvement and psoriatic arthritis ($P = 0.03$), palmoplantar psoriasis ($P < 0.001$), and psoriasis severity as indicated by the use of systemic treatment ($P = 0.003$) [3].

7.2.4 Other Factors

NP affects up to 80% of patients with psoriatic arthritis [6]. A meta-analysis of 21 articles found that 66% of individuals with psoriatic arthritis had nail changes [7].

7.3 Risk Factors

Risk factors for NP are not entirely clear. In a case-control study by Peng et al. [1] including 929 NP patients compared to 2,991 patients with cutaneous psoriasis but no nail involvement, those with nail involvement more often were active smokers, had a family history of psoriasis, drug allergies, light sensitivity, and comorbidities including diabetes, cardiovascular disease, and rheumatic disease ($P < 0.001$ for all) [1].

7.4 Clinical Features

In individuals with cutaneous psoriasis, nail symptoms typically appear later than skin manifestations, with an average delay of 9–11.5 years [8]. Nail matrix psoriasis presents with pitting, leukonychia, chromonychia, and nail crumbling, and less commonly Beau's lines, onychomadesis, trachyonychia, and total nail plate dystrophy [2]. Nail bed psoriasis presents with onycholysis, oil drops, splinter hemorrhages, and subungual hyperkeratosis [2]. Many patients will have psoriasis involving both the nail matrix and nail bed. In a retrospective study of 87 patients with isolated NP, the most common features were onycholysis (79%), nail pitting (70%), splinter hemorrhage (28%), and nail thickening (28%) [9]. In the aforementioned case-control study by Peng et al. [1], involvement of the scalp, palmoplantar regions, genitals, and presence of psoriatic arthritis was more common in the group with nail involvement (OR 3.10 (95% CI:2.58–3.71; $P < 0.001$), 3.63 (95% CI:3.07–4.30; $P < 0.001$), 3.40 (95% CI:2.80–4.12; $P < 0.001$), and 2.51 (95% CI:1.83–3.45; $P < 0.001$)), respectively [1]. With dermoscopy, the most common features of nail matrix and plate involvement were pitting (70.7%) and onycholysis (57.8%), respectively [6].

7.5 Clinical Features in Skin of Color

In a retrospective study of 87 patients with NP, 82% were of Fitzpatrick skin types I–III, while only 18% were of types IV–VI. Patients with skin types IV-VI had a longer time to diagnosis vs. patients with skin types I-III (59 vs. 24 months; $P = 0.009$), and had higher average nail psoriasis severity index scores (6 vs. 5; $P = 0.029$). There were similar clinical findings, including onycholysis (79% vs. 71%) and pitting (68% vs. 75%) ($P > 0.05$ for all) in skin types IV-V vs. I-III, but patients with darker skin types more often had longitudinal melanonychia [10].

7.6 Requirements for Diagnosis

Diagnosis of NP is made clinically. Dermoscopy, videodermoscopy, and capillaroscopy may also be utilized to better visualize nail changes [11]. Patients may have signs of cutaneous psoriasis and should be asked about a history of joint pains. Nail clippings with histopathology will help differentiate NP from other nail dystrophies, including onychomycosis. Supportive histopathological features using a nail clipping include subungual parakeratosis and infiltration of neutrophils, with the absence of hyphae. While a nail biopsy is rarely required for diagnosis, it may be considered in challenging cases.

7.7 Cases

Figures 7.1, 7.2, 7.3, 7.4, 7.5, 7.6, and 7.7 demonstrate the presentation of nail psoriasis in a clinical setting.

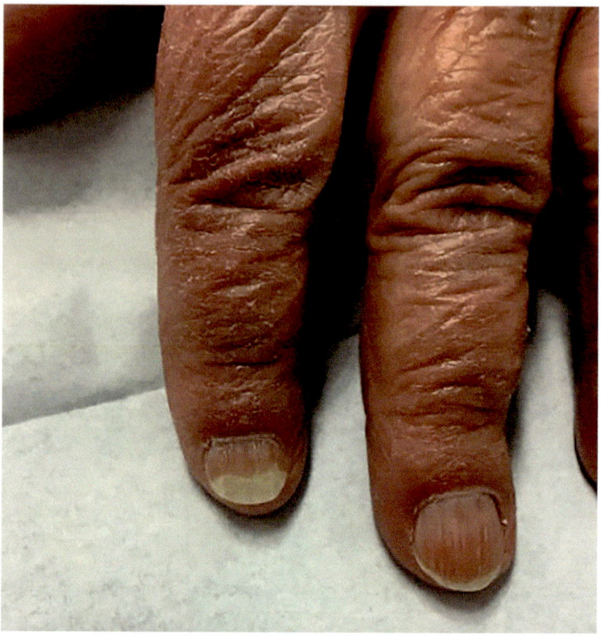

Fig. 7.1 87-Year-old female, Fitzpatrick type II, nail psoriasis, with onycholysis on the left second fingernail and an oil drop on the left third fingernail

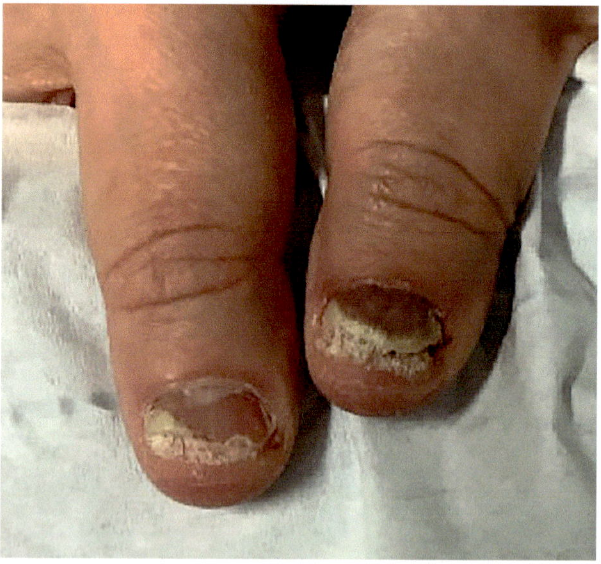

Fig. 7.2 51-Year-old female, Fitzpatrick type II, nail psoriasis, with onycholysis and nail bed hyperkeratosis on the bilateral thumbnails

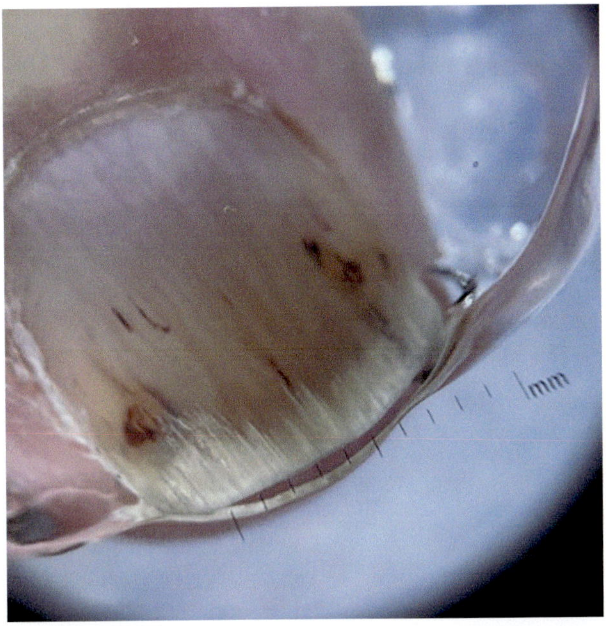

Fig. 7.3 60-Year-old male, Fitzpatrick type II, nail psoriasis, with dermoscopy showing onycholysis and splinter hemorrhages

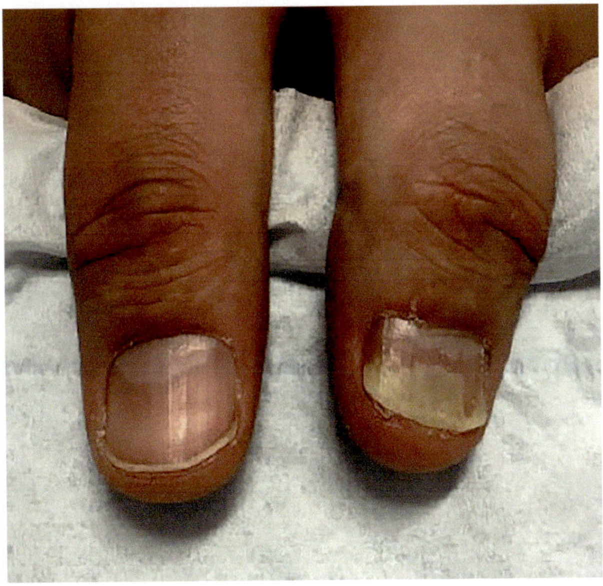

Fig. 7.4 40-Year-old male, Fitzpatrick type III, nail psoriasis, with onycholysis and nail bed hyperkeratosis of the left thumbnail

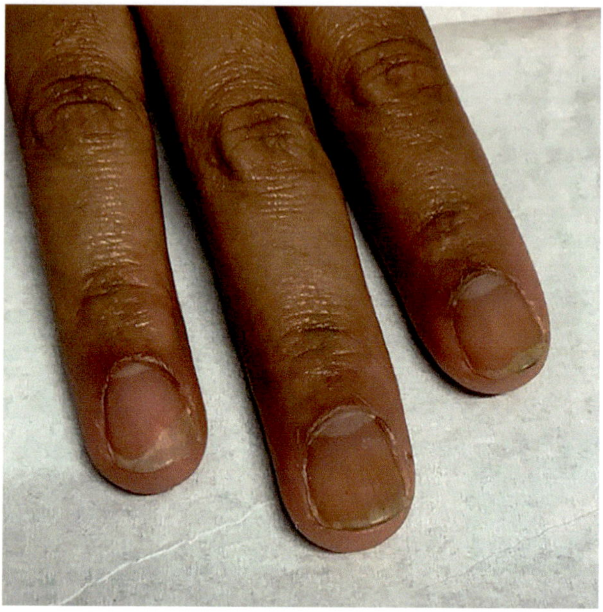

Fig. 7.5 45-Year-old female, Fitzpatrick type III, nail psoriasis, with onycholysis of the left second and fourth fingernails and an oil drop of the left second and third fingernails

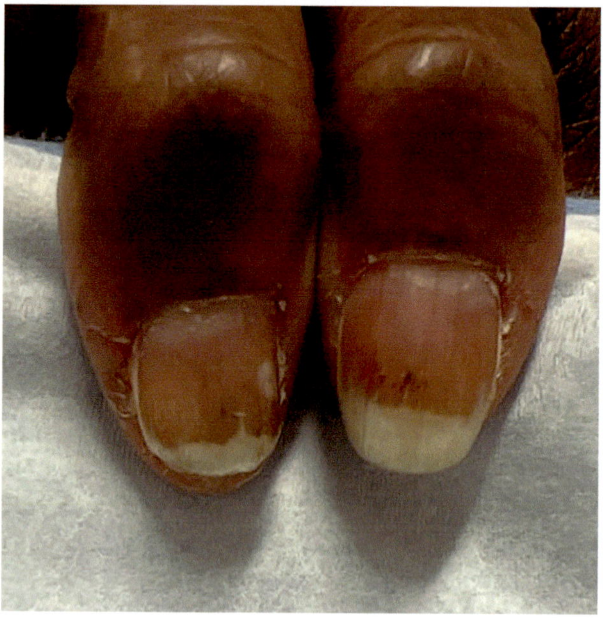

Fig. 7.6 61-Year-old female, Fitzpatrick type V, nail psoriasis, with onycholysis, oil drops, and splinter hemorrhages of the bilateral thumbnails

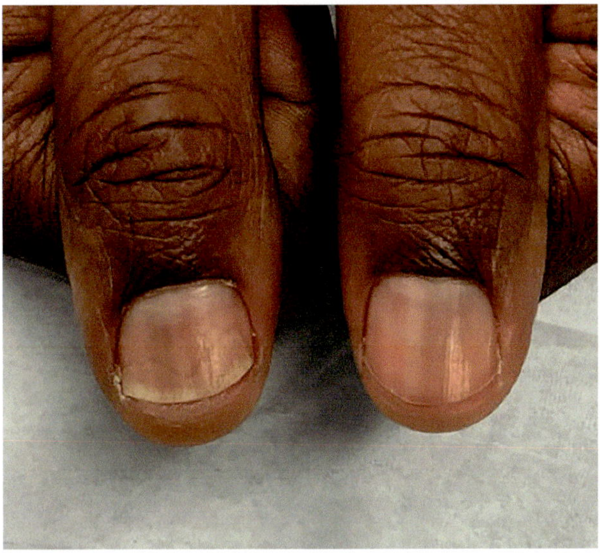

Fig. 7.7 59-Year-old male, Fitzpatrick type V, nail psoriasis, with nail pitting and onycholysis on the right thumbnail and longitudinal melanonychia on the bilateral thumbnails

References

1. Peng YT, Yu RT, Chen AJ, et al. Predicting the risk of nail involvement in psoriasis patients: development and assessment of a predictive nomogram. Diagnostics (Basel). 2023;13(4). https://doi.org/10.3390/diagnostics13040633.
2. Rigopoulos D, Baran R, Chiheb S, et al. Recommendations for the definition, evaluation, and treatment of nail psoriasis in adult patients with no or mild skin psoriasis: a dermatologist and nail expert group consensus. J Am Acad Dermatol. 2019;81(1):228–40. https://doi.org/10.1016/j.jaad.2019.01.072.
3. Pourchot D, Bodemer C, Phan A, et al. Nail psoriasis: a systematic evaluation in 313 children with psoriasis. Pediatr Dermatol. 2017;34(1):58–63. https://doi.org/10.1111/pde.13028.
4. Augustin M, Reich K, Blome C, Schäfer I, Laass A, Radtke MA. Nail psoriasis in Germany: epidemiology and burden of disease. Br J Dermatol. 2010;163(3):580–5. https://doi.org/10.1111/j.1365-2133.2010.09831.x.
5. Egeberg A, See K, Garrelts A, Burge R. Epidemiology of psoriasis in hard-to-treat body locations: data from the Danish skin cohort. BMC Dermatol. 2020;20(1):3. https://doi.org/10.1186/s12895-020-00099-7.
6. Ji C, Wang H, Bao C, et al. Challenge of nail psoriasis: an update review. Clin Rev Allergy Immunol. 2021;61(3):377–402. https://doi.org/10.1007/s12016-021-08896-9.
7. Sandre MK, Rohekar S. Psoriatic arthritis and nail changes: exploring the relationship. Semin Arthritis Rheum. 2014;44(2):162–9. https://doi.org/10.1016/j.semarthrit.2014.05.002.
8. Dogra A, Arora AK. Nail psoriasis: the journey so far. Indian J Dermatol. 2014;59(4):319–33. https://doi.org/10.4103/0019-5154.135470.
9. Chang MJ, Lee D, Desai AD, Lipner SR. The untold burden of isolated nail psoriasis: delayed diagnosis and significant risk of psoriatic arthritis in a retrospective study at an academic center. J Am Acad Dermatol. 2023;88(5):1192–4. https://doi.org/10.1016/j.jaad.2022.12.031.
10. Chang MJ, Lee D, Desai AD, Lipner SR. Disparities in time to diagnosis and disease severity in skin of colour patients with nail psoriasis: a retrospective analysis. J Eur Acad Dermatol Venereol. 2023;37. https://doi.org/10.1111/jdv.19110.
11. Haneke E. Nail psoriasis: clinical features, pathogenesis, differential diagnoses, and management. Psoriasis (Auckl). 2017;7:51–63. https://doi.org/10.2147/ptt.S126281.

Trachyonychia

8

Eden Axler and Shari R. Lipner

8.1 Description of Disease

Trachyonychia does not cause permanent nail changes or pterygium, and approximately 50% of cases resolve spontaneously. In a prospective study of 12 patients with trachyonychia, 6 patients had total resolution within 6 years of follow-up, without treatment [1].

8.2 Epidemiology

Trachyonychia may occur at any age, with peak age of onset between 3 and 12 years old [2]. The exact prevalence is unknown. While trachyonychia may occur idiopathically, several dermatologic diseases have been associated with this condition, including alopecia areata, psoriasis, lichen planus, and atopic dermatitis [3, 4]. Shiny trachyonychia is estimated to affect 3.3% of adults and 12% of children with alopecia areata [5]. Nail changes may precede or occur after hair loss begins. Opaque trachyonychia is linked to psoriasis, and individuals with both psoriasis and trachyonychia may experience nail plate thickening [3, 6]. In a retrospective study including 14 patients with cutaneous lichen planus and concomitant nail changes, 50% of patients had trachyonychia [7]. In a cohort study including 24 pediatric atopic dermatitis patients with nail changes, 12.5% had trachyonychia. There was no association between the severity of atopic dermatitis and the development of nail disease ($P = 0.236$) [8].

8.3 Risk Factors

Risk factors for trachyonychia have not been well studied. Risk factors may include history of alopecia areata, psoriasis, lichen planus, or atopic dermatitis.

S. R. Lipner, *Atlas of Nail Disorders Across All Skin Colors*,
https://doi.org/10.1007/978-3-031-74272-9_8

8.4 Clinical Features

In a retrospective review of 122 trachyonychia patients, pitting (80.3%), koilonychia (45%), and hyperkeratosis (19.6%) were the most common features [9].

8.5 Clinical Features in Skin of Color

Trachyonychia may occur in individuals of any skin color. Patients with darker skin types often have longitudinal melanonychia along with classic nail findings.

8.6 Requirements for Diagnosis

A nail clipping with histopathology may show the presence or absence of psoriasis and onychomycosis. Since trachyonychia may be diagnosed clinically and has a benign course, a biopsy is often not required, though it may be considered in difficult cases [6]. Histologically, trachyonychia is characterized by a spongiotic pattern [10].

8.7 Cases

Figures 8.1, 8.2, 8.3, 8.4, 8.5, and 8.6 demonstrate the presentation of trachyonychia in a clinical setting.

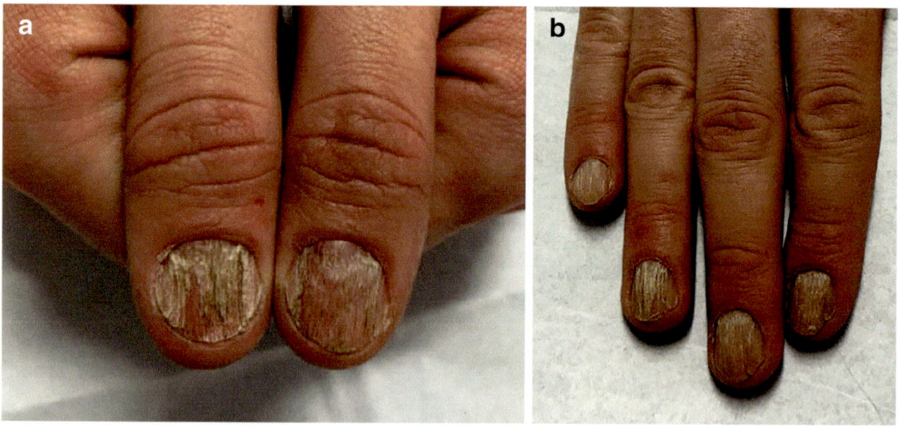

Fig. 8.1 (**a** and **b**) 31-Year-old male, Fitzpatrick type II, trachyonychia, with extensive longitudinal ridging of the thumbnails and fingernails

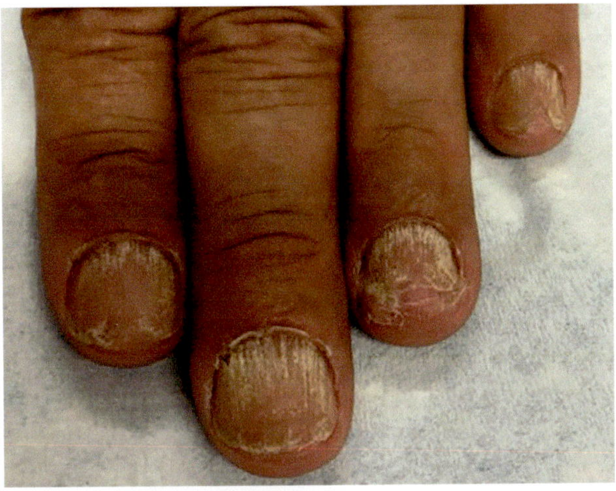

Fig. 8.2 58-Year-old male, Fitzpatrick type III, alopecia universalis and trachyonychia, with extensive ridging and onychoschizia of the fingernails (*from* Gupta et al. [11]; *with permission*)

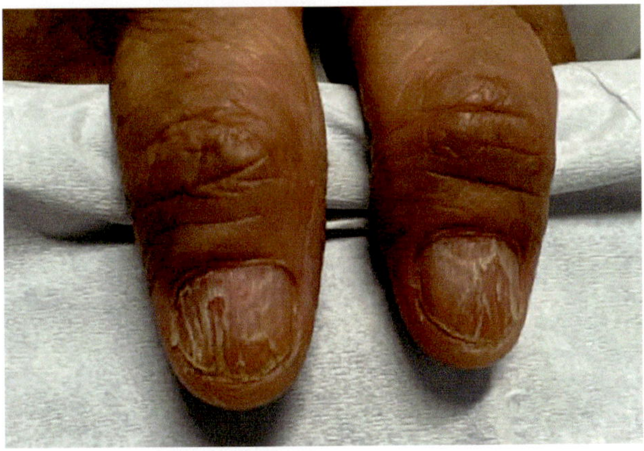

Fig. 8.3 54-Year-old female, Fitzpatrick type III, trachyonychia, with longitudinal ridging and onychoschizia of the bilateral thumbnails

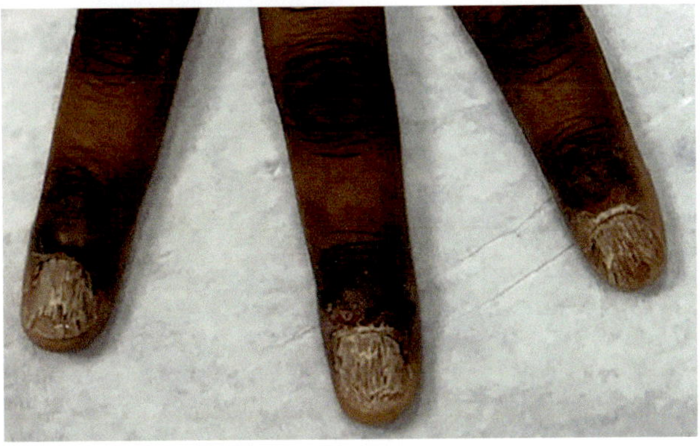

Fig. 8.4 39-Year-old female, Fitzpatrick type V, trachyonychia, with extensive longitudinal ridging of the fingernails

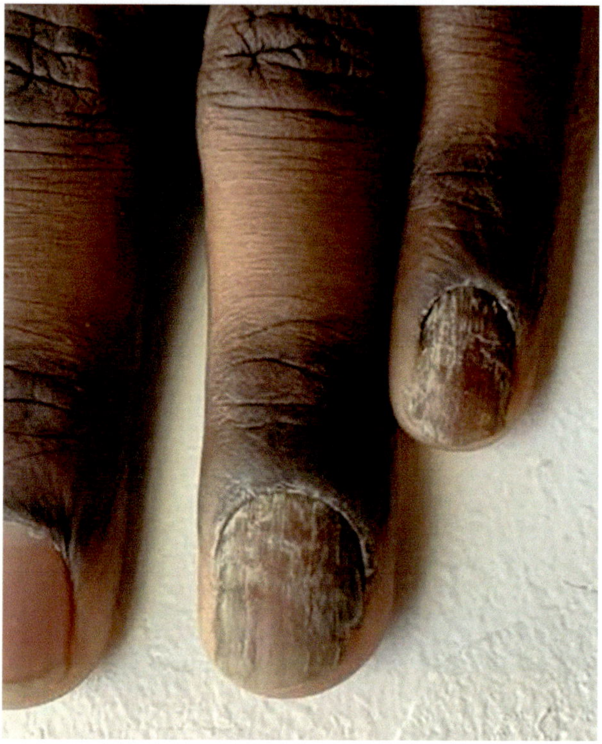

Fig. 8.5 34-Year-old female, Fitzpatrick type V, trachyonychia, with longitudinal ridging of the left fourth and fifth fingernails

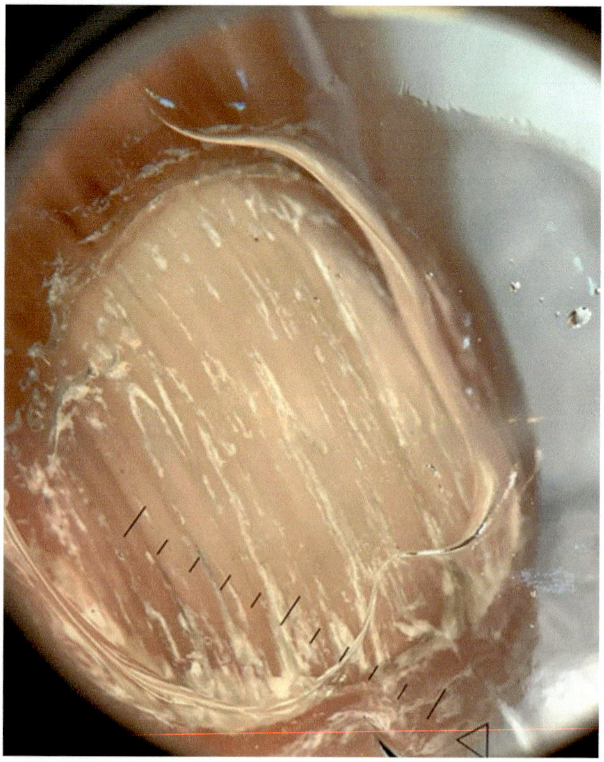

Fig. 8.6 Dermoscopy image of a 39-year-old female, Fitzpatrick type V, trachyonychia, with extensive longitudinal ridging of the left fourth fingernail

References

1. Sakata S, Howard A, Tosti A, Sinclair R. Follow up of 12 patients with trachyonychia. Australas J Dermatol. 2006;47(3):166–8. https://doi.org/10.1111/j.1440-0960.2006.00264.x.
2. Leung AKC, Leong KF, Barankin B. Trachyonychia. J Pediatr. 2020;216:239–239.e1. https://doi.org/10.1016/j.jpeds.2019.08.034.
3. Haber JS, Chairatchaneeboon M, Rubin AI. Trachyonychia: review and update on clinical aspects, histology, and therapy. Skin Appendage Disord. 2017;2(3–4):109–15. https://doi.org/10.1159/000449063.
4. Tosti A, Bardazzi F, Piraccini BM, Fanti PA. Idiopathic trachyonychia (twenty-nail dystrophy): a pathological study of 23 patients. Br J Dermatol. 1994;131(6):866–72. https://doi.org/10.1111/j.1365-2133.1994.tb08591.x.
5. Tosti A, Bardazzi F, Piraccini BM, Fanti PA, Cameli N, Pileri S. Is trachyonychia, a variety of alopecia areata, limited to the nails? J Invest Dermatol. 1995;104(5 Suppl):27s–8s. https://doi.org/10.1038/jid.1995.47.
6. Gordon KA, Vega JM, Tosti A. Trachyonychia: a comprehensive review. Indian J Dermatol Venereol Leprol. 2011;77(6):640–5. https://doi.org/10.4103/0378-6323.86470.
7. Wechsuruk P, Bunyaratavej S, Kiratiwongwan R, Suphatsathienkul P, Wongdama S, Leeyaphan C. Clinical features and treatment outcomes of nail lichen planus: a retrospective study. JAAD Case Rep. 2021;17:43–8. https://doi.org/10.1016/j.jdcr.2021.09.015.
8. Chung BY, Choi YW, Kim HO, Park CW. Nail dystrophy in patients with atopic dermatitis and its association with disease severity. Ann Dermatol. 2019;31(2):121–6. https://doi.org/10.5021/ad.2019.31.2.121.
9. Starace M, Alessandrini A, Bruni F, Piraccini BM. Trachyonychia: a retrospective study of 122 patients in a period of 30 years. J Eur Acad Dermatol Venereol. 2020;34(4):880–4. https://doi.org/10.1111/jdv.16186.
10. Rubin AI, Haneke E. A fresh look at the histopathology of trachyonychia. J Cutan Pathol. 2021;48(3):349–50. https://doi.org/10.1111/cup.13968.
11. Gupta MK, Geizhals S, Lipner SR. Intralesional triamcinolone matrix injections for treatment of trachyonychia. J Am Acad Dermatol. 2020;82(4):e121–2. https://doi.org/10.1016/j.jaad.2019.09.060. Epub 2019 Oct 4.

Part III

Benign Nail Tumors

Glomus Tumor

9

Rachel C. Hill and Shari R. Lipner

9.1 Description of Disease

Glomus tumors are benign tumors derived from neuromyoarterial glomus bodies, which play a role in thermoregulation and regulation of vascular flow [1, 2]. They are composed of a combination of glomus cells, smooth muscle cells, and blood vessels. Glomus tumors are most common in the digits and subungual region, since these anatomic areas are densely populated by glomus bodies [2, 3]. It is estimated that 75% of glomus tumors occur in the subungual region [4]. Glomus tumors may also be found in the dermis of the palms and forearms, and solid organs, including the stomach, pancreas, and the gastrointestinal tract [5]. There are three variants of glomus tumors: (1) solid, which is composed mainly of glomus cells (2) glomangioma, which is composed mainly of blood vessels, and (3) glomangiomyoma, which is composed mainly of smooth muscle cells [6]. Glomangiomyoma is the rarest variant of glomus tumor, comprising approximately 2–5% of all glomus tumors [7].

9.2 Epidemiology

9.2.1 Sex

While glomus tumors in general do not show a sex predilection, subungual glomus tumors may be more common in females [2, 5, 6, 8, 9]. In a 14-year retrospective review of clinical and histopathological-proven glomus tumors at a single academic center, 80% of glomus tumors involving the digits (44/55 cases) were in females [6].

S. R. Lipner, *Atlas of Nail Disorders Across All Skin Colors*,
https://doi.org/10.1007/978-3-031-74272-9_9

9.2.2 Age

Subungual glomus tumors most often affect individuals between the ages of 30 and 60 years old, with a mean age of 42 years in two retrospective studies of 75 cases and 110 cases of digital glomus tumors at single-center academic institutions [2, 3, 10]. Subungual glomangiomyomas have been described in children as young as three years old in case series of familial generalized multiple glomangiomyomas [8].

9.2.3 Other Factors

Multiple glomus tumors are highly associated with Neurofibromatosis I and are due to biallelic inactivation of NF1, a tumor suppressor gene [11–13]. Notably, sporadic cases of glomus tumors are not associated with inactivation of NF1 [14]. In a case-control study of 21 patients with glomus tumors of the hand diagnosed 1995–2010 and 200 randomly selected controls who had ganglion cyst excision procedures in the same time period, six patients in the glomus tumor group were diagnosed with Neurofibromatosis I, while none in the control group had glomus tumors. The odds ratio for glomus tumor among patients with Neurofibromatosis I was 168:1 [11]. Another retrospective cohort study of 42 glomus tumors in 34 individuals included six patients with Neurofibromatosis I who had a total of 12 glomus tumors, and recurrent tumors and multifocal tumors were more common vs. controls, although this did not reach statistical significance ($p > 0.05$) [12].

9.3 Risk Factors

Risk factors for glomus tumors have not been definitively established, but older age and female sex are likely risk factors.

9.4 Clinical Features

Glomus tumors typically present as small, solitary lesions (<1 cm). A blue nodule may be visible through the nail plate or localized longitudinal erythronychia may be appreciated on physical examination. Other nail findings include longitudinal grooves, onycholysis, onychoschizia, splinter hemorrhages, and nail plate thinning [2, 15–20]. The classic clinical features are a triad of cold sensitivity, intermittent pain, and pinpoint tenderness [10, 20]. The Love test, Hildreth test, and cold sensitivity tests may be used to elicit this clinical triad. The Love test involves applying pinpoint pressure to the area of the suspected tumor, which will result in extreme pain to the area affected by the tumor, with no pain affecting the surrounding parts of the nail [21]. The Hildreth test involves applying a tourniquet to the limb with the affected digit and is positive if inflation decreases pain in the nail [22]. The cold sensitivity test involves submerging the affected hand/foot in cold water to elicit pain upon exposure [2]. Transillumination can be used as a physical examination maneuver to aid in clinical diagnosis, as the tumor may become visible as light is transmitted through the nail plate [23]. On dermoscopy, the presence of a purple-red subungual spot and longitudinal erythronychia are highly specific for a glomus tumor [1]. Other dermoscopic findings are localized erythema with blue-white patchy areas, and a "candy-cane" appearance [15].

9.5 Clinical Features in Skin of Color

Clinical features of glomus tumors in patients with skin of color have not been previously described. In addition to classical features, longitudinal melanonychia may be present, which can obscure erythronychia and blue discoloration and complicate the diagnosis.

9.6 Requirements for Diagnosis

Although glomus tumors may be diagnosed clinically, the gold standard remains histopathologic testing to definitively confirm the diagnosis. Histopathology accompanied by total excision of the tumor is required for patients to improve symptoms and prevent tumor recurrence [2]. Advanced imaging, such as MRI and Doppler ultrasound, can be helpful in confirming the clinical diagnosis in equivocal cases, and in performing pre-surgical planning [3, 24, 25]. X-ray may detect bone erosions but is highly insensitive for diagnosis [26].

9.7 Cases

Figures 9.1, 9.2, 9.3, 9.4, 9.5, 9.6, and 9.7 demonstrate the presentation of glomus tumors in a clinical setting.

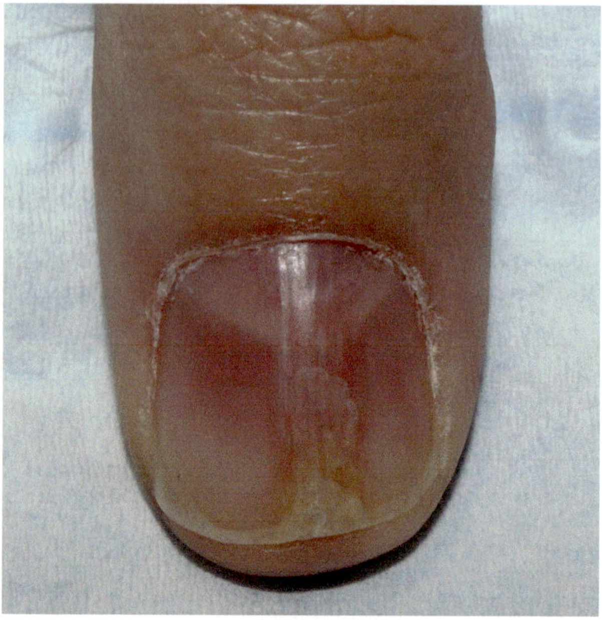

Fig. 9.1 40-Year-old female, Fitzpatrick type II, glomus tumor, with longitudinal erythronychia and onycholysis involving left thumbnail (*from* Curtis et al. [27]; CC-BY 4.0)

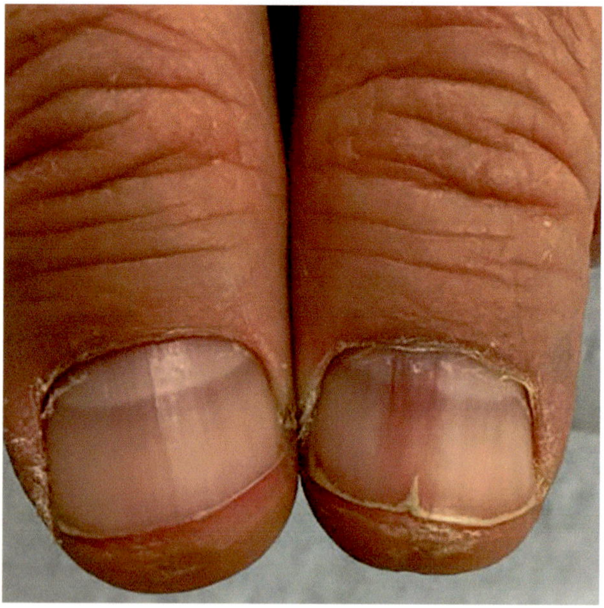

Fig. 9.2 53-Year-old male, Fitzpatrick type II, glomus tumor, with longitudinal erythroynchia and distal split involving left thumbnail

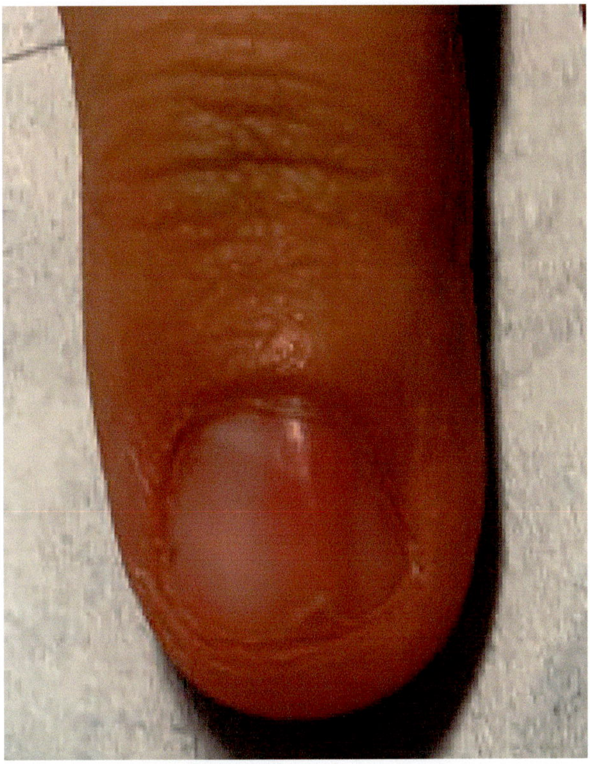

Fig. 9.3 33-Year-old female, Fitzpatrick type II, glomus tumor, with longitudinal erythronychia and longitudinal ridge affecting left second fingernail

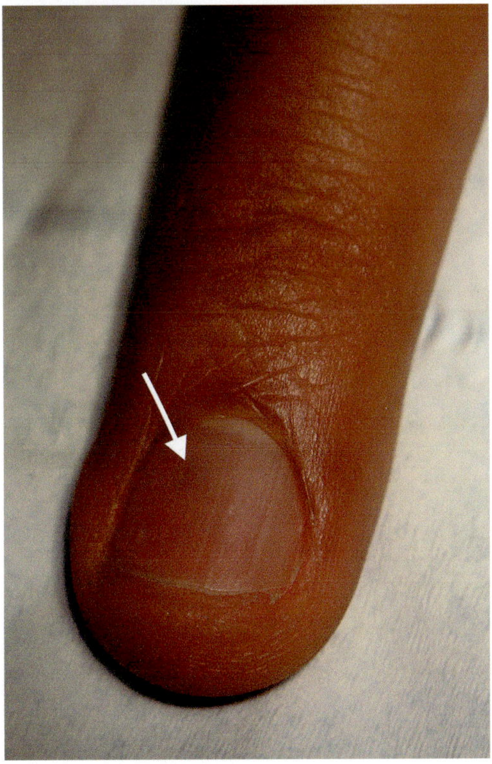

Fig. 9.4 51-Year-old male, Fitzpatrick type III, glomus tumor, with subtle blue discoloration visible through the nail plate of the right fourth fingernail

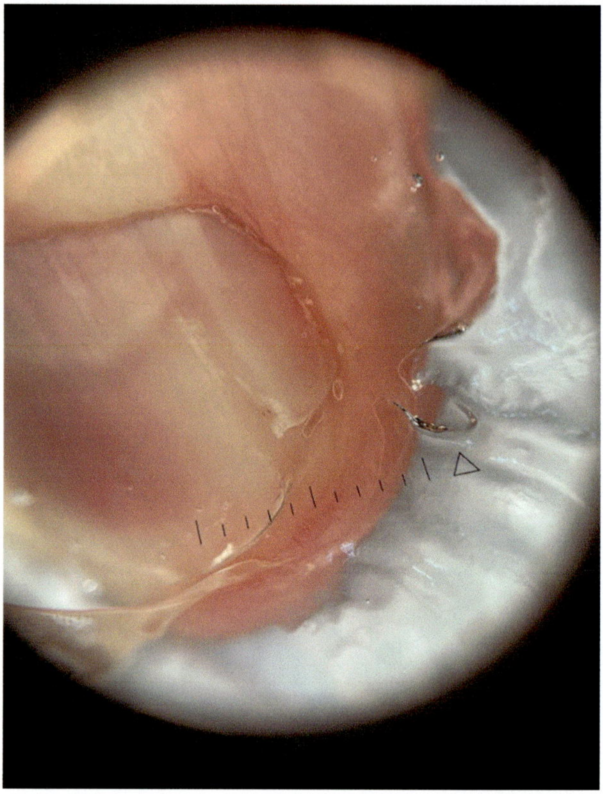

Fig. 9.5 51-Year-old female, Fitzpatrick type III, glomus tumor, with left thumbnail dystrophy including longitudinal red line appreciated with dermoscopy

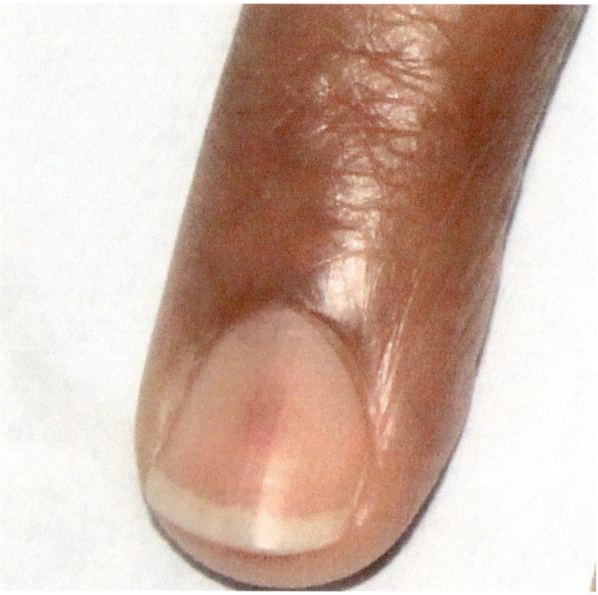

Fig. 9.6 67-Year-old female, Fitzpatrick type V, glomus tumor, with erythronychia involving right fourth fingernail

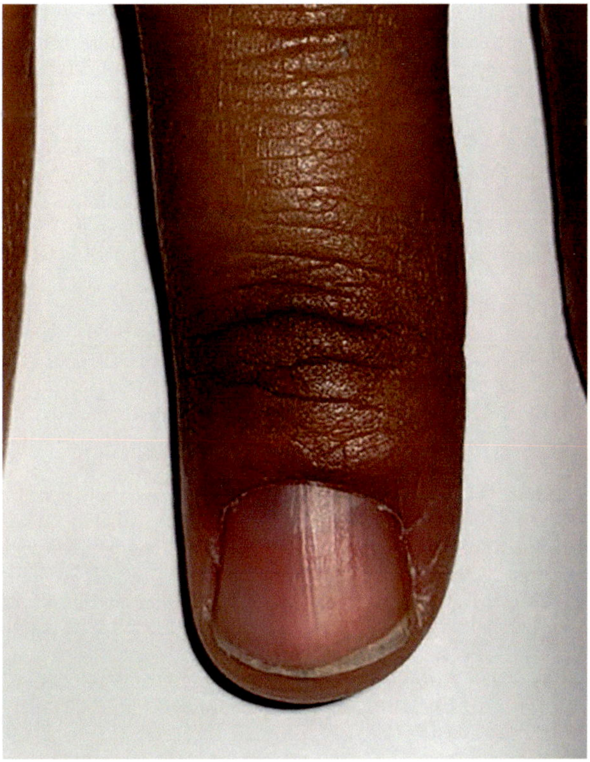

Fig. 9.7 33-Year-old female, Fitzpatrick type V, glomus tumor, with bluish discoloration involving right third fingernail

References

1. Álvarez-Salafranca M, Bañuls J, Thomas L, et al. Dermoscopy of glomus tumour: a cross-sectional study of 86 cases. J Eur Acad Dermatol Venereol. 2022;36(11):2016–24. https://doi.org/10.1111/jdv.18432.
2. Lipner SR, Scher RK. Longitudinal erythronychia of the fingernail. JAMA Dermatol. 2016;152(11):1271–2. https://doi.org/10.1001/jamadermatol.2016.2747.
3. Lin YC, Hsiao PF, Wu YH, Sun FJ, Scher RK. Recurrent digital glomus tumor: analysis of 75 cases. Dermatologic Surg. 2010;36(9):1396–400. https://doi.org/10.1111/j.1524-4725.2010.01647.x.
4. Morey VM, Garg B, Kotwal PP. Glomus tumours of the hand: review of literature. J Clin Orthop Trauma. 2016;7(4):286–91. https://doi.org/10.1016/j.jcot.2016.04.006.
5. Folpe AL, Fanburg-Smith JC, Miettinen M, Weiss SW. Atypical and malignant glomus tumors: analysis of 52 cases, with a proposal for the reclassification of glomus tumors. Am J Surg Pathol. 2001;25(1):1–12. https://doi.org/10.1097/00000478-200101000-00001.
6. Mravic M, LaChaud G, Nguyen A, Scott MA, Dry SM, James AW. Clinical and histopathological diagnosis of glomus tumor: an institutional experience of 138 cases. Int J Surg Pathol. 2015;23(3):181–8. https://doi.org/10.1177/1066896914567330.
7. Alkhateb O, Daaboul O, Daaboul B, Abouharb R, Alazmeh MA, Hamed G. Glomangiomyoma of the stomach: case report. Case Rep Gastroenterol. 2023;17(1):185–90. https://doi.org/10.1159/000529044.

8. Calduch L, Monteagudo C, Martínez-Ruiz E, et al. Familial generalized multiple glomangiomyoma: report of a new family, with immunohistochemical and ultrastructural studies and review of the literature. Pediatr Dermatol. 2002;19(5):402–8. https://doi.org/10.1046/j.1525-1470.2002.00114.x.
9. Takata H, Ikuta Y, Ishida O, Kimori K. Treatment of subungual glomus tumour. Hand Surg. 2001;6(1):25–7. https://doi.org/10.1142/s0218810401000394.
10. Lee DW, Yang JH, Chang S, et al. Clinical and pathological characteristics of extradigital and digital glomus tumours: a retrospective comparative study. J Eur Acad Dermatol Venereol. 2011;25(12):1392–7. https://doi.org/10.1111/j.1468-3083.2011.03979.x.
11. Harrison B, Moore AM, Calfee R, Sammer DM. The association between glomus tumors and neurofibromatosis. J Hand Surg Am. 2013;38(8):1571–4. https://doi.org/10.1016/j.jhsa.2013.05.025.
12. Kumar MG, Emnett RJ, Bayliss SJ, Gutmann DH. Glomus tumors in individuals with neurofibromatosis type 1. J Am Acad Dermatol. 2014;71(1):44–8. https://doi.org/10.1016/j.jaad.2014.01.913.
13. Lipner SR, Scher RK. Subungual glomus tumors: underrecognized clinical findings in neurofibromatosis 1. J Am Acad Dermatol. 2021;84(6):e269. https://doi.org/10.1016/j.jaad.2020.08.129.
14. Brems H, Park C, Maertens O, et al. Glomus tumors in neurofibromatosis type 1: genetic, functional, and clinical evidence of a novel association [published correction appears in Cancer Res. 2009 Oct 15;69(20):8216. Messia, Ludwine [corrected to Messiaen, Ludwine]]. Cancer Res. 2009;69(18):7393–401. https://doi.org/10.1158/0008-5472.CAN-09-1752.
15. Grover C, Jayasree P, Kaliyadan F. Clinical and onychoscopic characteristics of subungual glomus tumor: a cross-sectional study. Int J Dermatol. 2021;60(6):693–702. https://doi.org/10.1111/ijd.15358.
16. Wollstein A, Wollstein R. SUBUNGUAL GLOMANGIOMYOMA—A CASE REPORT. Hand Surg. 2012;17(2):271–3. https://doi.org/10.1142/S021881041272032X.
17. Demirdag HG, Akay BN, Kirmizi A, Serel S, Heper AO. Subungual Glomangiomyoma. J Am Podiatr Med Assoc. 2020;110(2):Article_13. https://doi.org/10.7547/19-051.
18. Kang TW, Lee KH, Park CJ. A case of subungual glomangiomyoma with myxoid stromal change. Korean J Dermatol. 2008;46(4):550–3.
19. Vega SML, Ruiz SJA, Ramírez CS, et al. Subungual glomangiomyoma: a case report. Dermatología Cosmética, Médica y Quirúrgica. 2022;20(2):258–62.
20. Hwang JK, Lipner SR. Blue nail discoloration: literature review and diagnostic algorithms. Am J Clin Dermatol. 2023;24(3):419–41. https://doi.org/10.1007/s40257-023-00768-6.
21. Hazani R, Houle JM, Kasdan ML, Wilhelmi BJ. Glomus tumors of the hand. Eplasty. 2008;8:e48.
22. Giele H. Hildreth's test is a reliable clinical sign for the diagnosis of glomus tumours. J Hand Surg Br. 2002;27(2):157–8. https://doi.org/10.1054/jhsb.2001.0724.
23. Tsiogka A, Belyayeva H, Sianos S, Rigopoulos D. Transillumination: a diagnostic tool to assess subungual glomus tumors. Skin Appendage Disord. 2021;7(3):231–3. https://doi.org/10.1159/000514011.
24. Baek HJ, Lee SJ, Cho KH, et al. Subungual tumors: clinicopathologic correlation with US and MR imaging findings. Radiographics. 2010;30(6):1621–36. https://doi.org/10.1148/rg.306105514.
25. Patel T, Meena V, Meena P. Hand and foot glomus tumors: significance of MRI diagnosis followed by histopathological assessment. Cureus. 2022;14(10):e30038. https://doi.org/10.7759/cureus.30038.
26. Dhami A, Vale SM, Richardson ML, Schachtel AK, Fleckman P. Comparing ultrasound with magnetic resonance imaging in the evaluation of subungual glomus tumors and subungual myxoid cysts. Skin Appendage Disord. 2023;9(4):262–7. https://doi.org/10.1159/000530397.
27. Curtis KL, Ho B, Jellinek NJ, Rubin AI, Tosti A, Lipner SR. Diagnosis and management of longitudinal erythronychia: a clinical review by an expert panel. J Am Acad Dermatol. 2024;91(3):480–9.

10 Onychomatricoma

Rachel C. Hill and Shari R. Lipner

10.1 Description of Disease

Onychomatricoma is a fibroepithelial tumor of nail matrix origin that was first described in 1992 [1–6]. It forms due to disruption in nail matrix differentiation and has been described as the only type of tumor that independently produces a nail plate [3]. It is typically painless and grows slowly [7]. In 2019, less than 200 cases had been reported [8]. Onychomatricoma is composed of finger-like projections arising from the nail matrix that are best seen when the nail is avulsed. These filiform projections form longitudinally arranged cavities within the nail plate that are visible from the distal edge of the nail [9, 10]. They most commonly affect the fingernails, although toenail involvement has been described [7, 11, 12].

10.2 Epidemiology

10.2.1 Sex

Based on the available literature, onychomatricoma affects women more frequently than men, with estimates of female: male ratios 1.3–2.16:1 [11]. However, in a case series of 34 onychomatricoma 2004–2013 at a single center by Lesort et al., the male: female ratio was 1.06 [13].

10.2.2 Age

In a study of 30 patients with pathology-confirmed onychomatricoma by Di Chiacchio et al., the average age was 47.9 years (range: 21–70 years) [11]. In Lesort et al.'s study of 34 onychomatricoma cases, the average age was 58.4 (Range: 27–85 years) [13]. While most cases are reported in middle and older individuals,

S. R. Lipner, *Atlas of Nail Disorders Across All Skin Colors*,
https://doi.org/10.1007/978-3-031-74272-9_10

children may also be affected, as in a case report in a four-year-old girl of Pakistani origin [7, 14].

10.2.3 Race

Onychomatricoma affects patients of all races and ethnic backgrounds, although to date more cases have been described in white patients than patients with skin of color [11, 15–18]. In a retrospective study of 30 patients in Miami and Brazil, 24/30 cases were described in non-skin-of-color patients, which is notable given the significant representation of individuals of African descent in these areas. This difference may be related to the underdiagnosis of the condition in patients with skin of color [11].

10.3 Risk Factors

In a genome-wide association study, onychomatricomas were characterized by losses on chromosome 11, which merits further study [3]. Cases of co-occurring onychomatricoma and onychomycosis have been reported, all involving the toenails, suggesting that the nail plate may become susceptible to a fungal infection when onychomatricoma is present [19, 20]. Trauma has also been suggested as a potential risk factor for developing onychomatricoma [21, 22].

10.4 Clinical Features

The classic clinical features associated with onychomatricoma include increased transverse curvature of the nail plate, a thickened and yellow longitudinal band accompanied by ridging, and splinter hemorrhages. Finger-like projections originate proximally and continue along the length of the nail plate, indicative of a matricial tumor, which becomes more apparent once the nail plate has been avulsed. The distal margin of the nail plate typically contains holes, which have been described as cavitations, honey-combs, or woodworm-like cavities [11, 22]. In the retrospective study of 30 patients with pathology-proven onychomatricoma, 85% had increased nail plate thickening, 80% had splinter hemorrhages, 73% had xanthonychia, and 50% had increased transverse nail plate curvature [11]. In Lesort et al.'s retrospective study of 34 pathology-confirmed cases of onychomatricoma, longitudinal parallel white and gray lines, splinter hemorrhages, dark dots at the distal edge of the nail plate, sharp and parallel lateral edges, and thickening were the most frequent dermoscopic features [13]. Dermoscopy may also show tortuous hairpin blood vessels [13, 23].

Other clinical variants include "pigmented onychomatricoma" and giant onychomatricoma [12, 17, 21, 24]. Pigmented onychomatricoma presents as a thickened brown-black longitudinal band, sometimes with yellowing of the distal nail plate. Pigmented onychomatricoma may be more common in men, patients with skin of color, and in the toenails vs. fingernails [17, 22]. It is thought that pigment formation is a result of melanocyte activation in the nail matrix [17, 22]. The giant variant is an onychomatricoma that encompasses the entire nail plate, causing extensive onychodystrophy. Giant onychomatricoma has been associated with repetitive trauma to a pre-existing onychomatricoma [10].

10.5 Clinical Features in Skin of Color

The pigmented variant of onychomatricoma may be more common in patients with darker skin tones [17]. In a case series of four patients with pigmented onychomatricoma, all patients were of Fitzpatrick skin types III or IV [22].

10.6 Requirements for Diagnosis

Because onychomatricoma uniquely induces an altered nail plate, nail clippings may be used as a method for diagnosis, although they are usually not diagnostic. Clippings may show a thickened nail plate with cavitations of various shapes and sizes that are filled with serous fluid and lined by epithelium [25]. Ultrasound and magnetic resonance imaging may show finger-like projections that affect the nail plate, although larger studies are needed to substantiate these findings [4]. Excision with histopathology remains the gold standard for diagnosis [4, 8].

10.7 Cases

Figures 10.1, 10.2, 10.3, 10.4, and 10.5 demonstrate the presentation of onychomatricoma in a clinical setting.

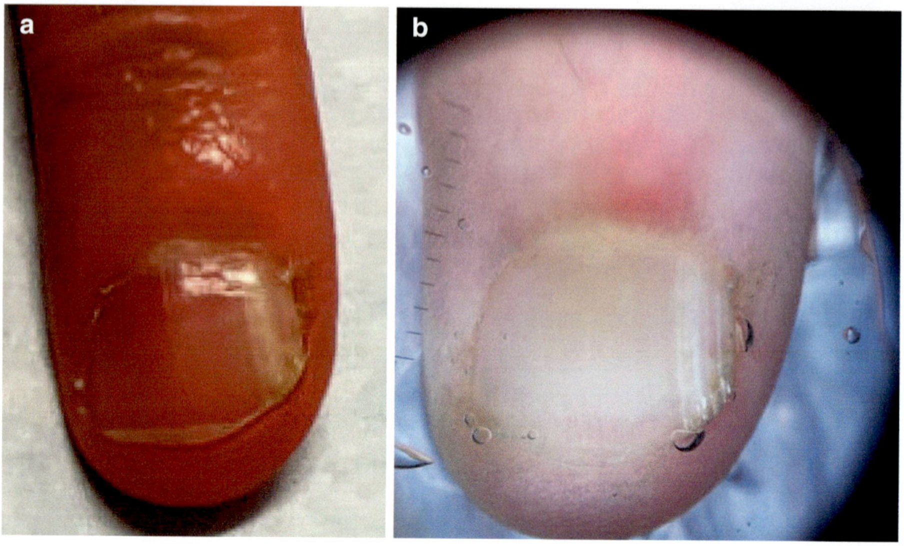

Fig. 10.1 (**a**) A 39-Year-old female, Fitzpatrick type I, onychomatricoma, with a thickened yellow band involving the right third fingernail. (**b**) With dermoscopy, capillaries could be appreciated at the proximal nail fold along with channels at the distal edge of the nail

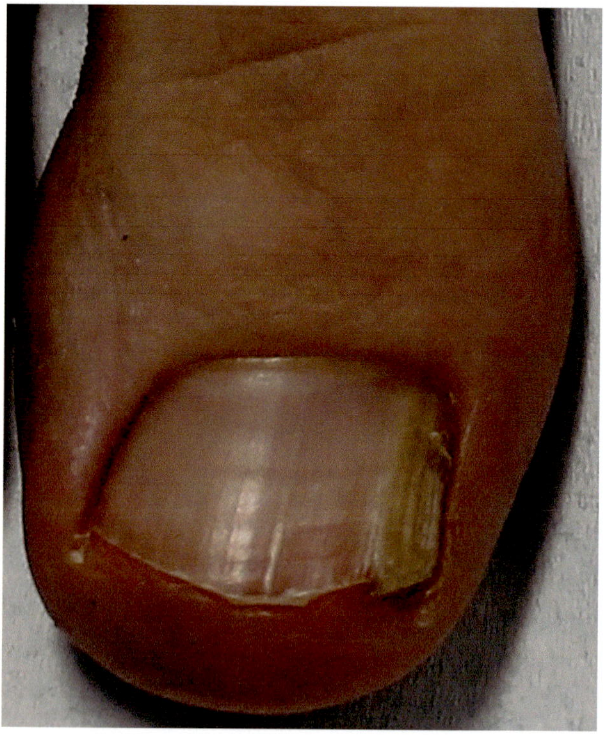

Fig. 10.2 A 35-Year-old female, Fitzpatrick type II, onychomatricoma, with a thickened linear yellow band involving the right great toenail. Channels were appreciated at the distal edge of the nail

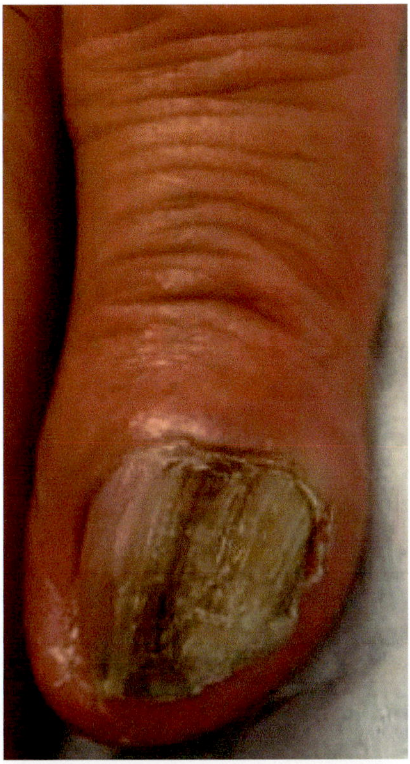

Fig. 10.3 A 68-Year-old male, Fitzpatrick type II, onychomatricoma, with a yellow, thickened band involving the left fifth fingernail. Splinter hemorrhages were better seen with dermoscopy. Channels were appreciated at the distal edge of the nail with dermoscopy

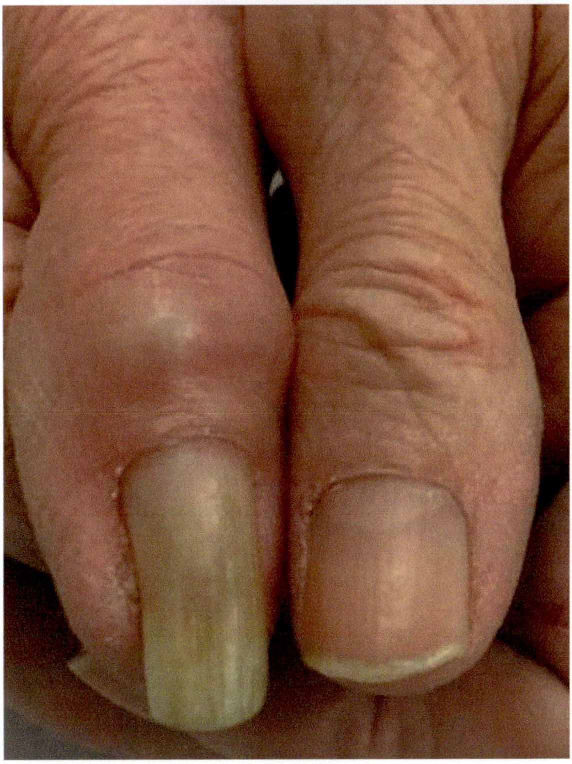

Fig. 10.4 A 72-Year-old male, Fitzpatrick type II, onychomatricoma, with a yellow, thickened band and increased transverse curvature forming a pincer nail affecting the right thumbnail. On dermoscopy, channels were seen at the distal edge of the nail

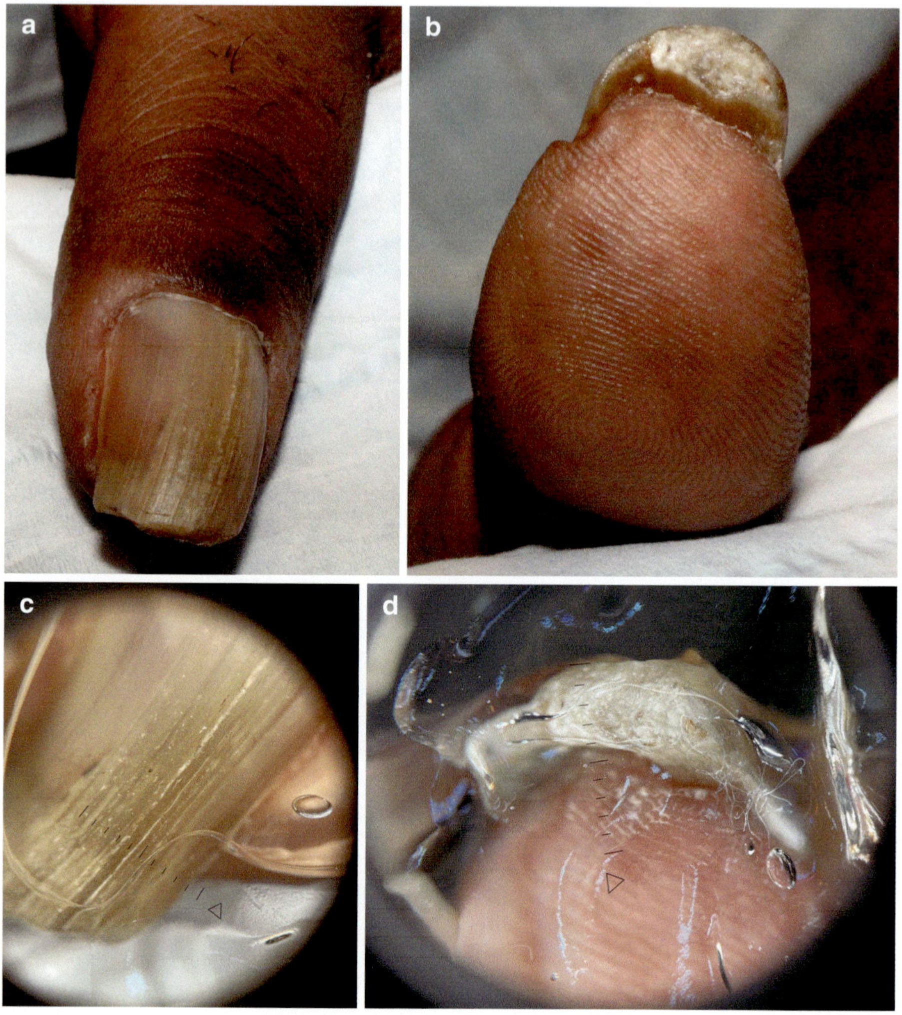

Fig. 10.5 (**a** and **b**) A 64-Year-old male, Fitzpatrick type V, onychomatricoma, with thickened, linear yellow nail plate, increased transverse curvature, and splinter hemorrhages involving the left thumbnail. Thickening is appreciated at the distal nail plate. (**c** and **d**) On dermoscopy, channels were seen at the distal edge of the nail

References

1. Becerro de Bengoa R, Gates JR, Losa Iglesias ME, Alija Martinez B. Rare toenail onychomatricoma: surgical resolution of five cases. Dermatologic Surg. 2011;37(5):709–11. https://doi.org/10.1111/j.1524-4725.2011.01969.x.
2. Haneke E, Fränken J. Onychomatricoma. Dermatologic Surg. 1995;21(11):984–7. https://doi.org/10.1111/j.1524-4725.1995.tb00538.x.
3. Cañueto J, Santos-Briz Á, García JL, Robledo C, Unamuno P. Onychomatricoma: genome-wide analyses of a rare nail matrix tumor. J Am Acad Dermatol. 2011;64(3):573–8, 578.e1. https://doi.org/10.1016/j.jaad.2009.07.051.

4. Cinotti E, Veronesi G, Labeille B, et al. Imaging technique for the diagnosis of onychomatricoma. J Eur Acad Dermatol Venereol. 2018;32(11):1874–8. https://doi.org/10.1111/jdv.15108.
5. Gaertner EM, Gordon M, Reed T. Onychomatricoma: case report of an unusual subungual tumor with literature review. J Cutan Pathol. 2009;36(Suppl 1):66–9. https://doi.org/10.1111/j.1600-0560.2008.01218.x.
6. Baran R, Kint A. Onychomatrixoma. Filamentous tufted tumour in the matrix of a funnel-shaped nail: a new entity (report of three cases). Br J Dermatol. 1992;126(5):510–5. https://doi.org/10.1111/j.1365-2133.1992.tb11827.x.
7. Lam C, Weyant GW, Billingsley EM. Longitudinal melanonychia of the toenail. JAMA Dermatol. 2014;150(4):449–50. https://doi.org/10.1001/jamadermatol.2013.8358.
8. Charfi O, Jaber K, Khammouma F, et al. Magnetic resonance imaging in the diagnosis of onychomatricoma: a case report. Skin Appendage Disord. 2019;5(4):246–50. https://doi.org/10.1159/000496474.
9. Okon LG, Saedi N, Schwartz L, Lee JB. A case of onychomatricoma: classic clinical, dermoscopic, and nail-clipping histologic findings. J Am Acad Dermatol. 2017;76(2s1):S19–s21. https://doi.org/10.1016/j.jaad.2016.04.041.
10. Estrada-Chavez G, Vega-Memije ME, Toussaint-Caire S, Rangel L, Dominguez-Cherit J. Giant onychomatricoma: report of two cases with rare clinical presentation. Int J Dermatol. 2007;46(6):634–6. https://doi.org/10.1111/j.1365-4632.2007.03300.x.
11. Di Chiacchio N, Tavares GT, Tosti A, et al. Onychomatricoma: epidemiological and clinical findings in a large series of 30 cases. Br J Dermatol. 2015;173(5):1305–7. https://doi.org/10.1111/bjd.13900.
12. Fierro-Arias L, Corrales-Rosas B, Mercadillo-Pérez P, Medina-Castillo D, Peniche-Castellanos A. Giant onychomatricoma in third toe: exceptional condition with surgical resolution. J Eur Acad Dermatol Venereol. 2016;30(3):525–7. https://doi.org/10.1111/jdv.12923.
13. Lesort C, Debarbieux S, Duru G, Dalle S, Poulhalon N, Thomas L. Dermoscopic features of onychomatricoma: a study of 34 cases. Dermatology. 2015;231(2):177–83. https://doi.org/10.1159/000431315.
14. Piraccini BM, Antonucci A, Rech G, Starace M, Misciali C, Tosti A. Onychomatricoma: first description in a child. Pediatr Dermatol. 2007;24(1):46–8. https://doi.org/10.1111/j.1525-1470.2007.00332.x.
15. Kamath P, Wu T, Villada G, Zaiac M, Elgart G, Tosti A. Onychomatricoma: a rare nail tumor with an unusual clinical presentation. Skin Appendage Disord. 2018;4(3):171–3. https://doi.org/10.1159/000484577.
16. Joshi TP, Dunn C, Huttenbach YT, Kim SJ. Onychomatricoma in a patient with skin of color. JAAD Case Rep. 2023;41:44–5. https://doi.org/10.1016/j.jdcr.2023.08.046.
17. Grover C, Gaurav V, Sharma S, Sinha S. Pigmented onychomatricoma presenting as pachymelanonychia Striata: a case report and review of literature. Skin Appendage Disord. 2023;9(5):366–72. https://doi.org/10.1159/000529820.
18. Joo HJ, Kim MR, Cho BK, Yoo G, Park HJ. Onychomatricoma: a rare tumor of nail matrix. Ann Dermatol. 2016;28(2):237–41. https://doi.org/10.5021/ad.2016.28.2.237.
19. Kallis P, Tosti A. Onychomycosis and onychomatricoma. Skin Appendage Disord. 2016;1(4):209–12. https://doi.org/10.1159/000445908.
20. Fayol J, Baran R, Perrin C, Labrousse F. Onychomatricoma with misleading features. Acta Derm Venereol. 2000;80(5):370–2. https://doi.org/10.1080/000155500459330.
21. Park SJ, Hong JK, Hong SA, Li K. Pigmented onychomatricoma after trauma: a case report and review of literature. Ann Dermatol. 2022;34(6):482–4. https://doi.org/10.5021/ad.20.156.
22. Ocampo-Garza J, Di Chiacchio NG, Di Chiacchio N. Pigmented onychomatricoma: four cases. Australas J Dermatol. 2018;59(1):e66–9. https://doi.org/10.1111/ajd.12638.
23. Geizhals S, Magro CM, Lipner SR. Dermatoscopy of onychomatricoma: tortuous hairpin vessels. Skinmed. 2022;20(6):444.
24. Kameda E, Matsuzawa T, Togawa Y, Ikeda JI, Matsue H. Case of pigmented onychomatricoma: a relationship between dermoscopic and pathological findings. J Dermatol. 2022;49(10):e397–8. https://doi.org/10.1111/1346-8138.16474.
25. Miteva M, de Farias DC, Zaiac M, Romanelli P, Tosti A. Nail clipping diagnosis of onychomatricoma. Arch Dermatol. 2011;147(9):1117–8. https://doi.org/10.1001/archdermatol.2011.240.

Onychopapilloma

11

Rachel C. Hill and Shari R. Lipner

11.1 Description of Disease

Onychopapilloma is a common benign tumor involving the nail bed and nail matrix [1]. It was first described in 1995 by Baran and Perrin, at which time it was labeled "localized multinucleate distal keratosis," and later named "onychopapilloma" by the same authors in 2000 [2, 3]. Pathologically, these tumors are composed of layered subungual hyperkeratosis at the distal nail edge extending past the hyponychium, epidermal hyperplasia, and nail bed matrix metaplasia, with or without multinucleate keratinocytes and focal hemorrhage [4–8]. Onychopapilloma is typically painless, although patients may present with concerns about cosmetic appearance or interference with daily activities, including the nail catching on clothes or difficulty picking up or manipulating objects [4].

11.2 Epidemiology

11.2.1 Sex

Onychopapilloma has been reported more often in women compared to men in most studies to date. In a cross-sectional study of 39 patients ($n = 43$ onychopapilloma) with histology-confirmed onychopapilloma by Canella et al., the majority were female (84.6%) [9]. Similarly, in a retrospective review of 47 patients with pathologically confirmed onychopapilloma by Tosti et al., 33 patients were female (70.2%) [4]. However, in a retrospective study of 39 patients diagnosed with onychopapilloma in South Korea, 23 patients were male (59.0%) vs. 16 female (41.0%) [10].

S. R. Lipner, *Atlas of Nail Disorders Across All Skin Colors*,
https://doi.org/10.1007/978-3-031-74272-9_11

11.2.2 Age

Onychopapilloma may occur at any age, including children, but is most commonly reported in middle-aged individuals. In the cross-sectional study of 39 patients (n = 43 onychopapilloma) with histology-confirmed onychopapilloma by Canella et al., the average age was 56.1 years (range 26–74 years) [9]. Similarly, in a retrospective review of 17 biopsy-confirmed onychopapilloma cases, the average age was 56.3 years (range 23–81 years) [8]. In a retrospective analysis of 68 patients with pathology-confirmed onychopapilloma, there were two children, ages 9 and 11 [11].

11.3 Risk Factors

Older age and female sex may be risk factors for onychopapilloma, but this requires validation. In the cross-sectional study of 39 patients (n = 43 onychopapilloma) with clinically diagnosed onychopapilloma by Canella et al., only three patients (7.7%) had a history of trauma, suggesting that trauma is likely not a risk factor for onychopapilloma development [9].

11.4 Clinical Features

Onychopapilloma is typically painless and more commonly affects the fingernails than toenails, and most frequently the thumbnail [12, 13]. The most common presentation is a thin band of longitudinal erythronychia in a single digit that does not widen over time [4, 5, 13–16]. In the retrospective analysis of 47 pathology-confirmed onychopapilloma cases by Tosti et al., 25 patients presented with longitudinal erythronychia, and 24 cases involved the thumbnail [4]. In addition, patients often present with a characteristic V-shaped notch or onycholytic area at the distal edge of the nail, with an accompanying subungual hyperkeratotic mass [5, 9]. The mass can be appreciated using dermoscopy at the distal nail edge. Splinter hemorrhages are often present and may be best visualized with dermoscopy [4, 17]. Splinter hemorrhages may occur within the band, or independently if a band is not present [4, 5, 10].

Less frequently, patients may instead present with longitudinal leukonychia or melanonychia [5]. In a case series of 13 patients clinically diagnosed with onychopapilloma, 23% (n = 3) presented with leukonychia, and 15% (n = 2) presented with melanonychia [12]. Similarly, in the retrospective analysis of pathology-confirmed onychopapilloma in 47 patients by Tosti et al., 15% (n = 7) presented with leukonychia, and 9% (n = 4) presented with melanonychia [4].

A malignant variant of onychopapilloma was reported in four cases [18–20]. Patients presented with pain and rapidly changing nail dystrophy (n = 1), longitudinal melanonychia (n = 2), and widened longitudinal erythronychia (n = 1). The presence of these features warrants high clinical suspicion, with excision and histopathologic examination required for diagnosis [18, 20].

11.5 Clinical Features in Skin of Color

In the retrospective analysis of pathology-confirmed onychopapilloma in 47 patients by Tosti et al., those with Fitzpatrick types IV-VI ($n = 4$) presented with longitudinal melanonychia, while patients with Fitzpatrick types I-III more often presented with longitudinal erythronychia or leukonychia ($n = 32$), suggesting that longitudinal melanonychia may be more common in darker skin tones [4]. However, onychopapilloma presenting as longitudinal melanonychia has also been described in patients with Fitzpatrick skin types I–III [21].

11.6 Requirements for Diagnosis

Onychopapilloma may often be diagnosed clinically if characteristic features are present, such as a painless longitudinal erythronychia, nail plate distal notching, and a subungual hyperkeratotic mass [13]. Diagnosis is supported by the presence of splinter hemorrhages and visualization of the subungual hyperkeratotic mass at the distal free edge of the nail with dermoscopy [4]. Previous studies have explored the utility of ultrasound to diagnose onychopapilloma. In a retrospective study of 22 cases of pathologically confirmed onychopapillomas, the most common ultrasound features included a hypoechoic band in the nail bed, upward displacement of the nail plate, and thickening at the distal margin of the nail [16]. Similarly, in the cross-sectional study of 39 patients ($n = 43$ onychopapilloma) with histopathology diagnosed onychopapilloma by Canella et.al, high-frequency ultrasound showed avascular hyperechoic masses in the nail plate in 95% of cases ($n = 41$) [9]. Excision with histopathology is the gold standard for definitive diagnosis, but is often unnecessary, particularly for stable nail findings.

11.7 Cases

Figures 11.1, 11.2, 11.3, 11.4, 11.5, and 11.6 demonstrate the presentation of onychopapilloma in a clinical setting.

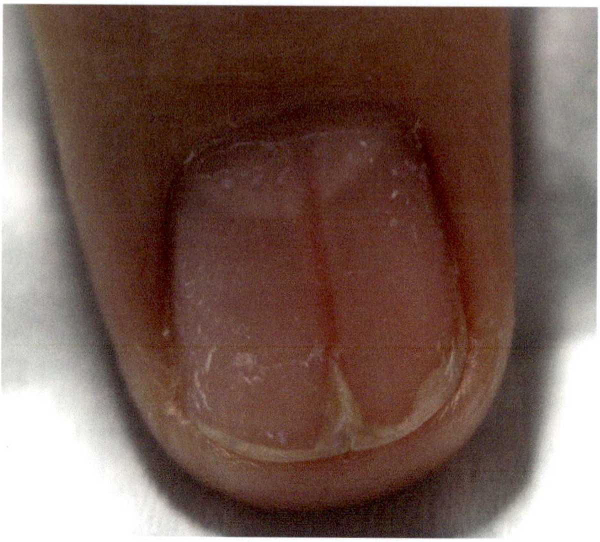

Fig. 11.1 34-Year-old female, Fitzpatrick type II, onychopapilloma, with longitudinal red band of the right thumbnail originating in the lunula with a distal split and hyperkeratotic papule at the hyponychium

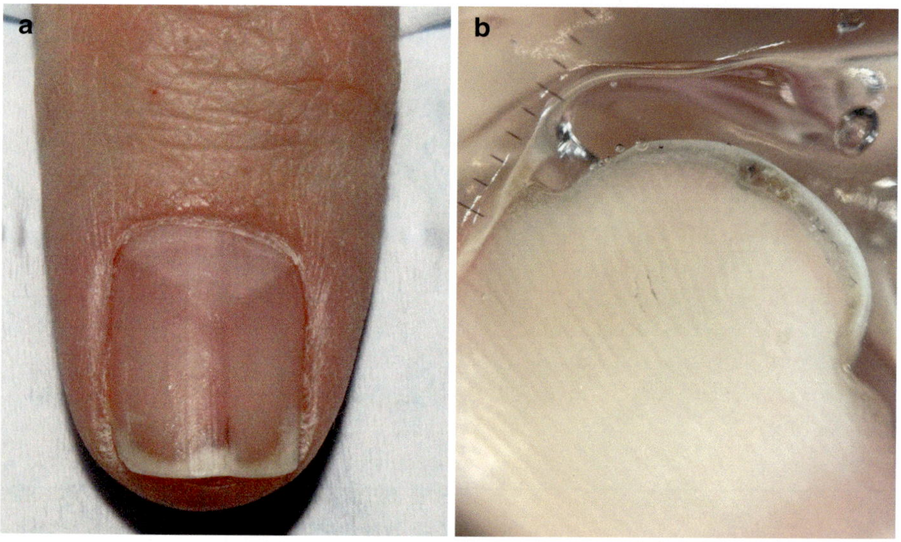

Fig. 11.2 (**a**) 29-Year-old female, Fitzpatrick type II, onychopapilloma, with longitudinal, white band proximally and red band distally involving the left first fingernail. Distal splinter hemorrhages were also present. (**b**) Dermoscopy showed the subungual papule clearly

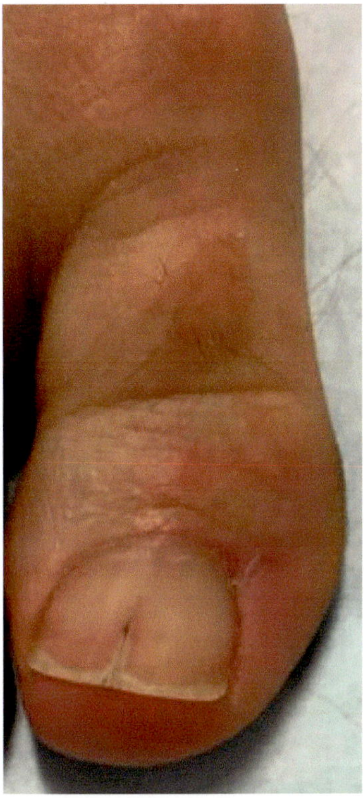

Fig. 11.3 45-Year-old female, Fitzpatrick type II, onychopapilloma, with longitudinal split and splinter hemorrhages involving the right first toenail

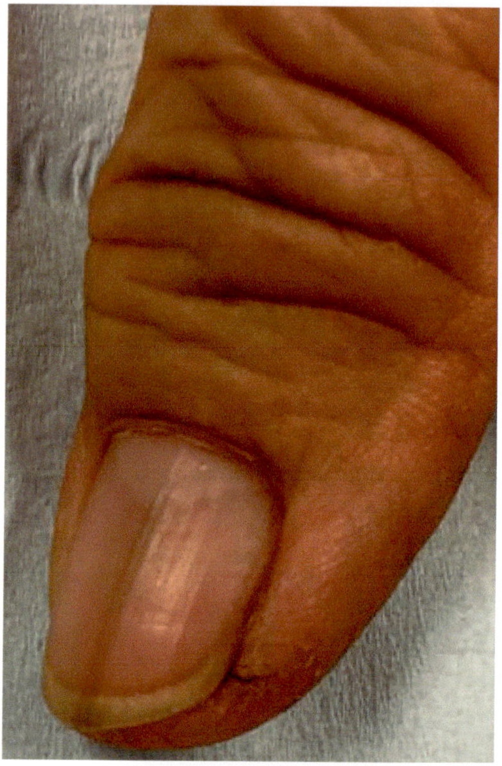

Fig. 11.4 81-Year-old female, Fitzpatrick type III, onychopapilloma, with 1 mm brown-grey longitudinal band of the left first fingernail originating in the lunula

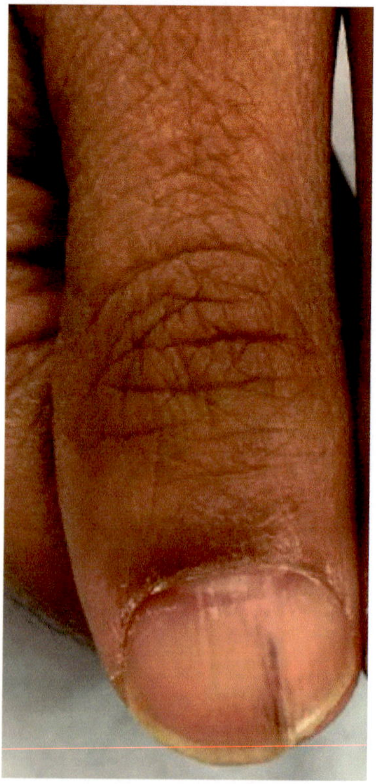

Fig. 11.5 34-Year-old male, Fitzpatrick type IV, onychopapilloma, with a longitudinal white band of the right first fingernail originating in the lunula with long splinter hemorrhages and a hyperkeratotic papule visible at the hyponychium

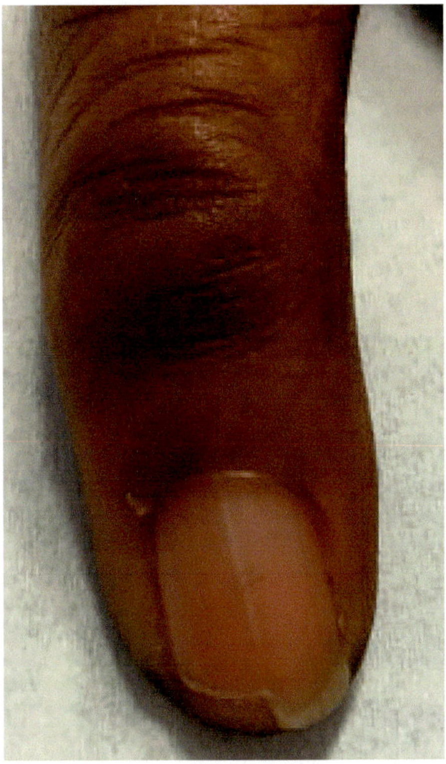

Fig. 11.6 57-Year-old female, Fitzpatrick type V, onychopapilloma, with longitudinal ridge and longitudinal white band of the right fifth fingernail

References

1. Hashimoto H, Ito T, Yamada Y, Oda Y, Furue M. Onychopapilloma presenting as longitudinal melanonychia: a case report and literature review. Australas J Dermatol. 2021;62(2):244–6. https://doi.org/10.1111/ajd.13543.
2. Baran R, Perrin C. Localized multinucleate distal subungual keratosis. Br J Dermatol. 1995;133(1):77–82. https://doi.org/10.1111/j.1365-2133.1995.tb02496.x.
3. Baran R, Perrin C. Longitudinal erythronychia with distal subungual keratosis: onychopapilloma of the nail bed and Bowen's disease. Br J Dermatol. 2000;143(1):132–5. https://doi.org/10.1046/j.1365-2133.2000.03602.x.
4. Tosti A, Schneider SL, Ramirez-Quizon MN, Zaiac M, Miteva M. Clinical, dermoscopic, and pathologic features of onychopapilloma: a review of 47 cases. J Am Acad Dermatol. 2016;74(3):521–6. https://doi.org/10.1016/j.jaad.2015.08.053.
5. Schneider SL, Tosti A. Tips to diagnose uncommon nail disorders. Dermatol Clin. 2015;33(2):197–205. https://doi.org/10.1016/j.det.2014.12.003.
6. Godse R, Rodriguez O, Ayoade KO, Rubin AI. Update on nail unit histopathology. Hum Pathol. 2023;140:214–32. https://doi.org/10.1016/j.humpath.2023.03.006.
7. Park HJ, Park HJ. A rare case of onychopapilloma presenting as a longitudinal erythronychia. Ann Dermatol. 2020;32(1):74–6. https://doi.org/10.5021/ad.2020.32.1.74.
8. Starace M, Alessandrini A, Ferrari T, Wong V, Baraldi C, Piraccini BM. Clinical and onychoscopic features of histopathologically proven onychopapillomas and literature update. J Cutan Pathol. 2022;49(2):147–52. https://doi.org/10.1111/cup.14119.
9. Canella C, Nakamura R, Leverone A, de Almeida CÁ, Iorizzo M, Yamada AF. Ultrasound imaging of onychopapilloma: evaluation of 43 cases. Eur J Radiol. 2023. https://doi.org/10.1016/j.ejrad.2023.111236.

10. Kim TR, Bae KN, Son JH, et al. Onychopapilloma: its clinical, dermoscopic and pathologic features. J Eur Acad Dermatol Venereol. 2022;36(11):2235–40. https://doi.org/10.1111/jdv.18461.
11. Delvaux C, Richert B, Lecerf P, André J. Onychopapillomas: a 68-case series to determine best surgical procedure and histologic sectioning. J Eur Acad Dermatol Venereol. 2018;32(11):2025–30. https://doi.org/10.1111/jdv.15037.
12. Fan X, Li T, Zhang X, et al. A new method to treat onychopapilloma with pulsed dye laser irradiation: a 13-case series report. J Dermatolog Treat. 2023;34(1):2213363. https://doi.org/10.1080/09546634.2023.2213363.
13. Hare AQ, Rich P. Nail tumors. Dermatol Clin. 2021;39(2):281–92. https://doi.org/10.1016/j.det.2020.12.007.
14. Jellinek NJ. Longitudinal erythronychia: suggestions for evaluation and management. J Am Acad Dermatol. 2011;64(1):167.e1. https://doi.org/10.1016/j.jaad.2009.10.047.
15. Jellinek NJ, Lipner SR. Longitudinal erythronychia: retrospective single-center study evaluating differential diagnosis and the likelihood of malignancy. Dermatologic Surg. 2016;42(3):310–9. https://doi.org/10.1097/DSS.0000000000000594.
16. Sechi A, Starace M, Piraccini BM, Wortsman X. Ultrasound features of onychopapilloma at high-frequency and ultra-high frequency. J Ultrasound Med. 2024;43(1):71–6. https://doi.org/10.1002/jum.16338.
17. Mattioli MA, Aromolo IF, Spigariolo CB, Marzano AV, Nazzaro G. Sonographic features of onychopapilloma: a single center retrospective observational study. J Clin Med. 2023;12(5):1795. https://doi.org/10.3390/jcm12051795.
18. Haneke E, Iorizzo M, Gabutti M, Beltraminelli H. Malignant onychopapilloma. J Cutan Pathol. 2021;48(1):174–9. https://doi.org/10.1111/cup.13904.
19. Rubin AI, Lee D, Baran R. Malignant onychopapilloma: a new nail unit clinicopathologic entity. J Cutan Pathol. 2021;48(3):347–8. https://doi.org/10.1111/cup.13941.
20. André J, Ewbank A, Moulonguet I, Richert B. Three atypical/malignant onychopapillomas in a 52-case series with immunohistochemical study. J Cutan Pathol. 2023;51:239. https://doi.org/10.1111/cup.14558.
21. Starace M, Ferrari T, Pezzetta S, et al. Pigmented onychopapilloma in Caucasians: a case series of six patients. Int J Dermatol. 2021;60(5):e192–4. https://doi.org/10.1111/ijd.15375.

Pyogenic Granuloma

12

Brianna Olamiju, Rachel C. Hill, and Shari R. Lipner

12.1 Description of Disease

Pyogenic granulomas (PGs) or lobular capillary hemangiomas are acquired benign vascular growths that can involve the periungual or subungual areas of the nail unit [1]. They are often painful and can bleed spontaneously due to the high vascularity of the nail unit [1]. PGs tend to grow rapidly and can be friable. In addition to PGs involving the nail, other common sites are the distal extremities, face, and gingiva [2].

12.2 Epidemiology

12.2.1 Sex

Both men and women may be affected by PG. In the largest systematic review of nail unit PGs, similar numbers of men (n = 129) and women (n = 132) were affected [1].

12.2.2 Age

PG is reported to be more frequent in the early decades of life [3]. However, in a retrospective study of 58 cases of nail PG, the mean age of adults was 48.4 years (range 7–86), suggesting patients of all ages may be affected, including children and older adults [4].

S. R. Lipner, *Atlas of Nail Disorders Across All Skin Colors*,
https://doi.org/10.1007/978-3-031-74272-9_12

12.3 Risk Factors

There are several risk factors documented in the literature for the development of PG including medications, such as oral and topical retinoids [5–9], chemotherapeutic medications, such as EGFR inhibitors [10–14], taxanes [15–17] 5-fluorouracil [18], and antiretroviral medications [19, 20]. Epidermal growth factor receptor (EGFR) inhibitors have been associated with the development of nail toxicities, including acute paronychia and co-occurring PG, in approximately 17% of patients receiving these medications [21, 22]. In a case series of 25 patients receiving EGFR therapy with 127 nails affected by paronychia, 60 nails were also affected by PG [21].

PG has also been associated with inflammatory skin diseases, such as sarcoidosis, psoriasis, and seronegative spondyloarthroarthritis [4]. Upper limb cast immobilization may also increase risk for PG [23–26]. Additionally, PG can occur following trauma and is associated with ingrown nails, retronychia, and friction [26]. PG is often associated with pregnancy, although the frequency with which pregnant women are affected is unknown [27]. The etiology of PG during pregnancy is hypothesized to be due to a tissue inflammatory response enhanced by female sex hormones [27].

12.4 Clinical Features

PGs present clinically as exophytic vascular papules or nodules [4]. Within the nail unit, they are most commonly found at periungual sites [1]. While most PGs are solitary, they may also occur in multiples. In a retrospective, observational study of 58 cases of periungual and subungual PG over a five year period, six patients developed multiple PGs during highly active antiretroviral therapy for HIV infection, seven patients developed multiple PGs during therapy for metastatic carcinoma, including EGFR inhibitors, capecitabine, and docetaxel, and three patients developed multiple PGs secondary to systemic inflammatory diseases [4]. In a cross-sectional study of 13 consecutive patients with PG, including five with PGs involving the fingers, the most common features were a reddish homogenous area (95%), white collarette (85%), intersecting "white rail" lines (31%), and ulceration (46%) [28].

12.5 Clinical Features in Skin of Color

Clinical features of PGs in patients with skin of color have not been previously described. Patients with skin of color are more likely to have physiologic melanonychia affecting the fingernails and toenails, which may accompany PG on physical examination and make diagnosis more difficult.

12.6 Requirements for Diagnosis

While PGs can be diagnosed clinically, histopathology may be required to confirm the diagnosis in equivocal cases, especially in solitary lesions. Ultrasound can also be performed, showing nodules that are hypoechoic compared with the subcutaneous fat, with slightly increased vascularization using color-doppler [29]. In cases of a single PG, especially involving the nail bed, performing a biopsy with histological examination is prudent to rule out a malignant neoplasm, including amelanotic melanoma, squamous cell carcinoma, and Kaposi sarcoma [3, 30–32]. Histologically, the pathological features of a mature PG show a polypoid exophytic ulcerated mass characterized by newly formed capillaries and venules in the edematous stroma and a mixed cell infiltrate with neutrophils scattered in the granulation tissue and in the lobules [4].

12.7 Cases

Figures 12.1, 12.2, 12.3, 12.4, 12.5, 12.6, and 12.7 demonstrate the presence of pyogenic granuloma in a clinical setting.

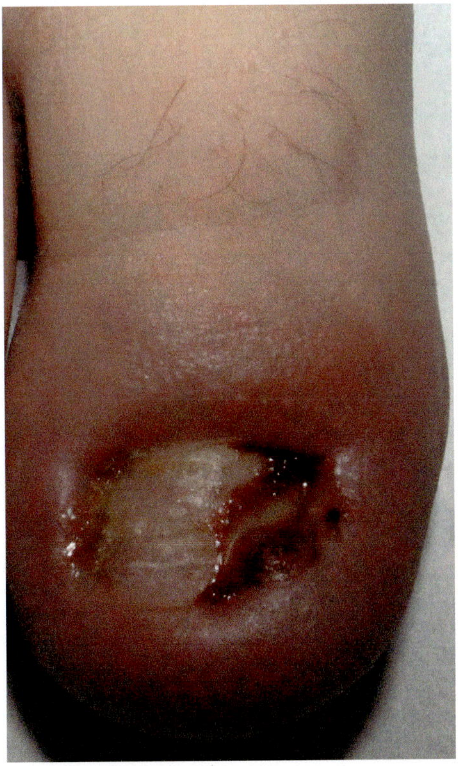

Fig. 12.1 13-Year-old female, Fitzpatrick type II, pyogenic granuloma, with erythematous friable nodule with purulent discharge involving the right great toenail

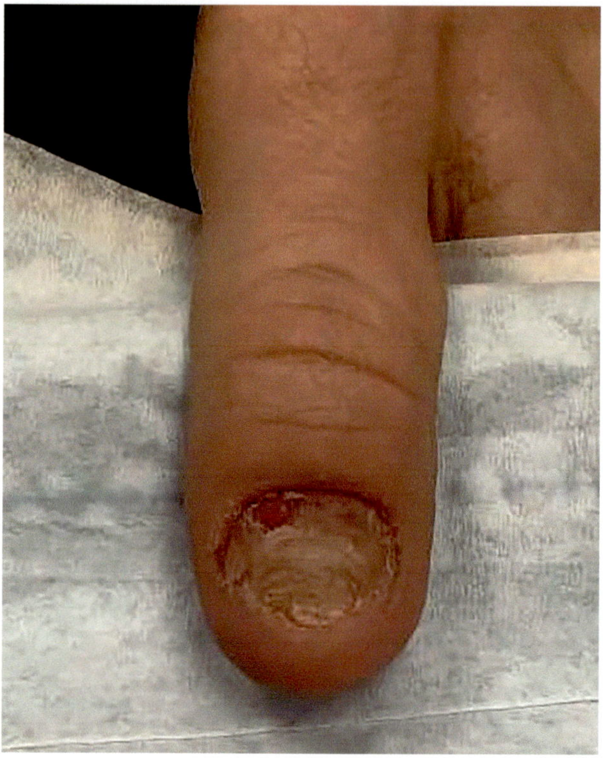

Fig. 12.2 39-Year-old male, Fitzpatrick type II, pyogenic granuloma, with circular area of the proximal nail plate missing and erythematous papule of the left thumbnail. The nail plate is severely dystrophic with ridges and grooves

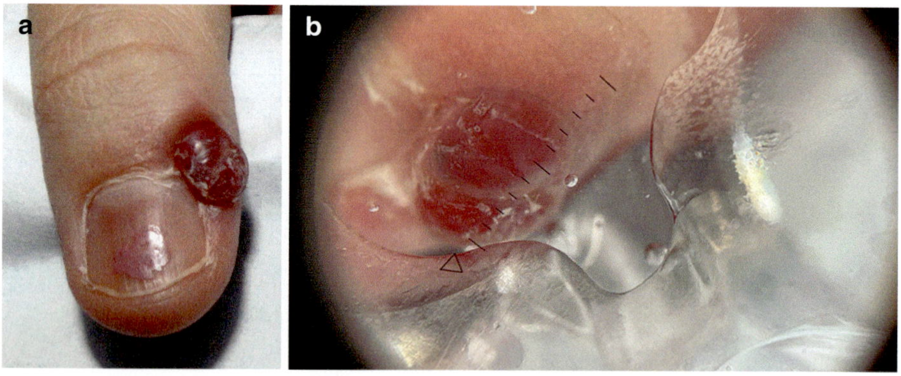

Fig. 12.3 (**a**) 33-Year-old female, Fitzpatrick type III, pyogenic granuloma, with an erythematous nodule of the lateral nail fold of the right thumb. (**b**) The nodule was better appreciated with dermoscopy, which revealed a reddish homogenous area. Note that the patient is wearing pink nail polish

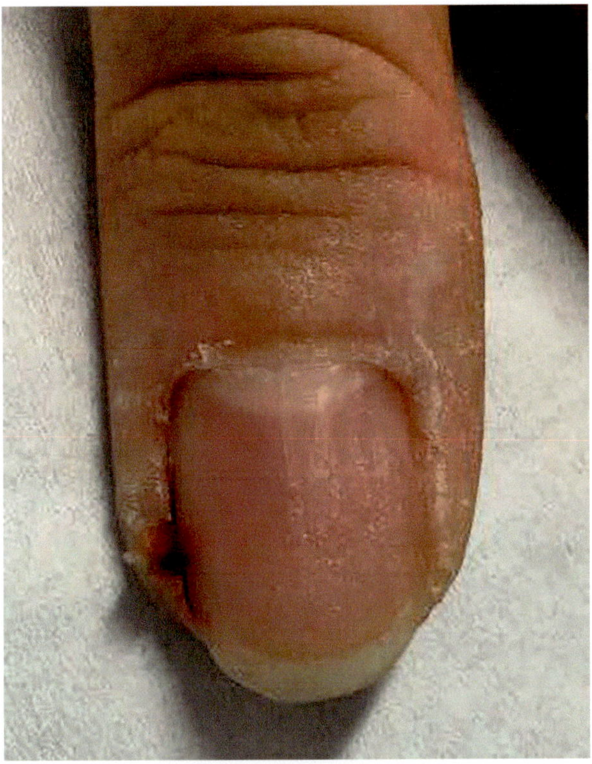

Fig. 12.4 28-Year-old female, Fitzpatrick type III, pyogenic granuloma, with 2 mm periungual pink papule and hemorrhagic crust involving the lateral nail fold of the left thumbnail

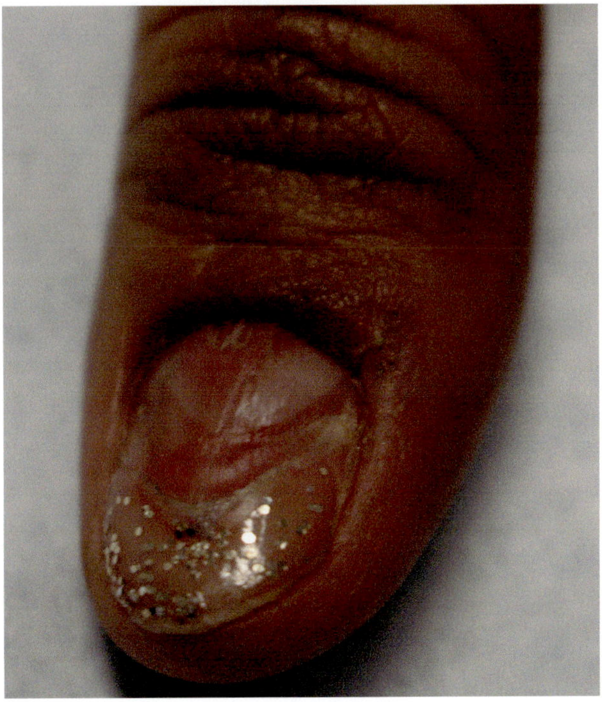

Fig. 12.5 43-Year-old female, Fitzpatrick type III, resolved pyogenic granuloma associated with pregnancy, with reddish discoloration of the lunula and separation of the proximal and distal nail plates of the left thumbnail. Note that the patient has nail polish on the distal nail plate

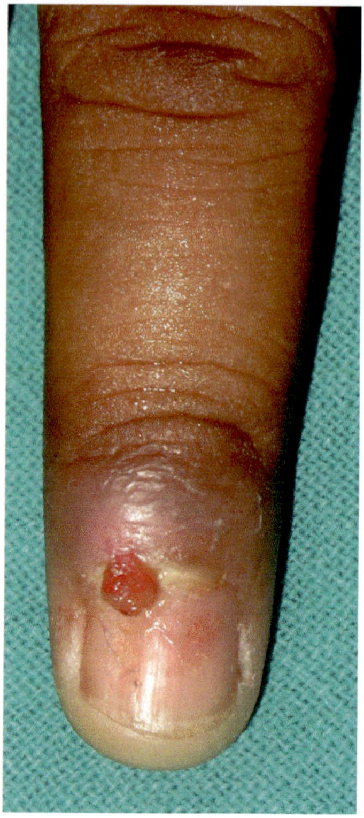

Fig. 12.6 Periungual pyogenic granuloma arising from the proximal nail fold in a middle-aged Indian male patient (Fitzpatrick type IV). The proximal nail fold swelling and erythema preceded the onset of the friable tumoral growth. The patient reported a history of recurrent episodes of bleeding on minor trauma (image *courtesy of* Chander Grover, MD, DNB)

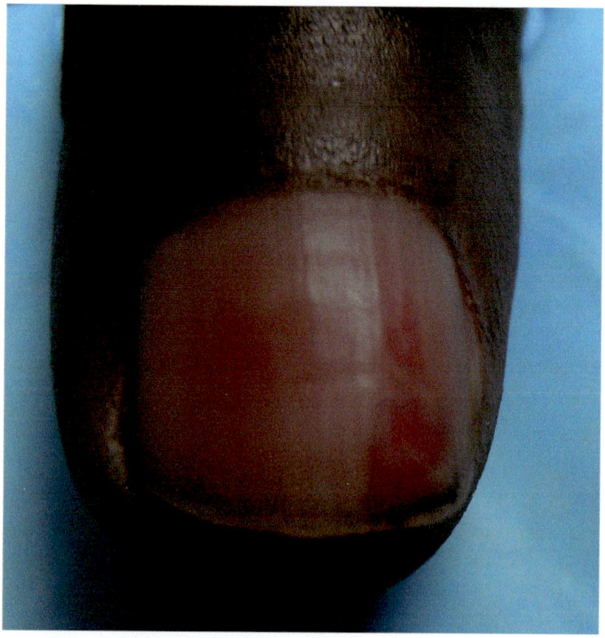

Fig. 12.7 Patient of unknown age and sex, Fitzpatrick type V, pyogenic granuloma, with an ill-defined, triangular, longitudinal band affecting the distal two-thirds of the nail plate (image *courtesy of* Antonella Tosti, MD)

References

1. Cascardo CA, Mansour MR, Mervak JE. Efficacy of available treatments for periungual and subungual pyogenic granulomas: a systematic review. JAAD Int. 2023;12:142–6.
2. Lopez-Castillo D, Curto-Barredo L, Sánchez-Schmidt JM, Pujol RM. Eruptive pyogenic granulomas on the proximal nail folds following cast immobilization: a case report with nail unit ultrasound findings. Acta Derm Venereol. 2020;100(6):adv00071.
3. Alessandrini A, Bruni F, Starace M, Piraccini BM. Periungual pyogenic granuloma: the importance of the medical history. Skin Appendage Disord. 2016;1(4):175–8.
4. Piraccini BM, Bellavista S, Misciali C, Tosti A, de Berker D, Richert B. Periungual and subungual pyogenic granuloma. Br J Dermatol. 2010;163(5):941–53.
5. Benedetto C, Crasto D, Ettefagh L, Nami N. Development of periungual pyogenic granuloma with associated paronychia following isotretinoin therapy: a case report and a review of the literature. J Clin Aesthet Dermatol. 2019;12(4):32–6.
6. Piraccini BM, Venturi M, Patrizi A. Periungual pyogenic granulomas due to topical tazarotene for nail psoriasis. G Ital Dermatol Venereol. 2014;149(3):363–6.
7. Armstrong K, Weinstein M. Pyogenic granulomas during isotretinoin therapy. J Dermatol Case Rep. 2011;5(1):5–7.
8. Thomas M, Shon W, Truong AK. Acitretin-induced periungual pyogenic granulomas and review. Dermatol Online J. 2021;27(7).
9. Figueiras Dde A, Ramos TB, Marinho AK, Bezerra MS, Cauas RC. Paronychia and granulation tissue formation during treatment with isotretinoin. An Bras Dermatol. 2016;91(2):223–5.
10. Sollena P, Mannino M, Tassone F, Calegari MA, D'Argento E, Peris K. Efficacy of topical beta-blockers in the management of EGFR-inhibitor induced paronychia and pyogenic granuloma-like lesions: case series and review of the literature. Drugs Context. 2019;8:212613.
11. Alamri A, Alghamdi Y, Alghamdi A, Albogami DB, Shahada O, AlHarbi A. Ibrutinib-induced paronychia and periungual pyogenic granuloma. Cureus. 2022;14(12):e32943.
12. Agematsu A, Kamata M, Namiki K, Yabuuchi Y, Nagata M, Tada Y. Usefulness of noninvasive management with the gutter method for epidermal growth factor receptor inhibitor-induced paronychia, pyogenic granuloma-like lesion, and ingrown nail. JAMA Dermatol. 2022;158(5):583–5.
13. Dika E, Barisani A, Vaccari S, Fanti PA, Ismaili A, Patrizi A. Periungual pyogenic granuloma following imatinib therapy in a patient with chronic myelogenous leukemia. J Drugs Dermatol. 2013;12(5):512–3.
14. Olamiju B, Bhullar S, Coleman EL, Leventhal JS. Management of paronychia with pseudo-pyogenic granulomas secondary to epidermal growth factor receptor inhibitors: an assessment of topical timolol and the need for multiple medical and procedural therapies. J Am Acad Dermatol. 2021;84(3):806–8.
15. Alessandrini A, Starace M, Cerè G, Brandi N, Piraccini BM. Management and outcome of taxane-induced nail side effects: experience of 79 patients from a single centre. Skin Appendage Disord. 2019;5(5):276–82.
16. Annunziata MC, Vastarella M, Marasca C, Panariello L, Donnarumma M, Fabbrocini G. Chemotherapy-induced periungual pyogenic granuloma: epidemiology and recurrence rates in our experience. Ital J Dermatol Venerol. 2022;157(2):198–9.
17. Devillers C, Vanhooteghem O, Henrijean A, Ramaut M, de la Brassinne M. Subungueal pyogenic granuloma secondary to docetaxel therapy. Clin Exp Dermatol. 2009;34(2):251–2.
18. Hare AQ, Rich P. Nail tumors. Dermatol Clin. 2021;39(2):281–92.
19. Williams LH, Fleckman P. Painless periungual pyogenic granulomata associated with reverse transcriptase inhibitor therapy in a patient with human immunodeficiency virus infection. Br J Dermatol. 2007;156(1):163–4.
20. Bouscarat F, Bouchard C, Bouhour D. Paronychia and pyogenic granuloma of the great toes in patients treated with indinavir. N Engl J Med. 1998;338(24):1776–7.

21. Panariello L, Donnarumma M, Cinelli E, Fabbrocini G. Case series showing the efficacy of 5-aminolaevulinic acid photodynamic therapy for epidermal growth factor receptor inhibitor-induced paronychia and pyogenic granuloma-like lesions. Br J Dermatol. 2019;180(3):676–7. https://doi.org/10.1111/bjd.17270.
22. Robert C, Sibaud V, Mateus C, et al. Nail toxicities induced by systemic anticancer treatments. Lancet Oncol. 2015;16(4):e181–9. https://doi.org/10.1016/S1470-2045(14)71133-7.
23. Baykal C, Kılıç S, Sezer S. Periungual pyogenic granuloma-like lesions following plaster cast immobilization: a case managed with symptomatic therapy. J Dtsch Dermatol Ges. 2018;16(1):74–5.
24. Thakur BK, Verma S, Mishra J. Pyogenic granuloma with onychomadesis following plaster cast immobilization. Indian J Dermatol Venereol Leprol. 2016;82(2):239.
25. Kılıç Sayar S, Sayar Y. Nail disorders associated with cast immobilization of the forearm and wrist: report of two cases and review of the literature. An Bras Dermatol. 2021;96(6):721–5.
26. Richert B, Lecerf P, Caucanas M, André J. Nail tumors. Clin Dermatol. 2013;31(5):602–17.
27. Pecci-Lloret MP, Linares-Pérez C, Pecci-Lloret MR, Rodríguez-Lozano FJ, Oñate-Sánchez RE. Oral manifestations in pregnant women: a systematic review. J Clin Med. 2024;13(3):707.
28. Zaballos P, Llambrich Á, Cuéllar F, Puig S, Malvehy J. Dermoscopic findings in pyogenic granuloma. Br J Dermatol. 2006;154(6):1108–11. https://doi.org/10.1111/j.1365-2133.2006.07193.x.
29. Lopez-Castillo D, Curto-Barredo L, Sánchez-Schmidt JM, Pujol RM. Multiple eruptive pyogenic granulomas on the proximal nail folds following cast immobilization: a case report with nail unit ultrasound findings. Acta Derm Venereol. 2020;100(6):adv00071.
30. Alkabbaa S, Alsaedan AM, Alammar AK. Pyogenic granuloma of the thumb mimicking squamous cell carcinoma of the nail subunit: case report and review of the literature. J Surg Case Rep. 2023;2023(3):rjad157.
31. Khullar G, Singh S, Saikia UN, Kumar A, Singh MP, Kanwar AJ. Squamous cell carcinoma of the nail fold masquerading as pyogenic granuloma. Indian J Dermatol Venereol Leprol. 2016;82(5):555–7.
32. Lee DY, Park SW. Kaposi sarcoma mimicking pyogenic granuloma below the toenail. Int J Dermatol. 2014;53(3):e202–4.

Subungual Exostosis

13

Rachel C. Hill and Shari R. Lipner

13.1 Description of Disease

Subungual exostosis is a benign, osseocartilaginous nail tumor that may affect the distal phalanx of the fingers and toes, and may be associated with a t(X;6)(q24–26;q15–21) chromosomal translocation [1–5]. On histology, subungual exostosis is characterized by the presence of trabecular bone, typically surrounded by a fibrocartilaginous cap, and represents a separate clinical entity from osteochondroma, which is characterized by a hyaline cartilage cap [4, 6, 7]. Because subungual exostosis may present either with or without pain and/or nail dystrophy, the differential diagnosis is broad and includes onychocryptosis, glomus tumor, amelanotic melanoma, traumatic onycholysis, onychogryphosis, pyogenic granuloma, and verruca [4, 8, 9].

13.2 Epidemiology

13.2.1 Sex

The sex distribution for subungual exostosis is roughly equal. In a six-year retrospective review of 19 patients with a sonographic diagnosis of subungual exostosis confirmed with histopathology, 63% were females ($n = 12$) [10]. Similarly, in a case series of 25 cases of histopathologic confirmed subungual exostosis or subungual osteochondroma by Göktay et al., including 14 cases of subungual exostosis, 64% ($n = 9$) of the subungual exostosis cases occurred in females [7]. In a case series of 48 cases of radiologic and histologic confirmed subungual exostosis by Chiheb et al., the male-to-female ratio was 1.1:1 (25 men and 23 women) [5]. In a systematic review by DaCambra et al., of 13 studies that included 287 cases of subungual exostosis of the toes, the male:female ratio was 146:143 [11].

S. R. Lipner, *Atlas of Nail Disorders Across All Skin Colors*,
https://doi.org/10.1007/978-3-031-74272-9_13

13.2.2 Age

Unlike most other types of nail tumors, which typically affect older adults, subungual exostosis more commonly occurs in young adults in the second and third decades of life, although any age group may be affected. Children and adolescents may also be affected [5, 8, 9, 11–15]. Of the 287 cases of toe subungual exostoses included in the systematic review by DaCambra et al., 55% of patients were under the age of 18 [11]. Similarly, in the case series of 48 patients with subungual exostosis by Chiheb et al., the average age of patients was 20 years old (range 6–93 years) [5].

13.3 Risk Factors

Subungual exostosis has been associated with a history of trauma to the affected digit but is subject to recall bias. In a case series of 21 subungual exostosis cases in children, 14% had a history of prior trauma [5, 11, 16–18]. In a case series of 16 patients who underwent surgery for exostosis, four patients (25%) recalled discrete trauma to the affected digit [18]. In the case series of 48 patients by Chiheb et al., 27 cases reported a history of trauma (56%) [5]. Repetitive microtrauma, such as wearing tight-fitting shoes, may also influence the development of exostosis. In the case series of 48 patients by Chiheb et al., eight patients (17%) reported wearing tight-fitting shoes [5]. In the systematic review by DaCambra et al., a history of infection in the affected digit was noted in 21 cases (14%) of 153 [11].

13.4 Clinical Features

Clinically, the presentation of subungual exostosis is varied. Patients may present with or without pain [7, 11, 19]. In the case series of 25 cases of subungual exostosis or osteochondroma by Göktay et al., including 14 cases of subungual exostosis, 50% of patients ($n = 7$) presented with pain [7]. In the systematic review of subungual exostosis of the toes by DaCambra et al., 193 of 250 patients (77%) presented with pain [11].

Similarly, nail dystrophy may or may not be present. Subungual exostosis typically begins as a firm, white nodule with a scale apparent below the distal edge of the nail, which becomes hyperkeratotic over time [11, 15, 17, 20]. In the series of 25 cases of subungual exostosis and osteochondroma by Göktay et al., including 14 cases of subungual exostosis, 50% of patients ($n = 7$) had a distal subungual mass on presentation, while 14.2% ($n = 2$) had a lateral subungual mass, and 14.2% ($n = 2$) had subungual hyperkeratosis and onycholysis [7]. In a case series of ten patients with radiologically and histologically confirmed subungual exostosis by Piccolo et al., nine of ten patients presented with a subungual nodule (90%) [21].

Subungual exostosis typically presents on the dorsomedial aspect of the distal phalanx [11, 17, 19]. The great toe is the most frequently affected digit, although any finger or toe may be involved [5, 7, 11, 18, 21, 22]. In the case series of 48 patients by Chiheb et al., subungual exostosis affected the first toe in 75% of cases (34/48) [5]. Similarly, in the case series of 25 cases of subungual exostosis and subungual osteochondroma by Göktay et al., of the 14 subungual exostosis cases, 12 cases (85.72%) involved the toes, 11 of which affected the first toe (91.67%) [7].

Vascular ectasia and onycholysis are the most common features of subungual exostosis on dermoscopy. In a case series of four patients with histopathologic confirmation of subungual exostosis, the most common features on dermoscopy were a yellow spot on the nail plate ($n = 4$) and onycholysis ($n = 2$) [22]. In the case series of ten patients with subungual exostosis by Piccolo et al., the most common features on dermoscopy were vascular ectasis (70%), hyperkeratosis (60%), onycholysis (40%), and ulceration (30%) [21].

13.5 Clinical Features in Skin of Color

Distinct clinical features of subungual exostosis in patients with skin of color have not been previously described. However, patients with darker skin tones may also have accompanying longitudinal melanonychia.

13.6 Requirements for Diagnosis

A clinical diagnosis of subungual exostosis may be confirmed with an X-ray, which will reveal a bony outgrowth arising from the dorsomedial aspect of the distal phalanx [5, 17]. Definitive diagnosis is made via excision with histology, showing trabecular bone surrounded by a fibrocartilaginous cap [4–7].

Subungual exostosis is treated with a localized excision of the tumor, although recurrences are common with incomplete excision [12]. In the systematic review of 287 cases of subungual exostosis of the toe by DaCambra et al., 124 cases included treatment information, of which five (4%) lesions recurred [11].

13.7 Cases

Figures 13.1, 13.2, 13.3, 13.4, 13.5, and 13.6 demonstrate the presentation of exostosis in a clinical setting.

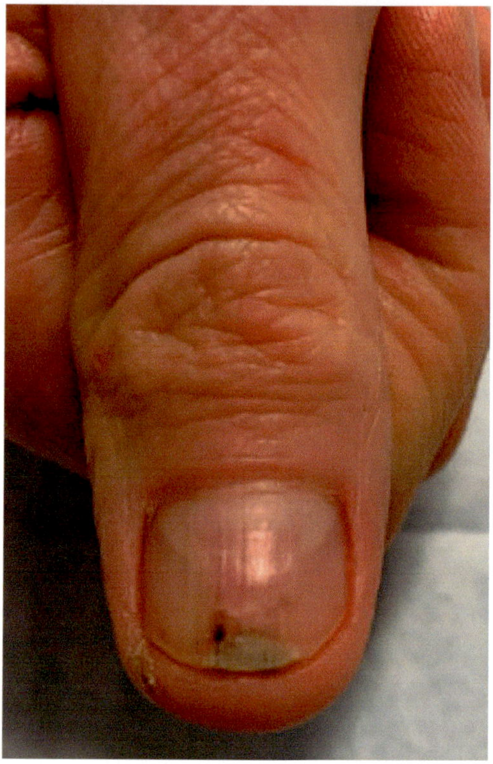

Fig. 13.1 43-Year-old male, Fitzpatrick type I, subungual exostosis, right thumbnail with 6 mm band of longitudinal erythronychia with splinter hemorrhages, originating in the distal lunula, with distal onycholysis

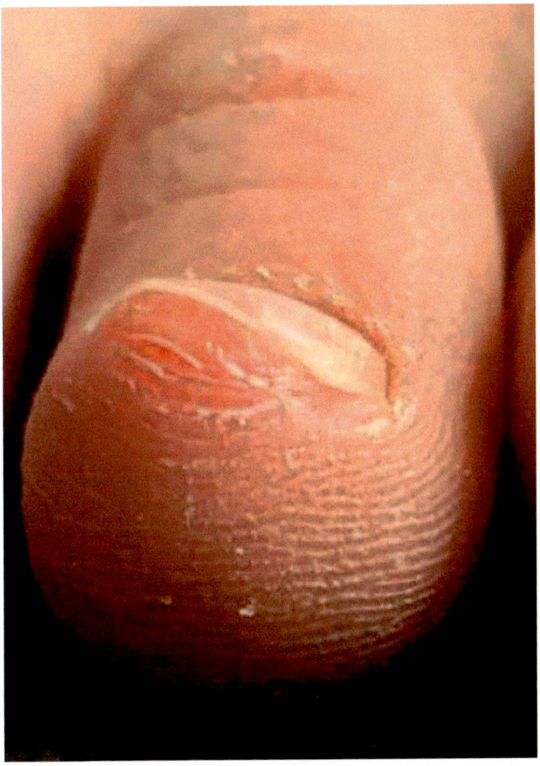

Fig. 13.2 14-Year-old female, Fitzpatrick type II, subungual exostosis, with flesh-colored, firm subungual papule and minimal onycholysis of the right second toenail

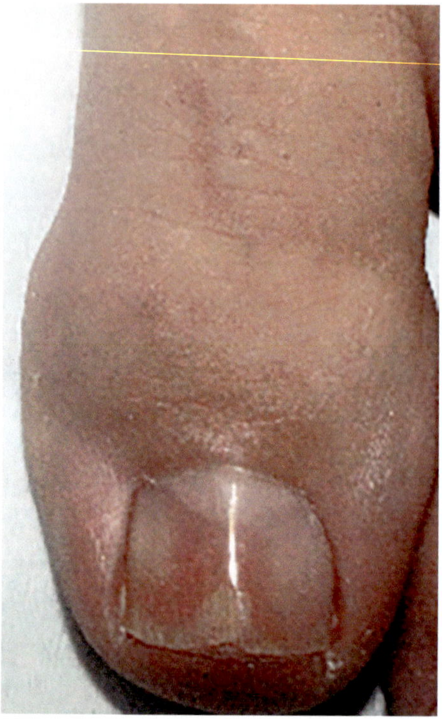

Fig. 13.3 57-Year-old female, Fitzpatrick type II, subungual exostosis left great toenail, with ridge and onycholysis overlying a firm hyperkeratotic papule

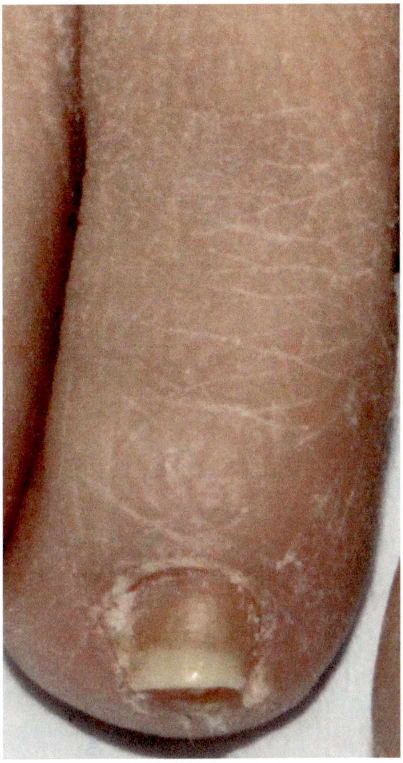

Fig. 13.4 58-Year-old female, Fitzpatrick type II, subungual exostosis, with firm hyperkeratotic papule of the distal left second toenail

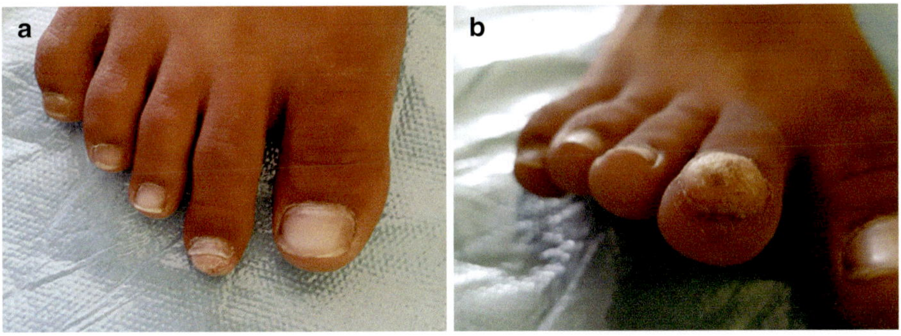

Fig. 13.5 (**a**, **b**) 12-year-old male, Fitzpatrick type IV, subungual exostosis, presenting with a firm, hyperkeratotic, subungual nodule affecting the right second toenail for 1.5 years (*from* Bennani et al. [23]; CC-BY 4.0, https://creativecommons.org/licenses/by/4.0)

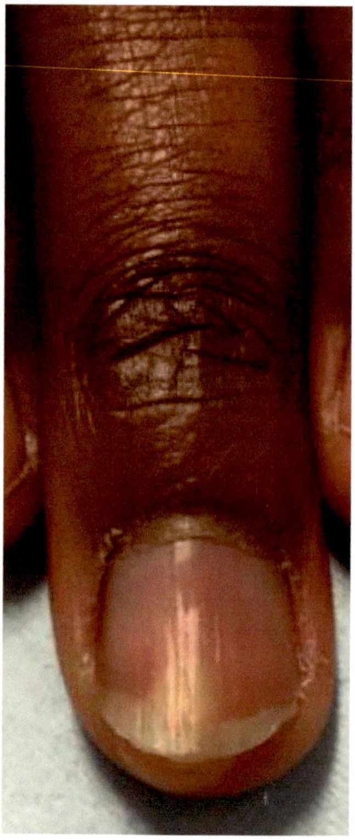

Fig. 13.6 39-Year-old male, Fitzpatrick type VI, subungual exostosis, with onycholysis overlying a firm, immobile bony, and nontender nodule of the left third fingernail

References

1. Storlazzi CT, Wozniak A, Panagopoulos I, et al. Rearrangement of the COL12A1 and COL4A5 genes in subungual exostosis: molecular cytogenetic delineation of the tumor-specific translocation t(X;6)(q13–14;q22). Int J Cancer. 2006;118(8):1972–6. https://doi.org/10.1002/ijc.21586.
2. Zambrano E, Nosé V, Perez-Atayde AR, et al. Distinct chromosomal rearrangements in subungual (Dupuytren) exostosis and bizarre parosteal osteochondromatous proliferation (Nora lesion). Am J Surg Pathol. 2004;28(8):1033–9. https://doi.org/10.1097/01.pas.0000126642.61690.d6.
3. Dal Cin P, Pauwels P, Poldermans LJ, Sciot R, Van den Berghe H. Clonal chromosome abnormalities in a so-called Dupuytren's subungual exostosis. Genes Chromosomes Cancer. 1999;24(2):162–4. https://doi.org/10.1002/(sici)1098-2264(199902)24:2<162::aid-gcc11>3.0.co;2-7.
4. Capasso G, Fabbrocini G, Marasca C. A subungual exostosis mimicking a periungual granuloma in a 9-year-old boy: an unexpected dermoscopic pattern. Skin Appendage Disord. 2021;7(6):483–5. https://doi.org/10.1159/000517199.
5. Chiheb S, Slimani Y, Karam R, Marnissi F, Hali F. Subungual exostosis: a case series of 48 patients. Skin Appendage Disord. 2021;7(6):475–9. https://doi.org/10.1159/000516660.
6. Guarneri C, Guarneri F, Risitano G, Lentini M, Vaccaro M. Solitary asymptomatic nodule of the great toe. Int J Dermatol. 2005;44(3):245–7. https://doi.org/10.1111/j.1365-4632.2004.02475.x.

7. Göktay F, Atış G, Güneş P, Macit B, Çelik NS, Gürdal Kösem E. Subungual exostosis and subungual osteochondromas: a description of 25 cases. Int J Dermatol. 2018;57(7):872–81. https://doi.org/10.1111/ijd.14003.
8. Yousefian F, Davis B, Browning JC. Pediatric subungual exostosis. Cutis. 2021;108(5):256–7. https://doi.org/10.12788/cutis.0380.
9. Hare AQ, Rich P. Nail tumors. Dermatol Clin. 2021;39(2):281–92. https://doi.org/10.1016/j.det.2020.12.007.
10. Whittle C, Aguirre J, Catalán V, Fajre X, Vargas F. Subungual exostosis: high-resolution ultrasound findings. J Diagn Med Sonogr. 2019;35(5):387–90. https://doi.org/10.1177/8756479319836943.
11. DaCambra MP, Gupta SK, Ferri-de-Barros F. Subungual exostosis of the toes: a systematic review. Clin Orthop Relat Res. 2014;472(4):1251–9. https://doi.org/10.1007/s11999-013-3345-4.
12. Russell JD, Nance K, Nunley JR, Maher IA. Subungual exostosis. Cutis. 2016;98(2):128–9.
13. Tiwari A, Agrawal N, Verma T, Lal H. Subungual osteochondroma: nail sparing excision. J Clin Orthop Trauma. 2016;7(Suppl 1):72–5. https://doi.org/10.1016/j.jcot.2016.06.014.
14. Dąbrowski M, Rusek D, Dańczak-Pazdrowska A, Litowińska A. The influence of clinical factors on treatment outcome and a recurrence of surgically removed protruded subungual osteochondroma and subungual exostosis. J Clin Med. 2023;12(19):6413. https://doi.org/10.3390/jcm12196413.
15. Womack ME, Fisher OJ, Landrum MR, Rose RA. Subungual exostosis of the hand: a case report in a 5-year-old boy and literature review. J Am Acad Orthop Surg Glob Res Rev. 2022;6(3):e21.00239. https://doi.org/10.5435/JAAOSGlobal-D-21-00239.
16. Letts M, Davidson D, Nizalik E. Subungual exostosis: diagnosis and treatment in children. J Trauma. 1998;44(2):346–9. https://doi.org/10.1097/00005373-199802000-00020.
17. Fox R, Katsarma E, Tiffin N, Singh M. Subungual exostosis presenting as a pyogenic granuloma-like lesion with reactive myofibroblastic proliferation in two young women. Dermatopathology (Basel). 2022;9(2):196–202. https://doi.org/10.3390/dermatopathology9020024.
18. Suga H, Mukouda M. Subungual exostosis: a review of 16 cases focusing on postoperative deformity of the nail. Ann Plast Surg. 2005;55(3):272–5. https://doi.org/10.1097/01.sap.0000174356.70048.b8.
19. Pascoal D, Balacó I, Alves C, Cardoso PS, Ling TP, Matos G. Subungual exostosis—treatment results with preservation of the nail bed. J Pediatr Orthop B. 2020;29(4):382–6. https://doi.org/10.1097/BPB.0000000000000723.
20. Orly J, Leducq S. Subungual exostosis of the toe. J Cutan Med Surg. 2022;26(6):646. https://doi.org/10.1177/12034754221102008.
21. Piccolo V, Argenziano G, Alessandrini AM, Russo T, Starace M, Piraccini BM. Dermoscopy of subungual exostosis: a retrospective study of 10 patients. Dermatology. 2017;233(1):80–5. https://doi.org/10.1159/000471800.
22. Demirdag HG, Tugrul Ayanoglu B, Akay BN. Dermoscopic features of subungual exostosis. Australas J Dermatol. 2019;60(2):e138–41. https://doi.org/10.1111/ajd.12911.
23. Bennani M, Assenhaji I, Baybay H, Elloudi S, Douhi S, Mernissi FZ. Subungual exostosis: unusual localization. J Clin Med Res. 2020;2(2):1–4.

Subungual Neurofibroma

14

Michael Ong and Shari R. Lipner

14.1 Description of Disease

Neurofibromas are peripheral nerve sheath tumors. They are composed of a mixture of cell types including Schwann cells, fibroblasts, and immune cells [1]. Neurofibromas are most commonly found in or near the skin, often extending along a nerve or involving multiple nerve fascicles [2]. Rarely, they may affect the digits and nails. Subungual neurofibromas may arise in association with neurofibromatosis I (NF1) or as solitary lesions [3] and are exceedingly rare with approximately 15 reported cases [4–7]. There are two main types of neurofibromas: cutaneous (cNF) and plexiform (pNF) [2]. cNF are benign, are found exclusively in the dermis, and are typically present during puberty. In contrast, pNF carries a risk for sarcomatous transformation and can be found deeper below the dermis. They are congenital and progress during childhood and adolescence. Subungual neurofibromas typically present as a myxoid histopathologic variant of cNF [8–10].

14.2 Epidemiology

14.2.1 Sex

While cutaneous neurofibromas affect men and women equally, subungual neurofibromas may be more common in females [4, 11]. There are only three reported cases of subungual neurofibromas in males [6, 12, 13].

S. R. Lipner, *Atlas of Nail Disorders Across All Skin Colors*,
https://doi.org/10.1007/978-3-031-74272-9_14

14.2.2 Age

Subungual neurofibromas most commonly affect middle-aged individuals with a mean age of 41 years based on a case report and literature review of nine other cases [7]. The youngest confirmed case is in a 13-year-old [14]. Subungual neurofibroma has also been described in a 34-year-old woman, who had recurrence after tumor resection at the age of eight years [15].

14.2.3 Other Factors

Neurofibromas are commonly solitary lesions, but about 10% of cases are associated with neurofibromatosis [11]. Neurofibromas result from a deletion in the NF1 gene in both sporadic and syndromic cases. The NF1 gene encodes neurofibromin, a negative regulator of Ras. Dysregulation of Ras can lead to increased cell proliferation and tumor formation [16]. In sporadic cases, only the lesional cells carry the NF1 mutation, whereas in syndromic cases, neurofibromas arise from a germline mutation in NF1 [16, 17]. No cases of subungual neurofibromas have been reported in association with NF1.

14.3 Risk Factors

Risk factors for subungual neurofibromas have not been definitively established, but older age and female sex are likely risk factors. Personal or family history of neurofibromatosis may also be a risk factor.

14.4 Clinical Features

Subungual neurofibromas typically present as small (<2 cm), solitary papules that are slow-growing. A white-pink nodular tumor may be appreciated on physical examination [5, 7]. Other nail findings include distal nail splitting, onychodystrophy, nail plate elevation and thickening, longitudinal riding, and increased nail plate convexity [4, 5, 7, 8, 13, 18, 19]. Dermoscopy findings have not been documented. Patients do not generally report preceding trauma. Although subungual neurofibromas lack distinct clinical features, they are usually not painful, which can aid in distinguishing them from other subungual tumors [5]. Only two reported cases have been associated with pain [18, 19]. Recurrence after surgical excision is rare [5, 18].

14.5 Clinical Features in Skin of Color

Clinical descriptions of subungual neurofibromas in patients with skin of color are limited. Case reports in Asian and White Hispanic individuals suggest that clinical findings may resemble those seen in White non-Hispanic individuals [12–14].

There are no reported cases of subungual neurofibromas in Black or African American patients.

14.6 Requirements for Diagnosis

Diagnosing subungual neurofibromas clinically is challenging due to its rarity and lack of pathognomonic symptoms [4]. Radiographic imaging is usually unremarkable but may reveal compression atrophy of the associated phalanx [7, 9, 14]. MRI may exhibit hyperintensity on T2 weighted image but is nonspecific for diagnosis [4, 5]. Confirming the diagnosis requires histological and immunochemical analysis. Histopathology may demonstrate a well-defined tumor comprised of elongated fusiform and spindle cells within a myxoid stroma, although these morphological features can overlap with solitary fibrous tumors [4–9, 12, 13, 18, 19]. Immunohistochemistry with S-100 is recommended since it serves as a specific marker for neurofibromas.

14.7 Cases

Figures 14.1, 14.2, 14.3, 14.4, and 14.5 demonstrate the presentation of subungual neurofibromas in a clinical setting.

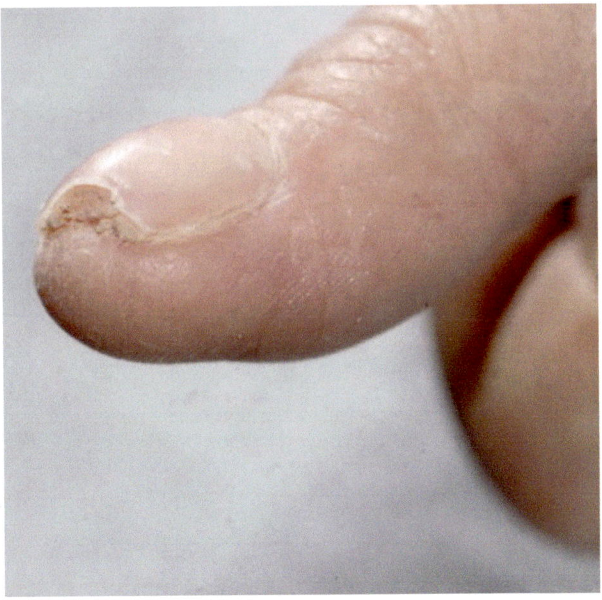

Fig. 14.1 Unknown age and sex, Fitzpatrick type II, subungual neurofibroma, with increased curvature of the nail with subungual hyperkeratosis (*from* Willard et al. [3]; *with permission*)

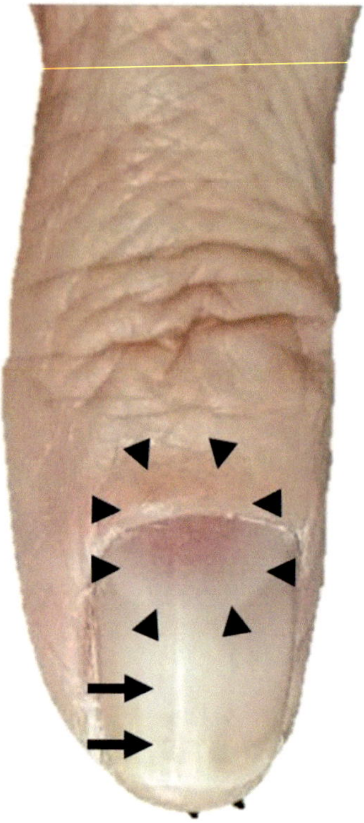

Fig. 14.2 62-Year-old female, Fitzpatrick type II, subungual neurofibroma, with reddish mass under the nail plate (triangles) and distal nail splitting (arrows) (*from* Suzuki et al. [5]; CC-BY 4.0, https://creativecommons.org/licenses/by/4.0)

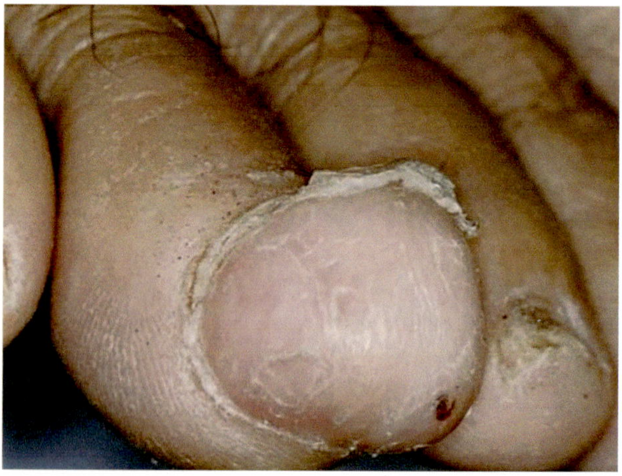

Fig. 14.3 51-Year-old man, Fitzpatrick type II, subungual neurofibroma, with a rounded, regular, normochromatic tumoral lesion in the subungual region of the right fourth toe (*from* Stolarczuk et al. [12]; CC-BY 4.0, https://creativecommons.org/licenses/by/4.0)

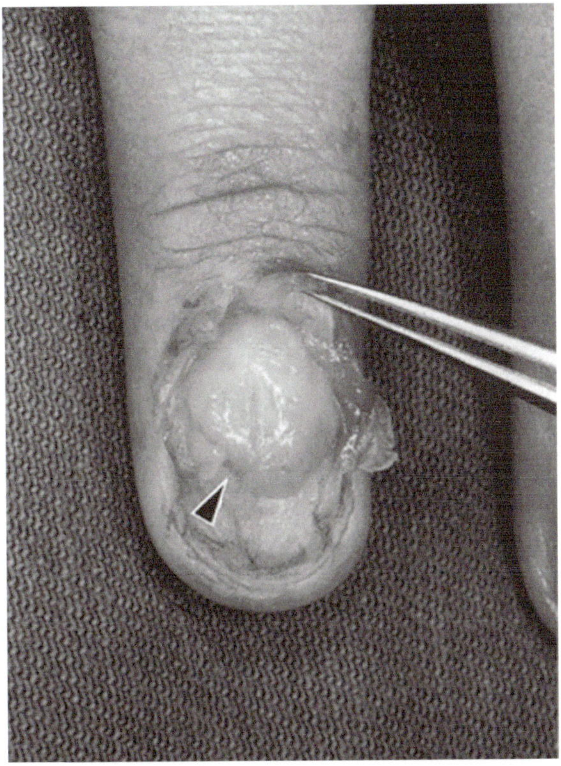

Fig. 14.4 13-Year-old Japanese female, unknown Fitzpatrick type, subungual neurofibroma, with a pale-yellow tumor (arrowhead) after ablation of the nail (*from* Niizuma and Iijima [14]; *with permission*)

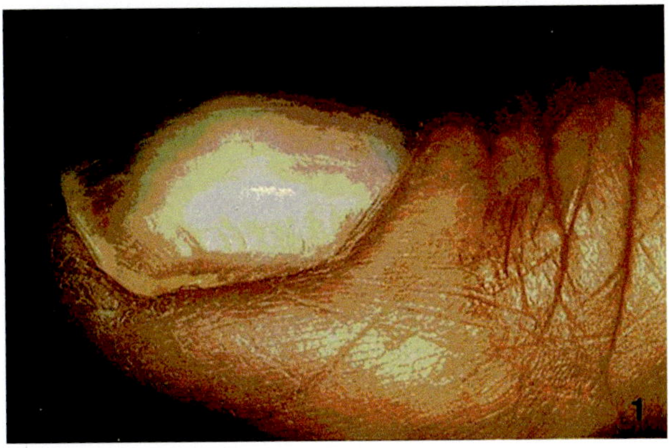

Fig. 14.5 60-Year-old female, Fitzpatrick type V, subungual neurofibroma, with marked overcurvature of the thumb (*from* Baran and Haneke [8]; CC-BY 4.0, https://creativecommons.org/licenses/by/4.0)

References

1. Jo VY, Fletcher CDM. WHO classification of soft tissue tumours: an update based on the 2013 (4th) edition. Pathology. 2014;46(2):95–104. https://doi.org/10.1097/PAT.0000000000000050.
2. Brosseau JP, Pichard DC, Legius EH, et al. The biology of cutaneous neurofibromas: consensus recommendations for setting research priorities. Neurology. 2018;91(2 Suppl 1):S14–20. https://doi.org/10.1212/WNL.0000000000005788.
3. Willard KJ, Cappel MA, Kozin SH, Abzug JM. Benign subungual tumors. J Hand Surg Am. 2012;37(6):1276–86. https://doi.org/10.1016/j.jhsa.2012.04.001.
4. Huajun J, Wei Q, Ming L, Chongyang F, Weiguo Z, Decheng L. Solitary subungual neurofibroma in the right first finger. Int J Dermatol. 2012;51(3):335–8. https://doi.org/10.1111/j.1365-4632.2011.05248.x.
5. Suzuki R, Hashimoto H, Okamoto O. Solitary subungual neurofibroma with glomus tumor-like appearance: a case report. Case Reports Plast Surg Hand Surg. 2020;7(1):43–5. https://doi.org/10.1080/23320885.2020.1750018.
6. Llamas-Velasco M, Espinosa P, Ovejero-Merino E, Pérez-González YC. Collision of subungual neurofibroma and onychomatricoma: S100 positivity as a clue. Am J Dermatopathol. 2019;41(9):649–51. https://doi.org/10.1097/DAD.0000000000001357.
7. Pertea M, Grosu OM, Terinte C, Poroch V, Velenciuc N, Lunca S. Nail bed solitary neurofibroma: a case report and literature review. Medicine (Baltimore). 2019;98(3):e14111. https://doi.org/10.1097/MD.0000000000014111.
8. Baran R, Haneke E. Subungual myxoid neurofibroma on the thumb. Acta Derm Venereol. 2001;81(3):210–1. https://doi.org/10.1080/000155501750376357.
9. Gmyrek RF, Beer R, Silvers DN, Reiffel R, Grossman ME. Periungual myxoid neurofibroma. Cutis. 2002;69(1):54–6.
10. Nagrani NS, Bhawan J. Histopathological variants of cutaneous neurofibroma: a compendious review. Dermatopathology. 2022;10(1):1–19. https://doi.org/10.3390/dermatopathology10010001.
11. Messersmith L, Krauland K. Neurofibroma. In: StatPearls. StatPearls Publishing; 2024. http://www.ncbi.nlm.nih.gov/books/NBK539707/.
12. Stolarczuk DDA, da Silva ALF, Filgueiras FM, Alves MFGS, Silva SCMC. Solitary subungual neurofibroma: a previously unreported finding in a male patient. An Bras Dermatol. 2011;86(3):569–72. https://doi.org/10.1590/s0365-05962011000300024.
13. Seo B-M, Lim J-S, Jung S-N, Yoo G, Byeon J-H. Solitary subungual myxoid neurofibroma of the thumb: a case report. J Korean Soc Plast Reconstr Surg. 2011;38(4):398–400.
14. Niizuma K, Iijima KN. Solitary neurofibroma: a case of subungual neurofibroma on the right third finger. Arch Dermatol Res. 1991;283(1):13–5. https://doi.org/10.1007/BF01207244.
15. Hocar O, Madhar M, Akhdari N, et al. Neurofibrome myxoïde du pouce. Chir Main. 2012;31(4):217–9. https://doi.org/10.1016/j.main.2012.07.007.
16. Ferner RE, Gutmann DH. Neurofibromatosis type 1 (NF1): diagnosis and management. Handb Clin Neurol. 2013;115:939–55. https://doi.org/10.1016/B978-0-444-52902-2.00053-9.
17. Tucker T, Riccardi VM, Brown C, et al. S100B and neurofibromin immunostaining and X-inactivation patterns of laser-microdissected cells indicate a multicellular origin of some NF1-associated neurofibromas. J Neurosci Res. 2011;89(9):1451–60. https://doi.org/10.1002/jnr.22654.

18. Roldan-Marin R, Dominguez-Cherit J, Vega-Memije ME, Toussaint-Caire S, Hojyo-Tomoka MT, Dominguez-Soto L. Solitary subungual neurofibroma: an uncommon finding and a review of the literature. J Drugs Dermatol. 2006;5(7):672–4.
19. Dangoisse C, Andre J, De Dobbeleer G, Van Geertruyden J. Solitary subungual neurofibroma. Br J Dermatol. 2000;143(5):1116–7. https://doi.org/10.1046/j.1365-2133.2000.03875.x.

Acquired Ungual Fibrokeratoma 15

Rachel C. Hill and Shari R. Lipner

15.1 Description of Disease

Acquired digital fibrokeratoma (ADFK) is a rare, benign, CD34-negative, or focally CD34-positive, fibrous tumor that may be localized to the nail unit, where it is termed an acquired ungual fibrokeratoma (AUFK) [1, 2]. AUFK typically arises from the proximal nail matrix or nail bed [3]. AUFK consists of dense collagen fibers with increased levels of fibroblasts and capillaries compared to the dermis, suggesting that the tumor may result from erroneous collagen formation by fibroblasts [1, 4]. Factor XIIIa, an intracellularly produced coagulation factor that stimulates the proliferation of fibroblasts, is expressed in ADFK and may play a role in its pathogenesis by acting as a growth factor promoting tumor development [5, 6]. Some studies cited herein refer to ADFK instead of AUFK due to the rarity of the latter. The reference to each study distinguishes whether the inclusion criteria included ADFK vs. AUFK specifically.

15.2 Epidemiology

15.2.1 Sex

Because AUFK is relatively uncommon and likely underreported, sex distribution is understudied. In a systematic review of AUFK cases by Ballan et al., including 103 articles and 78 tumors, the male:female ratio was 1:1 [7]. However, studies of ADFK instead suggest a greater prevalence in males vs. females. In a retrospective study of 50 cases of histopathologic confirmed ADFK by Kint et al., 29 patients were male and 21 were female [4]. In a retrospective study of 26 clinicopathologically confirmed cases of ADFK by Palaniappan, 21 patients were male, and 5 patients were female, with male:female ratio 4.2:1 [3]. In a retrospective study of 13 histopathological confirmed ADFK, including one AUFK, all patients were male [8].

S. R. Lipner, *Atlas of Nail Disorders Across All Skin Colors*,
https://doi.org/10.1007/978-3-031-74272-9_15

15.2.2 Age

Although AUFK typically affects adults in the third through seventh decades of life, it has been reported in children as young as six years old [9]. In a retrospective study of 20 patients with histopathologic confirmed AUFK by Hwang et al., the mean age was 41.2 years with a range of 15–79 years old [10]. In the retrospective study of 50 histopathologic confirmed ADFK by Kint et al., the mean age was 40 years, with a range of 12–77 years [4].

15.3 Risk Factors

Risk factors for AUFK may include trauma and repeated injury to the nail unit, but the data is sparse [12]. In the retrospective study of 50 histopathologic confirmed ADFK by Kint et al., one patient reported a history of trauma that occurred prior to tumor development [4]. In the retrospective study of 20 patients with AUFK by Hwang et al., four patients (20%) reported a history of preceding trauma [10]. ADFK has also been reported after staphylococcal infection in two case reports [1, 13, 14].

15.4 Clinical Features

Clinically, AUFK appears as a solitary, smooth, dome-shaped, or finger-like flesh-colored papule or nodule less than one cm in diameter [10, 12]. When ADFK or AUFK exceeds one cm, it is referred to as a "giant fibrokeratoma" [15–18]. Previous studies have classified AUFK into two types: type I, in which the tumor involves the nail plate, and type II, in which the tumor is periungual [19, 20].

Four clinical variants of AUFK tumors have been described, including dome-shaped, branching, flat, and rod-shaped [10]. The three ungual distributions of AUFK include periungual, intraungual, or subungual [10]. In the retrospective study of 20 patients with AUFK by Hwang et al., tumors were most frequently dome-shaped (8/20, 40%), followed by branching (5/20, 25%), flat (4/20, 20%), and rod-shaped (3/20, 20%), with the most frequent distribution periungual (15/20, 75%), followed by intraungual (4/20, 20%), or subungual (1/20, 5%) [10]. In some cases, the flat variant may expand to encompass the entire width of the nail unit [21].

The AUFK variant, size, and tumor location contribute to the clinical presentation [7]. Nail plate dystrophy likely occurs due to chronic pressure exerted on the nail matrix by the tumor [15]. In the study by Hwang et al., the most common nail findings were longitudinal groove (16/20, 80%), trachyonychia (8/20, 40%), chromonychia (4/20, 20%), onycholysis (4/20, 20%), subungual hyperkeratosis (3/20, 15%), and dissected nail plates (2/20, 10%) [10]. Other nail findings reported in the systematic review of AUFK by Ballan et al. included nail plate thinning and hemorrhagic crust [7].

AUFK may affect the toenails more commonly than fingernails [9, 10]. In the systematic review by Ballan et al., 67% and 33% of tumors affected the toenails and fingernails, respectively, with the great toenail and thumbnail most often affected (46% and 11%, respectively) [7]. In Hwang et al.'s study, toenails were more commonly involved than fingernails (16/20, 80% vs. 4/20, 20%, respectively) [10].

15.5 Clinical Features in Skin of Color

Although features of AUFK in skin of color patients have not been explicitly described, patients with skin of color are more likely to have physiologic melanonychia affecting the fingernails and toenails, which may obscure the clinical diagnosis.

15.6 Requirements for Diagnosis

Definitive diagnosis of AUFK is made via excision with histology, which shows hyperkeratosis and acanthosis of the epidermis with thick collagen fibers and dilated capillaries oriented along the longitudinal axis of the tumor in the dermis [10, 15, 19, 22]. In the systematic review of AUFK by Ballan et al., the overall recurrence rate after surgery was 15.5%, and more common when partial vs. complete surgical excision was performed (71.4% vs. 9.2%, $P < 0.001$) [7].

15.7 Cases

Figures 15.1, 15.2, 15.3, 15.4, 15.5, 15.6, and 15.7 demonstrate the presentation of AUFK in a clinical setting.

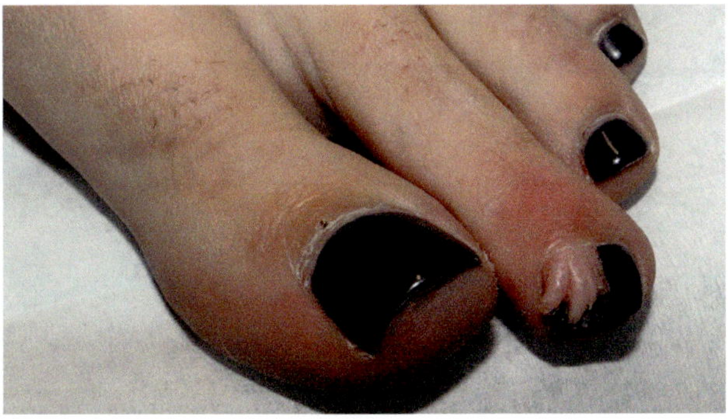

Fig. 15.1 38-Year-old female, Fitzpatrick type I, AUFK, with finger-like, flesh-colored projections involving the left second toenail

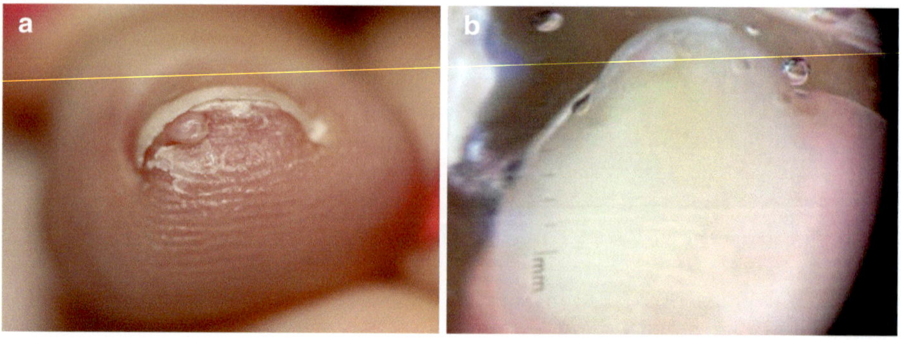

Fig. 15.2 (**a**) 35-Year-old female, Fitzpatrick type II, AUFK, with a subungual papule of the left third toenail. (**b**) The papule could be appreciated with dermoscopy when viewed end on

Fig. 15.3 41-Year-old male, Fitzpatrick type IV, AUFK, with conical papule with hyperkeratotic tip emerging from the proximal nail fold of the right thumbnail

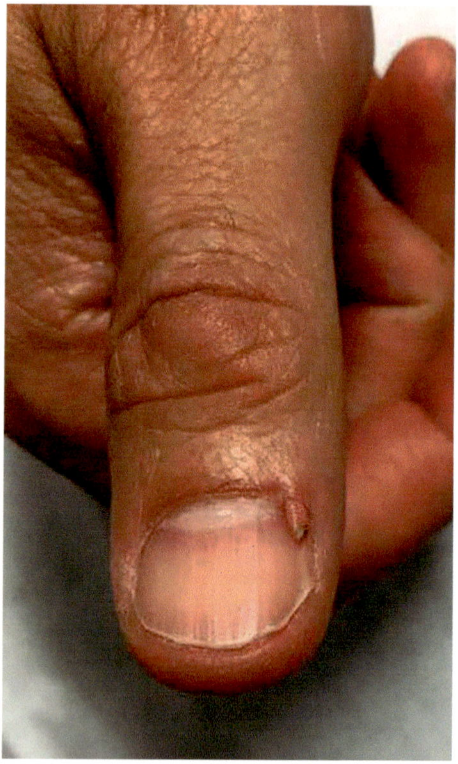

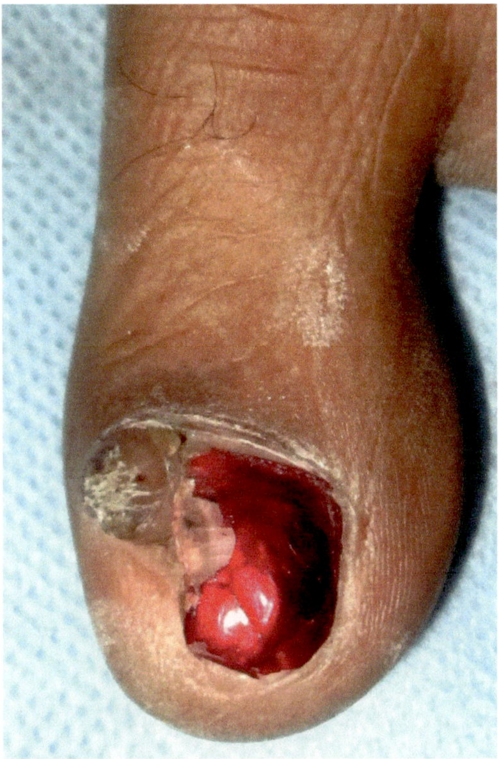

Fig. 15.4 41-year-old female, Fitzpatrick type IV, AUFK, with subungual papule involving the left great toenail (image *courtesy of* Chander Grover, MD, DNB)

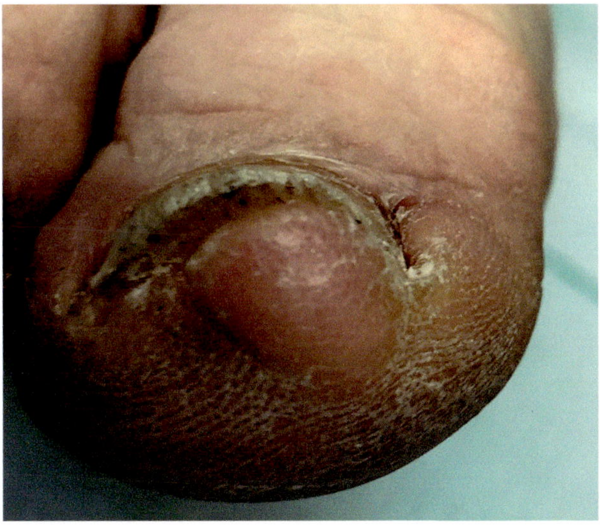

Fig. 15.5 72-Year-old female, Fitzpatrick type IV, AUFK, with subungual papule involving the right great toenail (image *courtesy of* Dr. Eckart Haneke, MD, PhD)

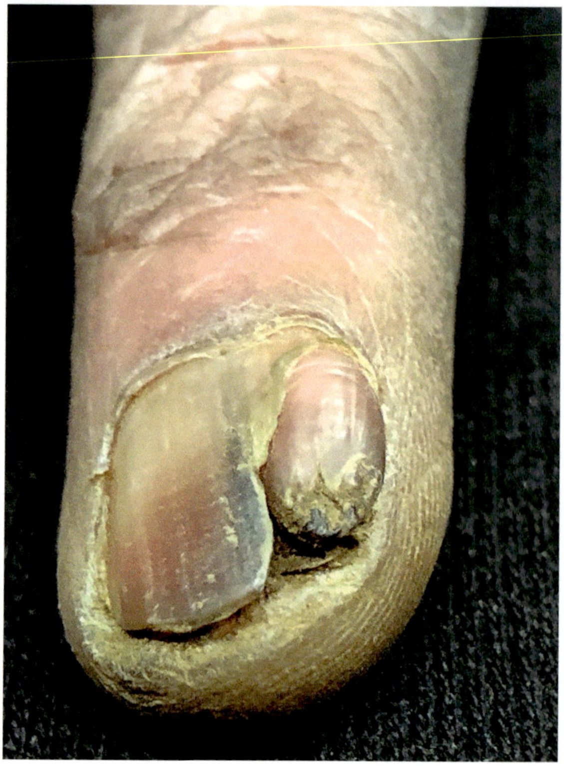

Fig. 15.6 62-Year-old female, Fitzpatrick type V, AUFK, with subungual papule involving the left second fingernail (image *courtesy of* Dr. Eckart Haneke, MD, PhD)

Fig. 15.7 17-Year-old male, Fitzpatrick type V, AUFK, with asymptomatic subungual papule involving the right fifth fingernail for more than 6 months. Total excision and histopathology confirmed the diagnosis (*from* Haneke et al. [23] with permission, photographed by Dr. Ranthilaka R. Ranawaka)

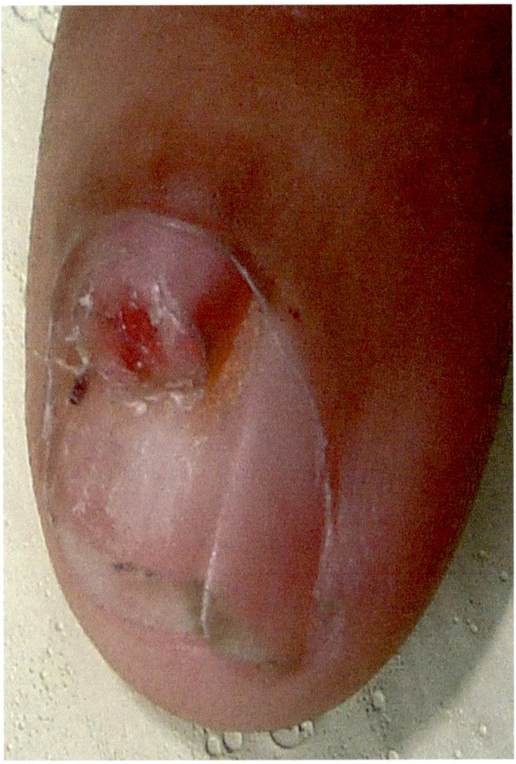

References

1. Shih S, Khachemoune A. Acquired digital fibrokeratoma: review of its clinical and dermoscopic features and differential diagnosis. Int J Dermatol. 2019;58(2):151–8. https://doi.org/10.1111/ijd.14046.
2. Cohen PR, Alpert RS, Calame A. Cellular digital fibroma: a comprehensive review of a CD34-positive acral lesion of the distal fingers and toes. Dermatol Ther (Heidelb). 2020;10(5):949–66. https://doi.org/10.1007/s13555-020-00418-3.
3. Palaniappan V, Sadhasivamohan A, Sankarapandian J, Karthikeyan K. Acquired fibrokeratoma: a retrospective study in a tertiary centre in South India. Indian J Dermatol. 2022;67(3):312. https://doi.org/10.4103/ijd.ijd_239_22.
4. Kint A, Baran R, De Keyser H. Acquired (digital) fibrokeratoma. J Am Acad Dermatol. 1985;12(5 Pt 1):816–21. https://doi.org/10.1016/s0190-9622(85)70101-6.
5. Nemeth AJ, Penneys NS. Factor XIIIa is expressed by fibroblasts in fibrovascular tumors. J Cutan Pathol. 1989;16(5):266–71. https://doi.org/10.1111/j.1600-0560.1989.tb00050.x.
6. Suh H-S, Choi J-H, Sung K-J, Koh J-K. A case of acquired digital fibrokeratoma: immunohistochemical stain with anti-factor XIIIa antibody. Korean J Dermatol. 1994;32:1131–5.
7. Ballan A, Zeinaty P, Tomb R, et al. Acquired ungual fibrokeratoma: a systematic review of the literature. Int J Dermatol. 2021;60(5):533–9. https://doi.org/10.1111/ijd.15278.
8. Baykal C, Buyukbabani N, Yazganoglu KD, Saglik E. Acquired digital fibrokeratoma. Cutis. 2007;79(2):129–32.
9. Venkatachalam K, Divya KS, Kinnera B, Babu KS. An interesting case report of acquired triradiate periungual fibrokeratoma and its dermoscopic features. Indian Dermatol Online J. 2023;14(2):266–7. https://doi.org/10.4103/idoj.idoj_224_22.

10. Hwang S, Kim M, Cho BK, Park HJ. Clinical characteristics of acquired ungual fibrokeratoma. Indian J Dermatol Venereol Leprol. 2017;83(3):337–43. https://doi.org/10.4103/0378-6323.193611.
11. Jahan N, Ashwini PK, Chethana SG, Betkerur J, Shastry V. Horn on the nail: acquired ungual fibrokeratoma. J Cutan Aesthet Surg. 2021;14(1):121–4. https://doi.org/10.4103/jcas.Jcas_71_19.
12. Sung KY, Lee S, Lee SY. An unusual presentation of acquired periungual fibrokeratoma: a mixed form of dome-shaped and branching type. Clin Case Rep. 2020;8(11):2129–31. https://doi.org/10.1002/ccr3.3073.
13. Amarouch H, Aitourghoui M, Ramli I, Zaouri H, Senouci K, Hassam B. Un fibrokératome digital acquis post-staphylococcique: une nouvelle observation [Post-staphylococcal acquired digital fibrokeratoma: a new case]. Presse Med. 2015;44(7–8):843–5. https://doi.org/10.1016/j.lpm.2015.03.015.
14. Sezer E, Bridges AG, Koseoglu D, Yuksek J. Acquired periungual fibrokeratoma developing after acute staphylococcal paronychia. Eur J Dermatol. 2009;19(6):636–7. https://doi.org/10.1684/ejd.2009.0771.
15. Mir MA, Vathulya M, Mahakalkar S, Manohar N. Acquired periungual fibrokeratoma looks like a supernumerary digit: an uncommon soft tissue tumor. J Cutan Aesthet Surg. 2020;13(3):261–3. https://doi.org/10.4103/jcas.Jcas_2_20.
16. Kakurai M, Yamada T, Kiyosawa T, Ohtsuki M, Nakagawa H. Giant acquired digital fibrokeratoma. J Am Acad Dermatol. 2003;48(5 Suppl):S67–8. https://doi.org/10.1067/mjd.2003.153.
17. Choi JH, Jung SY, Chun JS, et al. Giant acquired digital fibrokeratoma occurring on the left great toe. Ann Dermatol. 2011;23(1):64–6. https://doi.org/10.5021/ad.2011.23.1.64.
18. Hashiro M, Fujio Y, Tanaka M, Yamatodani Y. Giant acquired fibrokeratoma of the nail bed. Dermatology. 1995;190(2):169–71. https://doi.org/10.1159/000246671.
19. Moriue T, Yoneda K, Moriue J, Nakai K, Kubota Y. Multibranched acquired periungual fibrokeratoma. JAMA Dermatol. 2014;150(4):456–7. https://doi.org/10.1001/jamadermatol.2013.6631.
20. Yasuki Y. Acquired periungual fibrokeratoma—a proposal for classification of periungual fibrous lesions. J Dermatol. 1985;12(4):349–56. https://doi.org/10.1111/j.1346-8138.1985.tb02853.x.
21. Lencastre A, Richert B. Flat-pan nail-wide acquired epiungual fibrokeratoma: report of 4 cases. Skin Appendage Disord. 2019;5(2):111–3. https://doi.org/10.1159/000491582.
22. Kim YS, Lee JH, Park YM, Lee JY. Multiple acquired periungual fibrokeratoma. Ann Dermatol. 2016;28(4):513–4. https://doi.org/10.5021/ad.2016.28.4.513.
23. Haneke E, Ranawaka RR. Disorders of nails. In: Ranawaka RR, Kannangara AP, Karawita A, editors. Atlas of dermatoses in pigmented skin. Singapore: Springer; 2021. p. 723–64.

Ungual Fibromas

16

Rachel C. Hill and Shari R. Lipner

16.1 Description of Disease

Ungual fibromas are benign connective tissue tumors and present as multiple slow-growing, oval, or elongated flesh-colored papules or nodules on the proximal nail fold, lateral nail fold, or nail bed [1, 2]. They are also known as periungual fibromas, subungual fibromas, or, in the context of tuberous sclerosis complex (TSC), "Koenen tumors." Ungual fibromas may be symptomatic and can result in distortion of the nail plate with or without associated pain [3]. On histology, ungual fibromas are highly vascular, nonencapsulated, mainly fibrous lesions that are made up of stellate-shaped fibroblasts, dense collagen, and blood vessels [4].

16.2 Epidemiology

16.2.1 Sex

TSC is inherited in an autosomal dominant pattern, and therefore ungual fibromas associated with TSC are equally likely to affect men and women [5, 6]. The sex distribution of ungual fibromas caused by trauma is unknown.

16.2.2 Age

In the context of TSC, ungual fibromas typically occur by adolescence and become increasingly more common with age [5, 7]. Ungual fibromas typically appear in the second decade of life in patients with TSC but can have onset as late as the fifth decade [8]. In a cross-sectional study of 76 adult women with TSC (mean age 39 years, range 20–69 years), ungual fibromas were present in 61/76 patients (80%) [8]. In a retrospective study of 131 individuals with TSC, 0% of patients <5 years

S. R. Lipner, *Atlas of Nail Disorders Across All Skin Colors*,
https://doi.org/10.1007/978-3-031-74272-9_16

old, 23% of patients ages 5–14, 68% of patients 15–29, and 88% of patients ≥30 had ungual fibromas, suggesting that, ungual fibromas are more prevalent with increasing age in TSC patients [9].

16.2.3 Race

Previous studies have not reported on the association of ungual fibromas with race or ethnicity. Ungual fibromas can affect patients of all races and ethnicities [10].

16.3 Risk Factors

16.3.1 Tuberous Sclerosis Complex

Ungual fibromas are a diagnostic symptom of TSC, a multisystem disorder characterized by benign hamartomas involving the central nervous system, heart kidneys, lungs, and other organs [5, 6]. TSC results from an autosomal dominant mutation in the TSC1 or TSC2 genes. Mutations in these genes cause a defect in the formation of the hamartin-tuberin complex, leading to activation of the mTOR pathway, upregulation of vascular endothelial growth factor, and formation of benign hamartomas in multiple organs [3, 11]. However, up to two-thirds of TSC cases result from sporadic mutations [12–14]. It is estimated that 15–20% of patients with TSC will develop ungual fibromas [11, 15]. TSC can also manifest with epilepsy and cognitive deficits, in addition to a wide range of cutaneous findings and phenotypes [12].

16.3.2 Trauma

Sporadic ungual fibromas may also form secondary to trauma. In such cases, the ungual fibromas are more likely to be solitary or on a single digit and are not accompanied by other features indicative of TSC, such as facial angiofibromas [8, 16–18]. The frequency with which ungual fibromas secondary to trauma occur is unknown.

16.4 Clinical Features

When ungual fibromas occur in the context of TSC, they tend to be multiple vs. solitary [8]. Fibromas may be periungual or subungual, although the former is more common [8]. Unlike other types of benign nail tumors, the toenails are more frequently affected than the fingernails [8, 9, 19]. In the cross-sectional study of 76 adult women with TSC by Aldrich et al., periungual fibromas were more often localized to toenails compared to fingernails (282 vs. 86, $P < 0.001$). However, subungual fibromas were more common on the fingernails vs. toenails (71 vs. 45, $P = 0.016$) [8].

Other nail changes may be clinically apparent in patients with ungual fibromas, especially in the context of TSC. In the cross-sectional study by Aldrich et al., patients also exhibited splinter hemorrhages (46%), red comets (29%), and longitudinal leukonychia (18%) [8]. Longitudinal grooves in the nail may also form if the fibroma affects the nail matrix [8, 9]. Ungual fibromas may be painful if they are associated with significant onychodystrophy and can interfere with ambulation and mobility in severe cases [8, 20].

In patients with TSC, nail fibromas are accompanied by additional cutaneous features, including facial angiofibromas, hypomelanotic macules ("ash leaf spots"), confetti skin lesions, Shagreen patches, and fibrocephalic plaques [9, 21]. Hypomelanotic macules and fibrocephalic plaques may be observed earlier in life than ungual fibromas in patients with TSC [9].

16.5 Clinical Features in Skin of Color

Although features of ungual fibromas in patients with skin of color have not been explicitly described, patients with skin of color are more likely to have physiologic melanonychia affecting the fingernails and toenails, which may accompany ungual fibromas upon clinical presentation.

16.6 Requirements for Diagnosis

Because ungual fibromas typically occur in the context of TSC, the diagnostic criteria for TSC must be met for these tumors to be characterized as "Koenen tumors." For genetic criteria, the identification of a pathogenic variant in the TSC1 or TSC2 gene is sufficient for TSC diagnosis, regardless of the clinical features present in an individual patient [15]. Clinical manifestations of TSC, notably ungual fibromas, may not be clinically apparent until later in life, and thus genetic identification of a pathogenic variant of TSC allows for close monitoring of the development of clinical symptoms over time [15]. However, it is important to note that up to 15% of patients with clinically diagnosed TSC do not have a mutation identified via genetic testing, and thus a negative genetic test does not entirely rule out a diagnosis of TSC [15, 22]. For clinical diagnosis, patients must meet two major features or one major feature and two minor features to be definitively diagnosed with TSC; conversely, patients with one major feature or ≥ 2 minor features are diagnosed as "possible" TSC. Major criteria include: hypomelanotic macules (≥ 3; at least 5 mm diameter), angiofibroma (≥ 3), ungual fibromas of non-traumatic etiology (≥ 2), Shagreen patch, multiple retinal hamartomas, multiple cortical tubers, subependymal nodule (≥ 2), subependymal giant cell astrocytoma, cardiac rhabdomyoma, lymphangiomyomatosis, angiomyolipomas (≥ 2). Minor criteria include: "confetti" skin lesions; dental enamel pits (≥ 3), intraoral fibromas (≥ 2), retinal achromic patch, multiple retinal cysts, nonrenal hamartomas, and sclerotic bone lesions [15].

In equivocal cases or in the case of solitary lesions that are not concerning for TSC, excision with histopathology is the gold standard for definitive diagnosis. Histopathology is unnecessary for stable lesions.

16.7 Cases

Figures 16.1, 16.2, 16.3, 16.4, and 16.5 demonstrate the presentation of ungual fibromas in a clinical setting.

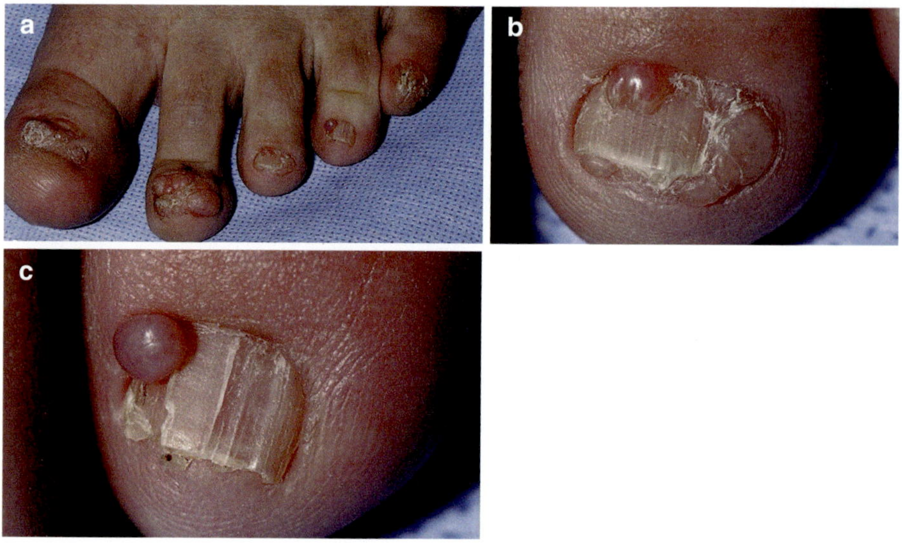

Fig. 16.1 (**a**) Patient of unknown age and sex, Fitzpatrick type II, ungual fibromas, with involvement of all nails. (**b**) The close-up of the third digit in *A* shows clove-like periungual, nail-like periungual fibroma, and subungual fibroma. (**c**) A close-up of the fourth digit in *A* shows globoid periungual fibroma and longitudinal groove without visible fibroma. Etiology: tuberous sclerosis (*from* Aldrich et al. [8]; *with permission*)

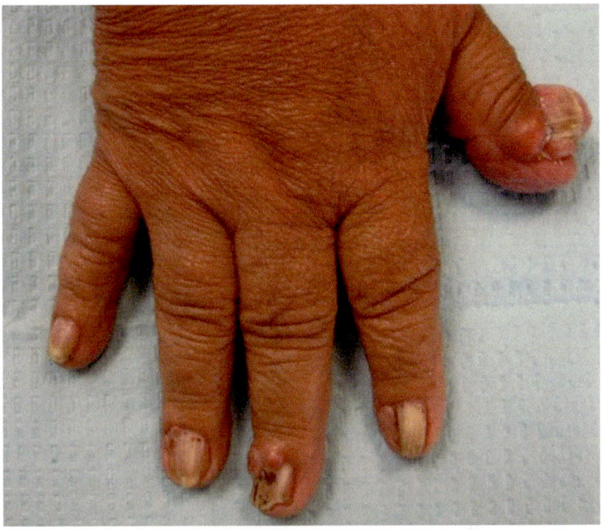

Fig. 16.2 20-Year-old female, Fitzpatrick type II, ungual fibromas, with involvement of the first to fourth digits causing severe dystrophy of the nails (*from* Nguyen et al. [5]; *with permission*)

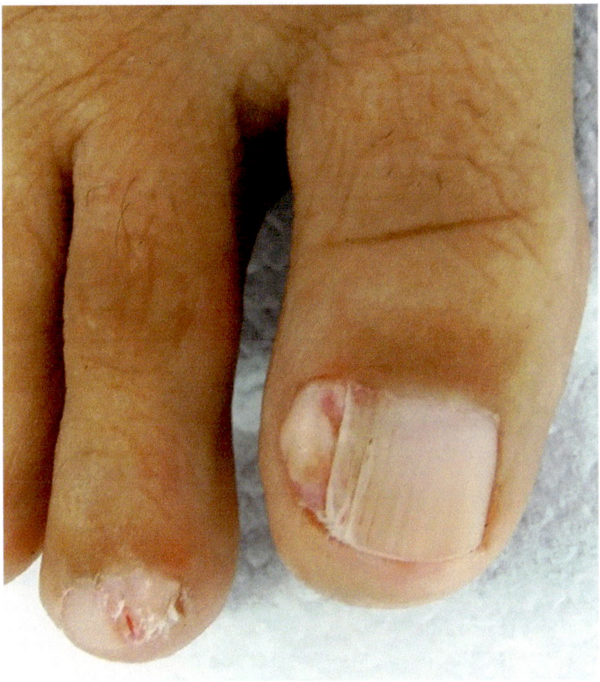

Fig. 16.3 Patient of unknown sex and age, Fitzpatrick type III, ungual fibromas, with involvement of the right first and second toenails. Etiology: tuberous sclerosis (*from* Haneke et al. [23]; *with permission*)

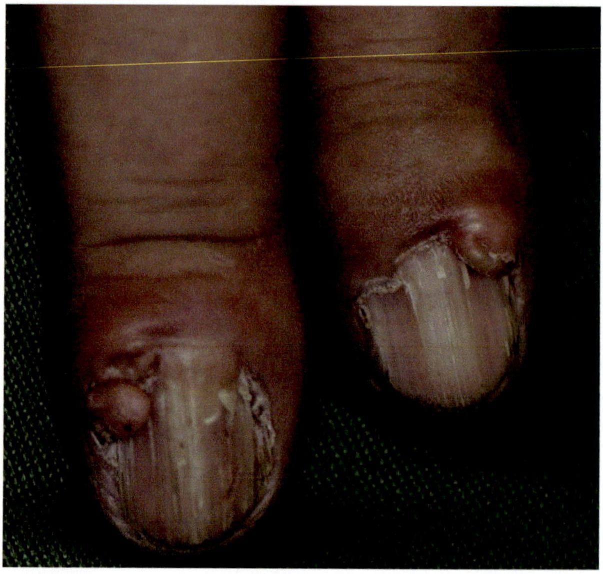

Fig. 16.4 Patient of unknown age and sex, Fitzpatrick type III, ungual fibromas, with periungual fibromas involving the left second and third digits, accompanied by severe longitudinal grooves. Etiology: tuberous sclerosis (*from* Northup et al. [15]; *with permission*)

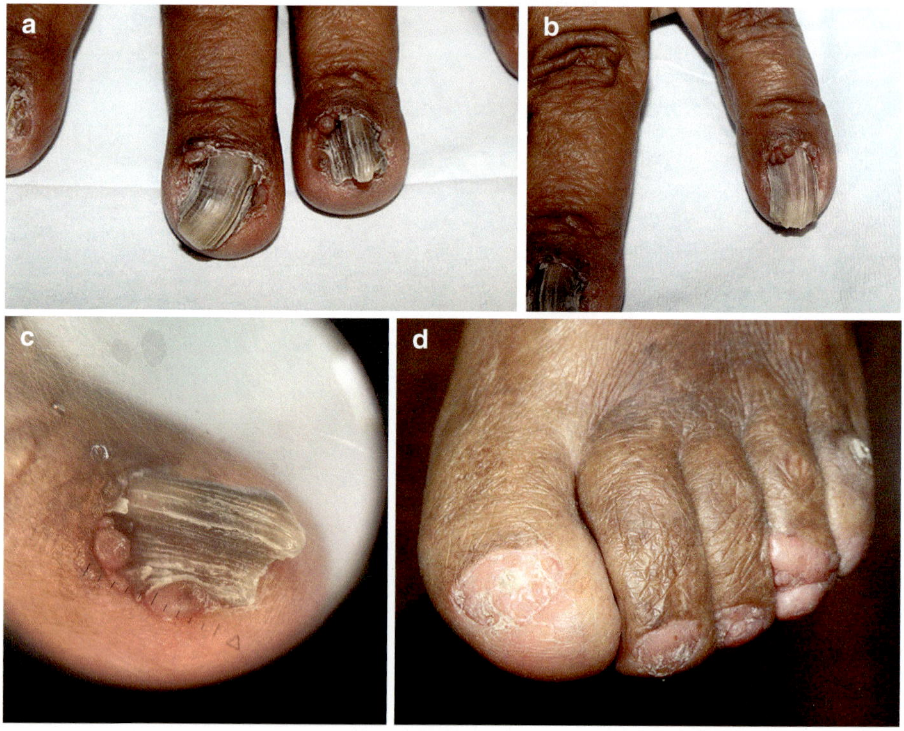

Fig. 16.5 (**a**–**d**) 78-Year-old female, Fitzpatrick type V, ungual fibromas, with thickening and parrot beak appearance of the fingernails, in addition to pink papules of the nail beds and nail folds (**a**, **b**). Ungual fibromas examined with dermoscopy demonstrating large and small papules and longitudinal ridging of the fingernails (**c**). Toenails appeared atrophic with accompanying ungual fibromas (**d**). Etiology: tuberous sclerosis

References

1. Abimelec P, Dumontier C. Chapter 24—Basic and advanced nail surgery (Part 2: Indications and complications). In: Scher RK, Tosti A, Elewski BE, Daniel CR, Fleckman P, Rich P, editors. Nails. 3rd ed. W.B. Saunders; 2005. p. 291–308.
2. Ortega-Quijano D, Pérez-García B, Vañó-Galván S. Tuberous sclerosis complex presenting as periungual fibromas and seizures in a 52-year-old woman. CMAJ. 2020;192(26):E714. https://doi.org/10.1503/cmaj.190449.
3. Muzic JG, Kindle SA, Tollefson MM. Successful treatment of subungual fibromas of tuberous sclerosis with topical rapamycin. JAMA Dermatol. 2014;150(9):1024–5. https://doi.org/10.1001/jamadermatol.2014.87.
4. Ma D, Darling T, Moss J, Lee CC. Histologic variants of periungual fibromas in tuberous sclerosis complex. J Am Acad Dermatol. 2011;64(2):442–4. https://doi.org/10.1016/j.jaad.2010.03.002.
5. Nguyen QD, DarConte MD, Hebert AA. The cutaneous manifestations of tuberous sclerosis complex. Am J Med Genet C Semin Med Genet. 2018;178(3):321–5. https://doi.org/10.1002/ajmg.c.31649.
6. Marchini M, Giglio E. Tuberous sclerosis complex. N Engl J Med. 2017;376(20):e42. https://doi.org/10.1056/NEJMicm1610501.
7. Tang CQY, Chia AQX, Sechachalam S. Symptomatic periungual fibroma of the hand. J Hand Microsurg. 2021;13(3):173–7. https://doi.org/10.1055/s-0040-1709099.
8. Aldrich CS, Hong CH, Groves L, Olsen C, Moss J, Darling TN. Acral lesions in tuberous sclerosis complex: insights into pathogenesis. J Am Acad Dermatol. 2010;63(2):244–51. https://doi.org/10.1016/j.jaad.2009.08.042.
9. Webb DW, Clarke A, Fryer A, Osborne JP. The cutaneous features of tuberous sclerosis: a population study. Br J Dermatol. 1996;135(1):1–5.
10. https://www.ninds.nih.gov/health-information/disorders/tuberous-sclerosis-complex.
11. Cardis MA, DeKlotz CMC. Cutaneous manifestations of tuberous sclerosis complex and the paediatrician's role. Arch Dis Child. 2017;102(9):858–63. https://doi.org/10.1136/archdischild-2016-312001.
12. Schwartz RA, Fernández G, Kotulska K, Jóźwiak S. Tuberous sclerosis complex: advances in diagnosis, genetics, and management. J Am Acad Dermatol. 2007;57(2):189–202. https://doi.org/10.1016/j.jaad.2007.05.004.
13. Jones AC, Shyamsundar MM, Thomas MW, et al. Comprehensive mutation analysis of TSC1 and TSC2—and phenotypic correlations in 150 families with tuberous sclerosis. Am J Hum Genet. 1999;64(5):1305–15. https://doi.org/10.1086/302381.
14. Consortium ECTS. Identification and characterization of the tuberous sclerosis gene on chromosome 16. Cell. 1993;75(7):1305–15.
15. Northrup H, Krueger DA, Northrup H, et al. Tuberous sclerosis complex diagnostic criteria update: recommendations of the 2012 International Tuberous Sclerosis Complex Consensus Conference. Pediatr Neurol. 2013;49(4):243–54. https://doi.org/10.1016/j.pediatrneurol.2013.08.001.
16. Bodensteiner JB, Narayanan V. Tuberous sclerosis complex. In: Johnson RT, Griffin JW, McArthur JC, editors. Current therapy in neurologic disease. 7th ed. Mosby; 2006. p. 103–7.
17. Zeller J, Friedmann D, Clerici T, Revuz J. The significance of a single periungual fibroma: report of seven cases. Arch Dermatol. 1995;131(12):1465–6. https://doi.org/10.1001/archderm.131.12.1465b.
18. Carlson RM, Lloyd KM, Campbell TE. Acquired periungual fibrokeratoma: a case report. Cutis. 2007;80(2):137–40.
19. Jóźwiak S, Schwartz RA, Janniger CK, Michałowicz R, Chmielik J. Skin lesions in children with tuberous sclerosis complex: their prevalence, natural course, and diagnostic significance. Int J Dermatol. 1998;37(12):911–7. https://doi.org/10.1046/j.1365-4362.1998.00495.x.
20. Aste N, Pau M, Aste N, Biggio P. Tuberous sclerosis with unusual giant ungual fibromas. J Eur Acad Dermatol Venereol. 2003;17(1):100–1. https://doi.org/10.1046/j.1468-3083.2003.00519_3.x.

21. Cascarino M, Leclerc-Mercier S. Histological patterns of skin lesions in tuberous sclerosis complex: a panorama. Dermatopathology (Basel). 2021;8(3):236–52. https://doi.org/10.3390/dermatopathology8030029.
22. Tyburczy ME, Dies KA, Glass J, et al. Mosaic and intronic mutations in TSC1/TSC2 explain the majority of TSC patients with no mutation identified by conventional testing. PLoS Genet. 2015;11(11):e1005637. https://doi.org/10.1371/journal.pgen.1005637.
23. Haneke E, Ranawaka RR. Disorders of nails. In: Ranawaka RR, Kannangara AP, Karawita A, editors. Atlas of dermatoses in pigmented skin. Singapore: Springer; 2021. p. 723–64.

Part IV

Malignant Nail Disorders

Nail Unit Melanoma

17

Rachel C. Hill and Shari R. Lipner

17.1 Description of Disease

Nail unit melanoma, also referred to as "subungual melanoma," is a form of cutaneous melanoma that develops in the nail matrix [1–3]. Nail unit melanoma is associated with a poor prognosis, often attributed to late recognition of advanced disease. Reported five-year survival rates are 16–87%, depending on the extent of disease at diagnosis [4, 5]. Nail unit melanoma is distinct from acral lentiginous melanoma, as the former is more often associated with KIT and KRAS mutations, while the latter is more often associated with BRAF and NRAS mutations [6].

17.2 Epidemiology

17.2.1 Sex

Nail unit melanoma may exhibit a female sex predilection, or female patients more often seek early medical advice compared to males. In a case series of 63 cases of nail unit melanoma in situ by Goettmann et al., 44 patients were female [7]. In a case series of 11 patients with melanoma in situ of the nail, 73% of patients were female ($n = 8$) [8]. Similarly, in a case series of seven patients with subungual melanoma, 71% of those affected were female ($n = 5$) [9]. In a case series of six patients with nail unit melanoma, two patients were male and four were female [10].

17.2.2 Age

Nail unit melanoma may be more common in patients in the fifth to seventh decades of life [2]. In the case series of 63 cases of nail unit melanoma in situ by Goettmann et al., the mean age was 51 years old (median 51 years, range 20–86 years), with 46

S. R. Lipner, *Atlas of Nail Disorders Across All Skin Colors*,
https://doi.org/10.1007/978-3-031-74272-9_17

of 63 cases in individuals over the age of 40 years [7]. Nail unit melanoma is exceedingly rare in children, but it may affect young adults [1, 11–16].

17.2.3 Race

While the absolute incidence and prevalence of nail unit melanoma is believed to be similar among patients who identify with various racial and ethnic groups, patients who identify as Black or African American and Asian likely experience a greater relative incidence and prevalence of nail unit melanoma. Nail unit melanoma accounts for 1–3% of melanomas in individuals who identify as White, whereas it may represent up to 35% of all melanomas in patients who identify as Black or African American patients and up to 58% of all melanomas in patients who identify as Asian [1, 5, 16, 17].

17.3 Risk Factors

Unlike other forms of cutaneous melanoma, sun exposure is likely not a risk factor for nail unit melanoma development [5, 18, 19]. Genetic risk may influence the development of nail unit melanoma. While acral lentiginous melanoma is recognized as a separate clinical entity from nail unit melanoma, previous studies have suggested a genetic predisposition, which may also be true for nail unit melanoma. In a case series of 978 patients with primary cutaneous melanoma at a single referral center, patients with acral lentiginous melanoma more often had a genetic predisposition to cancer vs. other types of primary cutaneous melanoma (22.1% vs. 7.1% with personal history of non-cutaneous malignancies, 58.1% vs. 36.4% with a first-degree relative with history of non-cutaneous neoplasia, respectively, $P < 0.001$ and $P = 0.004$, respectively) [19]. A population-based study, including 238,724 first-degree relatives of 46,091 melanoma patients from Nordic countries, found that family members of patients with acral melanoma were at increased risk for developing cutaneous melanoma (standard incidence ratio 4.0, 95% CI 1.5–8.8) [20]. Trauma has also been proposed as a risk factor for nail unit melanoma development. In a retrospective study of 87 cases of nail unit melanoma at a single center from 1998 to 2020, 71.8% of patients had a history of trauma preceding disease development ($n = 19$), and trauma-associated nail unit melanoma showed disease progression more frequently than non-trauma-associated nail unit melanoma within the cohort ($P = 0.034$) [21].

17.4 Clinical Features

Longitudinal melanonychia involving a single digit is by far the most common clinical feature of nail unit melanoma. The Hutchinson sign is defined as an extension of pigment onto the surrounding lateral or proximal nail folds or hyponychium, which is a common feature in invasive melanomas [2, 8]. In the case series of 63 patients with nail unit melanoma in situ by Goettmann et al., longitudinal melanonychia was present in 58 cases (92%), 40 of which were a solitary band (63%). Fingernails were more commonly affected than toenails ($n = 52$ vs. $n = 11$, respectively), and the thumb was the most common fingernail involved ($n = 28$). Of the 56 patients with detailed clinical history available, 46 had a history of changing longitudinal melanonychia, including widening and darkening of the band (82%), with rapid change reported in 23 of these cases (41%). The mean bandwidth in this case series was 3.45 mm with a median of 3 mm, while 22 patients presented with a narrow band of less than 3 mm in width. On clinical examination, heterochromic bands were more common than monochromic bands in the 50 cases with information on color available ($n = 47$ vs. $n = 3$, respectively), as were irregular borders than well-defined borders ($n = 34$ vs. $n = 12$, respectively, P-values not listed) [7]. In a retrospective study of 177 patients with longitudinal melanonychia, including 80 biopsy-confirmed cases of nail unit melanoma, nail unit melanoma cases more often appeared black ($n = 34$, 42.5%) vs. brown ($n = 21$, 26.25%) or multicolor ($n = 25$, 31.25%) compared to benign longitudinal melanonychia cases ($P < 0.001$). Nail unit melanoma cases also exhibited a wider band, and more were more often accompanied by nail plate splitting, Hutchinson sign, and history of band change compared to benign longitudinal melanonychia cases (all $P < 0.001$) [2]. In a retrospective observational study of 97 patients with nail unit melanoma, including 59 patients with in situ disease and 38 with invasive disease, total melanonychia, destruction of the nail plate, ulceration, and polychromia were more common in invasive disease vs. in situ disease (all $P < 0.05$) [22].

While nail unit melanoma is classically associated with darkly pigmented bands in the nail, some cases are amelanotic. Amelanotic melanoma might account for up to 25% of all nail melanomas and sometimes presents with an ulcerated and vascular nodule, similar in appearance to a pyogenic granuloma, with or without nail plate destruction [1, 23–25]. In a retrospective review of 140 nail unit melanoma cases at a tertiary referral center, amelanotic disease was associated with a greater risk for recurrence vs. melanotic disease (adjusted hazard ratio 5.69; 95% CI 1.16–27.84) [26].

Dermoscopic features of nail unit melanoma include the brown-black background color of the band(s) comprising the longitudinal melanonychia, with irregular lines (including color, spacing, parallelism, width irregularities) running longitudinally from the proximal nail fold [27–29]. There may be heterochromia evident within the bands. A "micro-Hutchinson sign" may be appreciated if pigment involving the periungual skin or hyponychium is visible on dermoscopy, but not otherwise appreciated with the naked eye [27, 30]. Dermoscopy also aids in defining the width of the band, with wider bands more frequently associated with nail unit melanoma vs. benign melanonychia [31]. A retrospective observational study by Benati et al. also defined granular pigmentation as a new criterion for nail unit melanoma, which consists of "fine light to dark brown granularity" apparent on dermoscopy. In their study including 82 histopathologic-diagnosed bands, 25 of which were nail unit melanomas, 40% of the melanoma cases exhibited granular pigmentation, which was more frequent than in benign lesions ($P < 0.001$) [32]. However, cases of patients diagnosed with nail unit melanoma who presented with dermoscopic features typically associated with benign longitudinal melanonychia have been reported, including regular lines on dermoscopy. This highlights the importance of considering the entire clinical picture when evaluating longitudinal melanonychia, and not relying solely on dermoscopy [10]. Dermoscopic features of amelanotic melanoma include a polymorphic vascular pattern accompanied by "milky-red" areas [27].

17.5 Clinical Features in Skin of Color

Explicit differences in clinical and dermoscopic features of nail unit melanoma in patients with skin of color have not been described. However, patients with nail unit melanoma and skin of color may present with benign longitudinal melanonychia involving other nails, which complicates the clinical picture and may delay diagnosis [33, 34]. Patients with skin of color may also experience increased widening of pigmented bands with age, which may result in an increased incidence of biopsies performed for benign lesions [35]. In a retrospective cohort study of 248 cases of benign longitudinal melanonychia, patients with darker vs. lighter skin types had higher bandwidth percentage and received a number of nail unit biopsies for benign lesions ($P = 0.0125$ and $P = 0.032$, respectively) [34].

17.6 Requirements for Diagnosis

Levit et al. reported on the ABCDEF criteria that can be used to assess the likelihood of a nail unit melanoma diagnosis, including age (peak incidence between fifth and seventh decades of life), brown to black pigmentation and breadth of band >3 mm with irregular borders, change in the nail appearance, digit (most commonly involved is the thumbnail followed by the great toenail), extension of pigment onto the periungual skin, and family or personal history of melanoma [36]. However, in a retrospective study of 84 consecutive patients who underwent nail matrix biopsy for longitudinal melanonychia, including 27 with complete data for the ABCDEF criteria ($n = 7$ with nail unit melanoma, $n = 20$ with benign longitudinal melanonychia), the average number of ABCDEF criteria met was 2.86 in the melanoma group vs. 2.45 criteria in the benign longitudinal melanonychia group ($P = 0.361$), suggesting that these criteria may not be useful in diagnosing nail unit melanoma. This study showed that the average width percentage in the nail unit melanoma group was 49.5% vs. 24.8% in the benign longitudinal melanonychia group ($P = 0.002$), with post hoc analysis suggesting that nail matrix biopsy might be considered for patients with bandwidth ≥40% of the width of the nail unit [29]. While clinical features may be indicative of nail unit melanoma, a definitive diagnosis of nail unit melanoma can only be rendered following nail matrix biopsy with histopathology [1].

17.7 Prognosis

The prognosis associated with nail unit melanoma depends on several factors, including age at diagnosis, Breslow thickness and presence of ulceration on diagnosis, amelanosis, vascular invasion, and stage, among others [37]. Detection of the disease with Breslow depth ≤0.5 mm and successful complete excision of the nail unit, including the nail matrix (en bloc excision), or Mohs micrographic surgery, increases the chance of survival [37]. Amputation is reserved for advanced disease. Notably, a meta-analysis found no difference in local recurrence of nail unit melanoma for patients treated with functional surgery, including en bloc excision of the nail unit, vs. amputation for in situ or minimally invasive disease (defined as Breslow thickness ≤0.5 mm) [38].

17.8 Cases

Figures 17.1, 17.2, 17.3, 17.4, and 17.5 demonstrate the presentation of exostosis in a clinical setting.

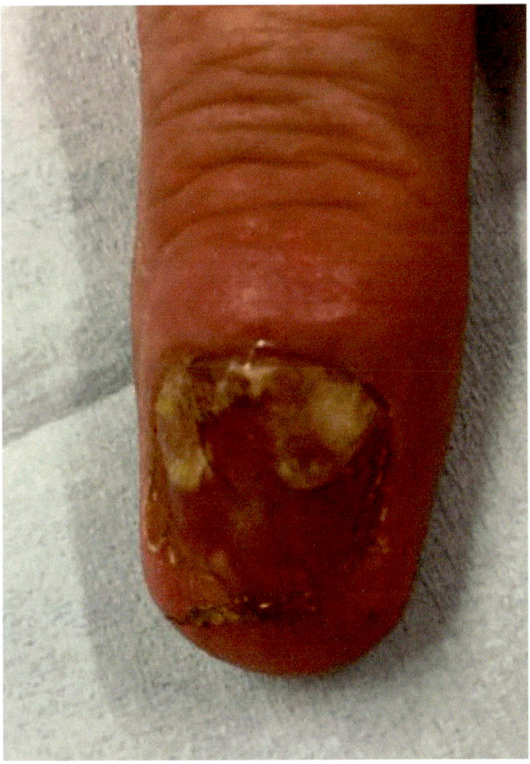

Fig. 17.1 60-Year-old female, Fitzpatrick type II, nail unit melanoma, presenting with severe onycholysis and oozing of the left second fingernail. Dermatopathology showed subungual amelanotic malignant melanoma, Breslow depth at least 1.18 mm, with ulceration

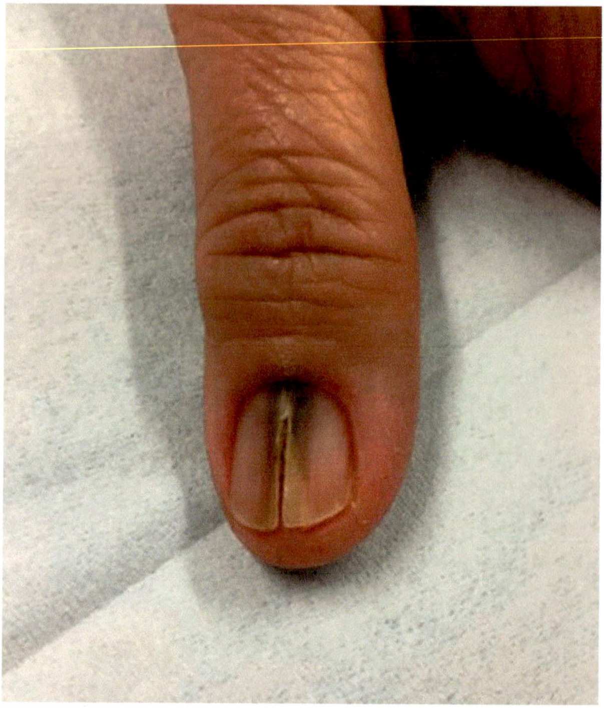

Fig. 17.2 61-Year-old female, Fitzpatrick type III, nail unit melanoma, with 3.5 mm brown-black longitudinal band of the left thumbnail, wider proximally compared to distally, with longitudinal split and subungual hyperkeratosis extending from hyponychium to lunula. Dermatopathology showed a nail unit melanoma involving the nail bed and hyponychium, Breslow depth 0.6 mm, and nail bed ulceration

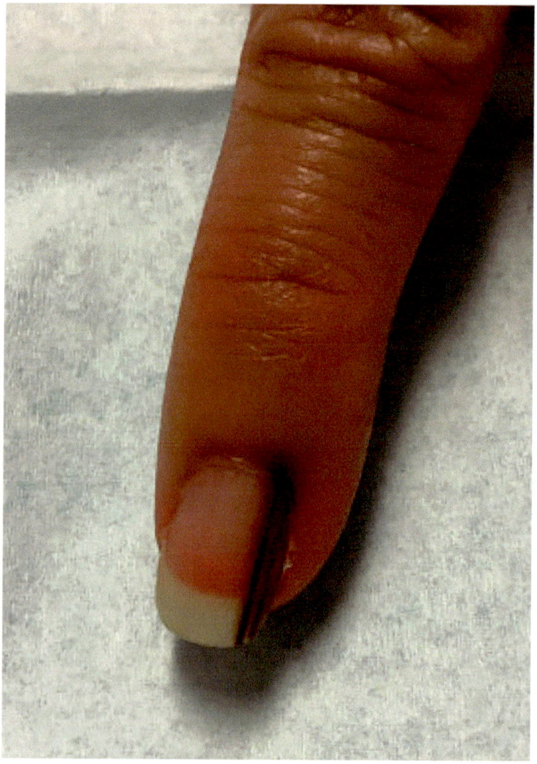

Fig. 17.3 61-Year-old female, Fitzpatrick type III, nail unit melanoma, presenting with a brown longitudinal band of the right fifth fingernail, 2 mm proximally, 1.8 mm distally, with irregular lines on dermoscopy and no pigment on hyponychium or nail folds. Dermatopathology showed nail unit melanoma in situ

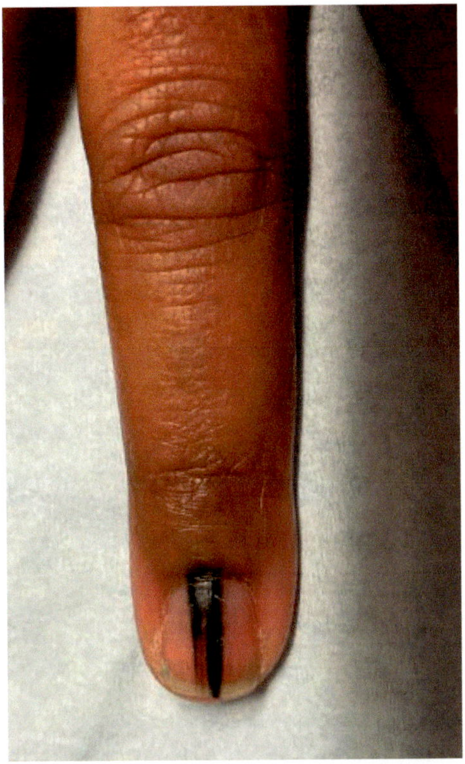

Fig. 17.4 52-Year-old female, Fitzpatrick type V, nail unit melanoma, presenting with a longitudinal black band of the left fourth fingernail. Dermatopathology showed nail unit melanoma in situ

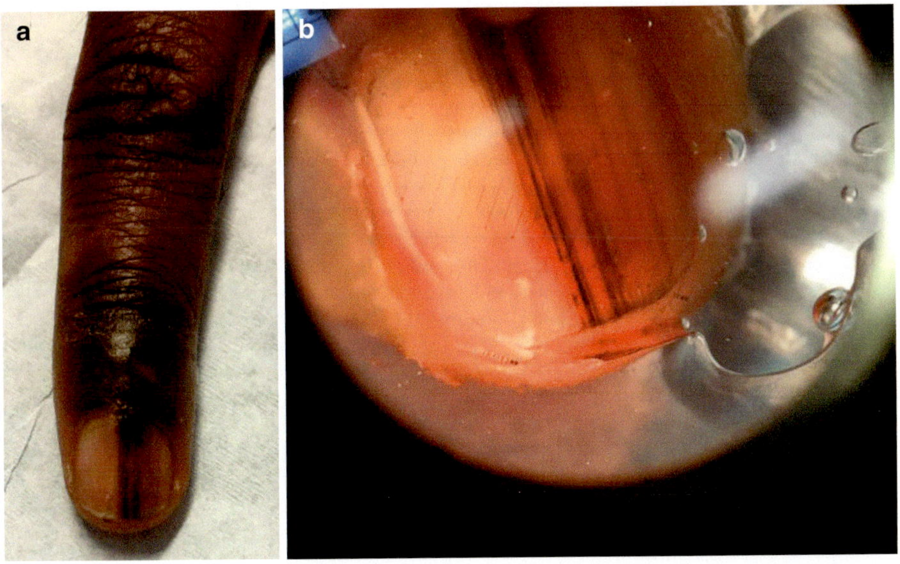

Fig. 17.5 (**a**) 39-Year-old female, Fitzpatrick type VI, nail unit melanoma, presenting with a 3 mm dark brown longitudinal band of the left second fingernail. (**b**) Dermoscopy showed a brown background with irregular brown lines in terms of spacing and color. Dermatopathology showed a nail unit melanoma in situ

References

1. Conway J, Bellet JS, Rubin AI, Lipner SR. Adult and pediatric nail unit melanoma: epidemiology, diagnosis, and treatment. Cells. 2023;12(6):964. https://doi.org/10.3390/cells12060964.
2. Lee SG, Oh BH, Chung KY, Roh MR. Looking beyond the Hutchinson sign: a retrospective study of clinical factors indicating the presence and invasiveness of nail unit melanoma in patients with longitudinal melanonychia. Dermatologic Surg. 2024;50(1):21–7. https://doi.org/10.1097/DSS.0000000000003982.
3. Le M, Gabrielli S, Zloty D. Mohs micrographic surgery is equivalent to nail unit excision or amputation for melanoma in situ of the nail unit: a systematic review and meta-analysis. Dermatologic Surg. 2023;49(8):755–8. https://doi.org/10.1097/DSS.0000000000003840.
4. https://dermatology.ca/public-patients/nails/subungual-melanoma/.
5. Cohen T, Busam KJ, Patel A, Brady MS. Subungual melanoma: management considerations. Am J Surg. 2008;195(2):244–8. https://doi.org/10.1016/j.amjsurg.2007.03.010.
6. Holman BN, Van Gulick RJ, Amato CM, et al. Clinical and molecular features of subungual melanomas are site-specific and distinct from acral melanomas. Melanoma Res. 2020;30(6):562–73. https://doi.org/10.1097/CMR.0000000000000688.
7. Goettmann S, Moulonguet I, Zaraa I. In situ nail unit melanoma: epidemiological and clinic-pathologic features with conservative treatment and long-term follow-up. J Eur Acad Dermatol Venereol. 2018;32(12):2300–6. https://doi.org/10.1111/jdv.15124.
8. Neczyporenko F, André J, Torosian K, Theunis A, Richert B. Management of in situ melanoma of the nail apparatus with functional surgery: report of 11 cases and review of the literature. J Eur Acad Dermatol Venereol. 2014;28(5):550–7. https://doi.org/10.1111/jdv.12131.
9. Sureda N, Phan A, Poulalhon N, Balme B, Dalle S, Thomas L. Conservative surgical management of subungual (matrix derived) melanoma: report of seven cases and literature review. Br J Dermatol. 2011;165(4):852–8. https://doi.org/10.1111/j.1365-2133.2011.10477.x.
10. Duarte AF, Correia O, Barros AM, Ventura F, Haneke E. Nail melanoma in situ: clinical, dermoscopic, pathologic clues, and steps for minimally invasive treatment. Dermatologic Surg. 2015;41(1):59–68. https://doi.org/10.1097/DSS.0000000000000243.
11. Lohman ME, McCalmont TH, Cordoro KM. An evidence-based approach to pediatric melanonychia. Dermatol Clin. 2022;40(1):37–49. https://doi.org/10.1016/j.det.2021.09.004.
12. Iorizzo M, Tosti A, Di Chiacchio N, et al. Nail melanoma in children: differential diagnosis and management. Dermatologic Surg. 2008;34(7):974–8. https://doi.org/10.1111/j.1524-4725.2008.34191.x.
13. Tosti A, Piraccini BM, Cagalli A, Haneke E. In situ melanoma of the nail unit in children: report of two cases in fair-skinned Caucasian children. Pediatr Dermatol. 2012;29(1):79–83. https://doi.org/10.1111/j.1525-1470.2011.01481.x.
14. Motta A, López C, Acosta A, Peñaranda C. Subungual melanoma in situ in a Hispanic girl treated with functional resection and reconstruction with onychocutaneous toe free flap. Arch Dermatol. 2007;143(12):1600–2. https://doi.org/10.1001/archderm.143.12.1600.
15. Leung AK, Robson WL, Liu EK, et al. Melanonychia striata in Chinese children and adults. Int J Dermatol. 2007;46(9):920–2. https://doi.org/10.1111/j.1365-4632.2007.03232.x.
16. Thai KE, Young R, Sinclair RD. Nail apparatus melanoma. Australas J Dermatol. 2001;42(2):71–83. https://doi.org/10.1046/j.1440-0960.2001.00486.x.
17. Mole RJ, MacKenzie DN. Subungual melanoma. In: StatPearls. Treasure Island, FL: StatPearls Publishing; 2023.
18. Möhrle M, Häfner HM. Is subungual melanoma related to trauma? Dermatology. 2002;204(4):259–61. https://doi.org/10.1159/000063354.
19. Nagore E, Pereda C, Botella-Estrada R, Requena C, Guillén C. Acral lentiginous melanoma presents distinct clinical profile with high cancer susceptibility. Cancer Causes Control. 2009;20(1):115–9. https://doi.org/10.1007/s10552-008-9221-y.
20. Fallah M, Pukkala E, Sundquist K, et al. Familial melanoma by histology and age: joint data from five Nordic countries. Eur J Cancer. 2014;50(6):1176–83. https://doi.org/10.1016/j.ejca.2013.12.023.

21. Choi ME, Cho H, Won CH, Chang SE, Lee MW, Lee WJ. Clinicopathologic characteristics of trauma-related nail apparatus melanoma: a comparative study according to the presence of trauma prior to melanoma development [published correction appears in Dermatology. 2023;239(1):174]. Dermatology. 2023;239(1):165–73. https://doi.org/10.1159/000525726.
22. Ohn J, Hur K, Cho Y, et al. Developing a predictive model for distinguishing invasive nail unit melanoma from nail unit melanoma in situ. J Eur Acad Dermatol Venereol. 2021;35(4):906–11. https://doi.org/10.1111/jdv.17036.
23. Lipner SR. Ulcerated nodule of the fingernail. JAMA. 2018;319(7):713–4. https://doi.org/10.1001/jama.2018.0179.
24. Ariel IM. Amelanotic melanomas: an analysis of 77 patients. Curr Surg. 1981;38(3):151–5.
25. Harrington P, O'Kelly A, Trail IA, Freemont AJ. Amelanotic subungual melanoma mimicking pyogenic granuloma in the hand. J R Coll Surg Edinb. 2002;47(4):638–40.
26. Oh BH, Lee S, Park JW, et al. Risk of recurrence of nail unit melanoma after functional surgery versus amputation. J Am Acad Dermatol. 2023;88(5):1017–23. https://doi.org/10.1016/j.jaad.2022.12.039.
27. Longo C, Pampena R, Moscarella E, et al. Dermoscopy of melanoma according to different body sites: head and neck, trunk, limbs, nail, mucosal and acral. J Eur Acad Dermatol Venereol. 2023;37(9):1718–30. https://doi.org/10.1111/jdv.19221.
28. Ko D, Oromendia C, Scher R, Lipner SR. Retrospective single-center study evaluating clinical and dermoscopic features of longitudinal melanonychia, ABCDEF criteria, and risk of malignancy [published correction appears in J Am Acad Dermatol. 2020 Jan;82(1):260]. J Am Acad Dermatol. 2019;80(5):1272–83. https://doi.org/10.1016/j.jaad.2018.08.033.
29. Piraccini BM, Alessandrini A, Starace M. Onychoscopy: dermoscopy of the nails. Dermatol Clin. 2018;36(4):431–8. https://doi.org/10.1016/j.det.2018.05.010.
30. Littleton TW, Murray PM, Baratz ME. Subungual melanoma. Orthop Clin North Am. 2019;50(3):357–66. https://doi.org/10.1016/j.ocl.2019.03.003.
31. Akay BN, Kirmizi A, Bostanci S, Okcu Heper A, Farabi B. Paediatric melanoma of the nail unit with rapid progression: a case report with dermatoscopic follow-up and intraoperative dermatoscopic images. Australas J Dermatol. 2020;61(1):46–8. https://doi.org/10.1111/ajd.13182.
32. Benati E, Ribero S, Longo C, et al. Clinical and dermoscopic clues to differentiate pigmented nail bands: an International Dermoscopy Society study. J Eur Acad Dermatol Venereol. 2017;31(4):732–6. https://doi.org/10.1111/jdv.13991.
33. Brunsgaard EK, Wu YP, Grossman D. Melanoma in skin of color: Part I. Epidemiology and clinical presentation. J Am Acad Dermatol. 2023;89(3):445–56. https://doi.org/10.1016/j.jaad.2022.04.056.
34. Lee DK, Chang MJ, Desai AD, Lipner SR. Clinical and dermoscopic findings of benign longitudinal melanonychia due to melanocytic activation differ by skin type and predict likelihood of nail matrix biopsy. J Am Acad Dermatol. 2022;87(4):792–9. https://doi.org/10.1016/j.jaad.2022.06.1165.
35. Singal A, Bisherwal K. Melanonychia: etiology, diagnosis, and treatment. Indian Dermatol Online J. 2020;11(1):1–11. https://doi.org/10.4103/idoj.IDOJ_167_19.
36. Levit EK, Kagen MH, Scher RK, Grossman M, Altman E. The ABC rule for clinical detection of subungual melanoma. J Am Acad Dermatol. 2000;42(2 Pt 1):269–74. https://doi.org/10.1016/S0190-9622(00)90137-3.
37. Lee DJR, Arbache ST, Quaresma MV, Nico MMS, Gabbi TVB. Nail apparatus melanoma: experience of 10 years in a single institution. Skin Appendage Disord. 2018;5(1):20–6. https://doi.org/10.1159/000488722.
38. Jo G, Cho SI, Choi S, Mun JH. Functional surgery versus amputation for in situ or minimally invasive nail melanoma: a meta-analysis. J Am Acad Dermatol. 2019;81(4):917–22. https://doi.org/10.1016/j.jaad.2019.06.012.

18 Nail Unit Squamous Cell Carcinoma

Rachel C. Hill and Shari R. Lipner

18.1 Description of Disease

Squamous cell carcinoma (SCC) of the nail unit is the most common type of nail malignancy. SCC of the nail unit is often slow-growing and may originate from the progression of Bowen's Disease, defined as SCC in situ [1]. It is estimated that there is a 3–5% risk of Bowen's Disease developing into invasive SCC [2]. In many cases, patients ultimately diagnosed with nail unit SCCs report that their affected nail(s) had been abnormal for several years, possibly even decades. Known as the "great mimicker," nail unit SCC has many different clinical presentations that resemble both benign and malignant lesions, and therefore diagnosis is often delayed [3, 4].

18.2 Epidemiology

18.2.1 Sex

Previous studies have shown that SCC is most often identified in male patients, with an estimated 2:1 (male:female) ratio [3]. In a retrospective study of 19 cases of nail unit SCC at an academic institution in South Korea by Lee et al., 13 patients were male (68.4%) [5]. In a retrospective study including 34 patients with 42 confirmed nail unit SCCs by Tang et al., 27 of 34 (79%) patients were male [6]. Similarly, in a retrospective study of 41 nail unit SCCs at a single institution by Dika et al., 24 patients (61.54%) were male [7]. In a retrospective study of 51 patients with 54 nail unit SCCs at a single center by Lecerf et al., 72.5% of patients were male [8].

S. R. Lipner, *Atlas of Nail Disorders Across All Skin Colors*,
https://doi.org/10.1007/978-3-031-74272-9_18

18.2.2 Age

Nail unit SCC typically affects patients >50 years old and peaks during the fifth to seventh decades of life [8–10]. In a retrospective study of 15 patients diagnosed with SCC of the nail unit and treated with Mohs surgery by Dika et al., the patients ranged in age from 29 to 89 years old, with a median age of 57 years [9]. In a separate retrospective study of 41 patients with nail unit SCC by Dika et al., the mean age was 64.7 years old, with a range of 24–93 years [11]. In the retrospective study of 51 patients with 54 nail unit SCCs by Lecerf et al., the mean age was 60.8 years old with a range of 21–83 years [8].

18.2.3 Race

Race is not reported in many nail unit SCC studies. In a retrospective review of 31 patients who underwent Mohs surgery for biopsy-proven SCC in situ of the nail unit at a single cancer center, 27 patients identified as white (87.1%), 3 patients identified as Hispanic (9.7%), and 1 patient identified as Black (3.2%) [12].

18.3 Risk Factors

There are several known factors for developing nail unit SCC. High-risk human papillomavirus (HPV) strains, including HPV-16, may increase the risk for nail unit SCC. In a case series of three patients with HPV and Bowen's Disease, with in situ hybridization and polymerase chain reaction (PCR) used to detect HPV in biopsy samples, two samples were positive for HPV-16 and one was positive for HPV-73 [13]. In a literature review of 74 cases of Bowen's Disease of the nail unit, in which HPV genotyping was performed by immunohistochemistry, in situ hybridization, and/or PCR, 23 cases were positive for HPV-16 (32.8% of those reviewed) [13]. Likewise, in the case series of 41 patients with nail unit SCC by Dika et al., 15 cases (36.6%) were HPV-16 positive [11]. In a case series including 23 in situ and invasive SCCs of the nail unit in patients with HPV at a single center and accompanying literature review of 51 cases of digital SCC associated with HPV, seven patients (10%) had a history of dysplasia or carcinoma of the genitals associated with the same HPV strain as their nail unit SCC [14]. In a case report of a 28-year-old human immunodeficiency virus-infected male who presented with multiple invasive SCCs involving his fingernails, the patient was also positive for HPV-26, indicating that other HPV strains may also predispose patients to nail unit SCC [15].

Trauma, exposure to ionizing radiation, and smoking are also risk factors for nail unit SCC. In the retrospective study of 15 patients with nail unit SCC and treated with Mohs by Dika et al., seven (46.7%) patients reported a history of trauma [9]. In a case series of 12 patients with subungual SCC at a large cancer center, five patients had chronic radiation exposure, four of which were occupational exposures (veterinarian $n = 2$, physician $n = 1$, dentist $n = 1$) [16].

Immunosuppression is also believed to play a role in the pathogenesis of nail unit SCC. In a retrospective study of 43 patients diagnosed with nail unit SCC at a tertiary nail referral center, seven patients (16%) had a history of immunosuppression, including chronic lymphoid leukemia and patients taking immunosuppressants for ≥ three years for bone marrow transplantation, renal transplantation, and rheumatoid arthritis [17]. The immunosuppressed group had a mean duration of symptoms of nine months vs. 65 months in the immunocompetent group ($P < 0.001$). Immunosuppressed patients also more commonly presented with involvement of multiple fingers (4/7 patients in the immunosuppressed group vs. 2/36 patients in the immunocompetent group, $P < 0.001$) [17]. It is hypothesized that a history of smoking may further increase the risk of nail unit SCC [18]. In the retrospective study including 34 patients with 42 confirmed nail unit SCCs by Tang et al., current or past tobacco use was reported in 27 of 34 patients (79%) [6].

18.4 Clinical Features

Nail unit SCC more commonly affects the fingernails than the toenails, especially the first, second, and third fingernails of the dominant hand, possibly due to increased likelihood of trauma or proximity to cigarettes in smokers [3, 19]. In the retrospective study of 15 patients who underwent Mohs surgery for nail unit SCC by Dika et al., the fingernails were affected in 14 cases (93.3%), with six cases (40%) involving the first digit [9]. In the retrospective study, including 34 patients with 42 confirmed nail unit SCCs by Tang et al., 39 SCCs (91%) were localized to the fingernails [6]. In the retrospective review of 51 patients with 54 nail unit SCCs by Lecerf et al., 53 cases (98%) involved the fingernails [8].

Nail unit SCC typically has an indolent and chronic course due to slow tumor growth [3]. SCC affecting the nail may arise from the nail bed, the proximal or lateral nail folds, or from the hyponychium [3]. In the retrospective review of 51 patients with 54 nail unit SCCs by Lecerf et al., 31 cases (57.4%) involved the nail bed, 17 (31.5%) involved the lateral or proximal nail folds, and six (11.1%) involved both the nail bed and the nail folds [8]. Onycholemmal carcinoma (OC) is a rare subtype of nail unit SCC in which the tumor originates from the epithelium of the nail bed [20].

There are several non-specific clinical features associated with nail unit SCC, which may make distinguishing it from other benign or malignant lesions of the nail unit difficult. The most common clinical appearance of nail unit SCC resembles a periungual verruca [7, 21]. In the retrospective study of 19 cases of nail unit SCC at an academic institution in South Korea by Lee et al., the most common symptoms included pain (84.2%), purulent discharge (57.8%), oozing (36.8%), and bleeding (21.1%). Notably, 79% of patients were initially misdiagnosed, most often with onychomycosis or viral warts [5]. In the retrospective study, including 34 patients with 42 confirmed nail unit SCCs by Tang et al., the most common symptoms were nail dystrophy ($n = 31$, 74%) and onycholysis ($n = 22$, 52%) [6]. In the retrospective study of 51 patients with 54 nail unit SCCs by Lecerf et al., subungual hyperkeratosis, onycholysis, oozing, and nail plate destruction were the most common clinical symptoms of nail unit SCC [8]. Rarely, nail unit SCC may present as an isolated longitudinal melanonychia [22–30].

Onychoscopy may be a useful adjunct to the physical examination when there is clinical suspicion for nail unit SCC. In a retrospective study of 44 subungual SCC cases, localized hyperkeratosis was more often seen on dermoscopy for SCCs compared to 34 cases of previously published onychomatricomas (OR 6.25, $P = 0.012$, 95% Confidence Interval 1.50–26.01) [31, 32]. In an observational study using intra-operative dermoscopy in 53 patients with nail unit SCC, the most common dermoscopic features were dotted, irregular, or curved vessels (92.5%, 88.7%, and 86.8%, respectively). Other features included pink background (84.9%), translucent structureless area (84.9%), sagittal vessels (84.9%), and whitish scaly areas (81.1%) [33]. Onycholysis, wart-like growths, irregular borders, splinter hemorrhages, and nail thickening may also be appreciated in nail unit SCC [3, 31]. Because these features may be appreciated on dermoscopy with other nail unit conditions, dermoscopy is not considered diagnostic.

18.5 Clinical Features in Skin of Color

Nail unit SCC in patients with skin of color may be more likely to manifest clinically as longitudinal melanonychia [22–30]. In a case series of two patients with Fitzpatrick types IV and V skin presenting with SCC in situ published in 2021, both patients presented with monodactylous longitudinal melanonychia. The authors of this case series stated that all cases of Bowen's disease manifesting with longitudinal melanonychia reported in the literature in the past 20 years involved patients with skin of color, but the editor has also diagnosed lighter-skinned patients with nail unit SCC that presented as longitudinal melanonychia [30].

18.6 Requirements for Diagnosis

An X-ray may be used to investigate bone involvement in cases of advanced nail unit SCC, while magnetic resonance imaging may be used to localize the extent of disease prior to surgery and to assist with staging [3]. Biopsy with histopathologic examination remains the gold standard for definitive diagnosis [3].

18.7 Prognosis

If recognized at an early stage, the prognosis for SCC of the nail unit is excellent due to typically slow tumor growth and rarity of metastasis [3, 4]. The treatment of choice for early-stage nail unit SCC is Mohs micrographic surgery [34]. If diagnosis is delayed, patients may experience local destruction of the nail unit and surrounding tissue, while more advanced disease may invade the bone. Bony invasion should be suspected in patients who present with concerning clinical features accompanied by pain [3]. Patients with evidence of bone invasion on X-ray imaging may require wide excision or amputation [3, 35].

18.8 Cases

Figures 18.1, 18.2, 18.3, 18.4, 18.5, 18.6, and 18.7 demonstrate the presentation of exostosis in a clinical setting.

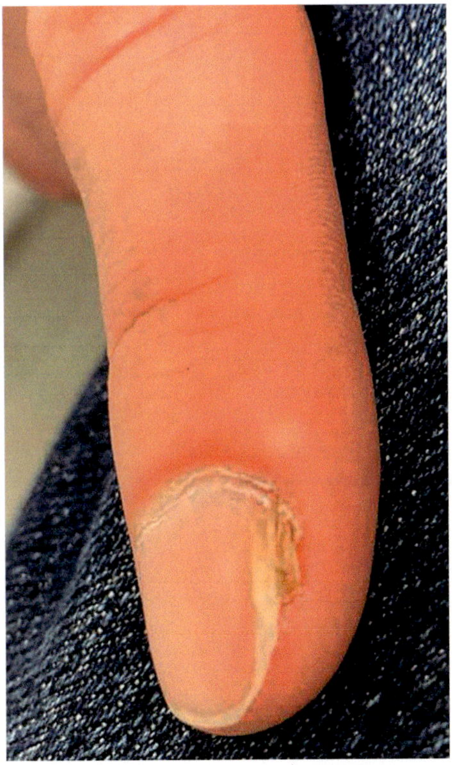

Fig. 18.1 40-Year-old male, Fitzpatrick type II, nail unit SCC, with lateral onycholysis and hyperkeratosis involving the right second fingernail

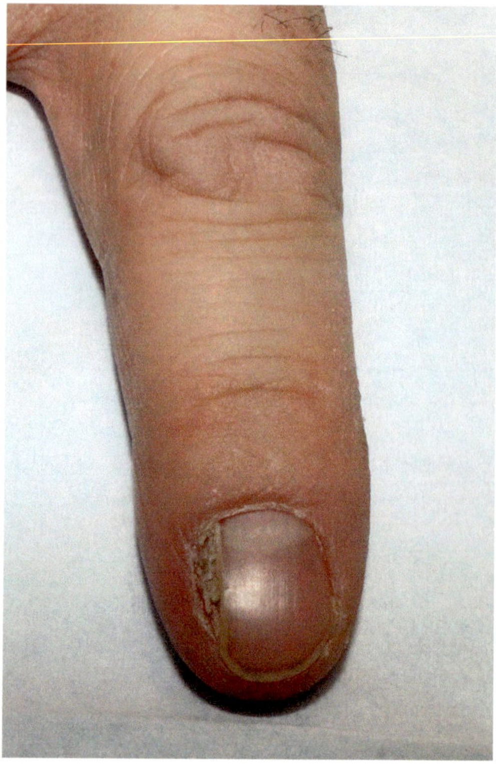

Fig. 18.2 40-Year-old male, Fitzpatrick type II, nail unit SCC, with hyperkeratosis laterally involving the right second fingernail

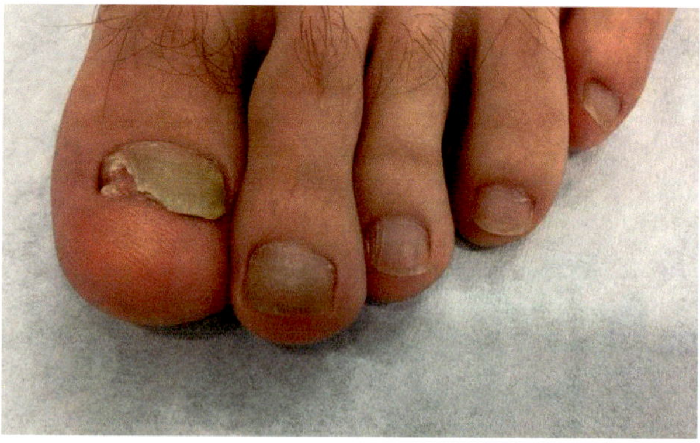

Fig. 18.3 30-Year-old male, Fitzpatrick type III, nail unit SCC, with nail plate thickening and hyperkeratosis medially of the left great toenail

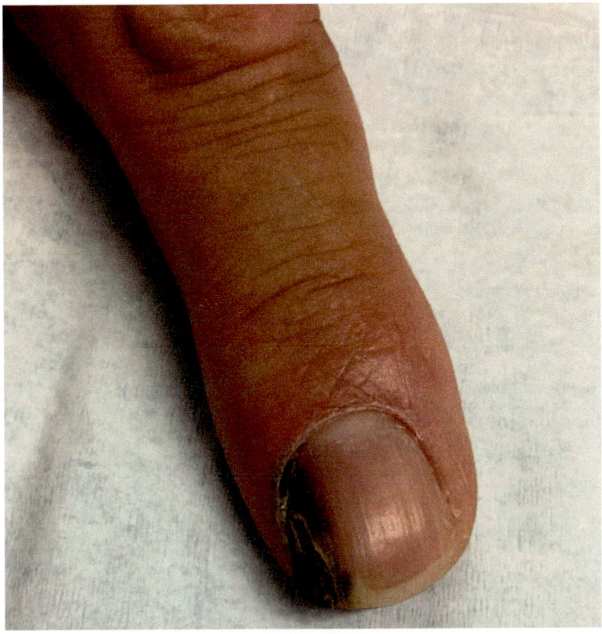

Fig. 18.4 65-Year-old male, Fitzpatrick type III, nail unit SCC, with 3 mm gray brown longitudinal band of the right second fingernail and onychoschizia

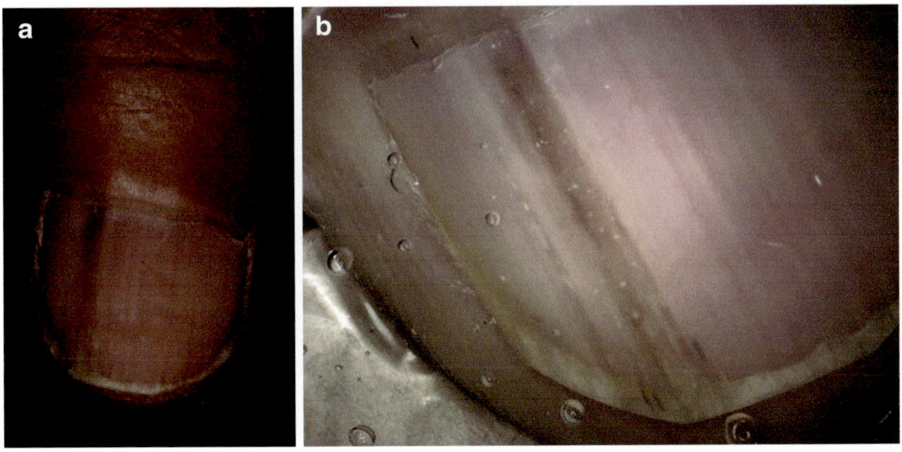

Fig. 18.5 72-Year-old male, Fitzpatrick type III, subungual Bowen disease, with 1.5 mm longitudinal melanonychia involving the left thumbnail (*from* Saito et al. [36]; *with permission*)

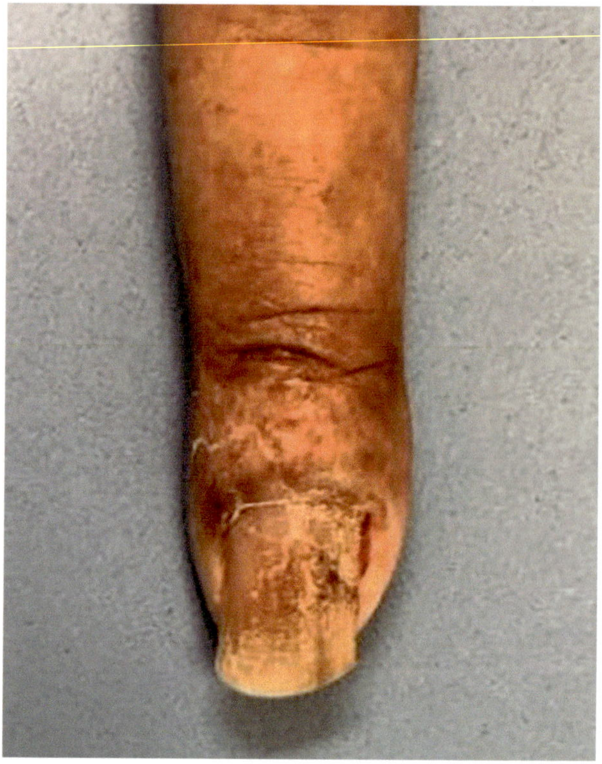

Fig. 18.6 87-Year-old female, Fitzpatrick type IV, nail unit SCC, with right third fingernail nail plate destruction and longitudinal melanonychia extending to the distal nail edge (*courtesy of* Thomas Knackstedt, MD, MPH, FACMS)

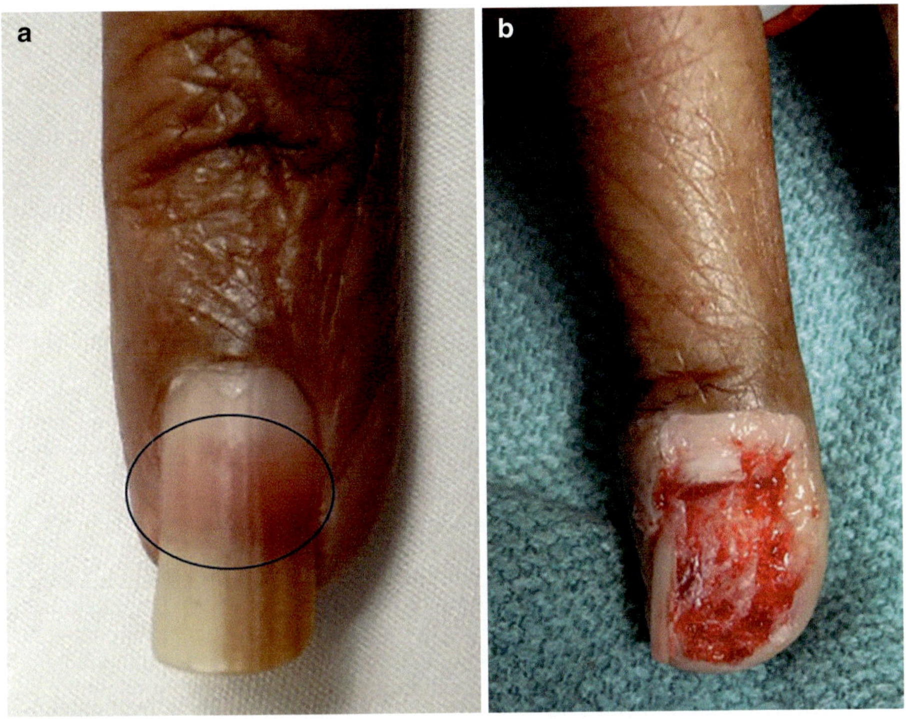

Fig. 18.7 (**a**, **b**) 88-Year-old female, Fitzpatrick type V, nail unit SCC, with erythema of the right fourth fingernail and extensive nail bed involvement revealed with Mohs surgery (*courtesy of* Thomas Knackstedt, MD, MPH, FACMS)

References

1. Haneke E. Important malignant and new nail tumors. J Dtsch Dermatol Ges. 2017;15(4):367–86. https://doi.org/10.1111/ddg.13223.
2. Neubert T, Lehmann P. Bowen's disease—a review of newer treatment options. Ther Clin Risk Manag. 2008;4(5):1085–95.
3. Starace M, Alessandrini A, Dika E, Piraccini BM. Squamous cell carcinoma of the nail unit. Dermatol Pract Concept. 2018;8(3):238–44. https://doi.org/10.5826/dpc.0803a17.
4. Dany M. Nail unit squamous cell carcinoma: updates on diagnosis, surgical approach, and the use of Mohs micrographic surgery. Cutis. 2020;106(5):E11–4. https://doi.org/10.12788/cutis.0122.
5. Lee TM, Jo G, Kim M, et al. Squamous cell carcinoma of the nail unit: a retrospective review of 19 cases in Asia and comparative review of Western literature. Int J Dermatol. 2019;58(4):428–32. https://doi.org/10.1111/ijd.14306.
6. Tang N, Maloney ME, Clark AH, Jellinek NJ. A retrospective study of nail squamous cell carcinoma at 2 institutions. Dermatologic Surg. 2016;42(Suppl 1):S8–S17. https://doi.org/10.1097/DSS.0000000000000521.
7. Dika E, Starace M, Patrizi A, Fanti PA, Piraccini BM. Squamous cell carcinoma of the nail unit: a clinical histopathologic study and a proposal for classification. Dermatologic Surg. 2019;45(3):365–70. https://doi.org/10.1097/DSS.0000000000001805.

8. Lecerf P, Richert B, Theunis A, André J. A retrospective study of squamous cell carcinoma of the nail unit diagnosed in a Belgian general hospital over a 15-year period. J Am Acad Dermatol. 2013;69(2):253–61. https://doi.org/10.1016/j.jaad.2013.02.008.
9. Dika E, Piraccini BM, Balestri R, et al. Mohs surgery for squamous cell carcinoma of the nail: report of 15 cases. Our experience and a long-term follow-up. Br J Dermatol. 2012;167(6):1310–4. https://doi.org/10.1111/j.1365-2133.2012.11129.x.
10. Dika E, Fanti PA, Patrizi A, Misciali C, Vaccari S, Piraccini BM. Mohs surgery for squamous cell carcinoma of the nail unit: 10 years of experience. Dermatologic Surg. 2015;41(9):1015–9. https://doi.org/10.1097/DSS.0000000000000452.
11. Dika E, Venturoli S, Patrizi A, et al. The detection of human papillomavirus-16 in squamous cell carcinoma of the nail unit: a case series. J Am Acad Dermatol. 2017;76(2):354–6. https://doi.org/10.1016/j.jaad.2016.08.063.
12. Aleissa S, Cowen E, Navarrete-Dechent C, et al. Squamous cell carcinoma in situ upstaging is not frequent in the nail unit: a tertiary cancer center experience. Arch Dermatol Res. 2022;314(1):89–93. https://doi.org/10.1007/s00403-020-02125-7.
13. Grundmeier N, Hamm H, Weissbrich B, Lang SC, Bröcker EB, Kerstan A. High-risk human papillomavirus infection in Bowen's disease of the nail unit: report of three cases and review of the literature. Dermatology. 2011;223(4):293–300. https://doi.org/10.1159/000335371.
14. Alam M, Caldwell JB, Eliezri YD. Human papillomavirus-associated digital squamous cell carcinoma: literature review and report of 21 new cases. J Am Acad Dermatol. 2003;48(3):385–93. https://doi.org/10.1067/mjd.2003.184.
15. Handisurya A, Rieger A, Bankier A, et al. Human papillomavirus type 26 infection causing multiple invasive squamous cell carcinomas of the fingernails in an AIDS patient under highly active antiretroviral therapy [published correction appears in Br J Dermatol. 2007 Dec;157(6):1304]. Br J Dermatol. 2007;157(4):788–94. https://doi.org/10.1111/j.1365-2133.2007.08094.x.
16. Attiyeh FF, Shah J, Booher RJ, Knapper WH. Subungual squamous cell carcinoma. JAMA. 1979;241(3):262–3.
17. Ormerod E, de Berker D. Nail unit squamous cell carcinoma in people with immunosuppression. Br J Dermatol. 2015;173(3):701–12. https://doi.org/10.1111/bjd.13860.
18. Barone H, Schaeffer M, Buckland M, LaFond AA, Krach K. Squamous cell carcinoma in situ of the nail unit: current evidence and recommendations for patient centered treatment. J Cutan Med Surg. 2023;27(1):51–9. https://doi.org/10.1177/12034754221134226.
19. Inkaya E, Sayit E, Sayit AT, Zan E, Bakirtas M. Subungual squamous cell carcinoma of the third finger with radiologic and histopathologic findings: a report of case. J Hand Microsurg. 2015;7(1):194–8. https://doi.org/10.1007/s12593-014-0152-4.
20. Waterton K, Magro CM, Lipner SR. Nail unit squamous cell carcinoma with onycholemmal features: case report and review of the literature. Skin Appendage Disord. 2023;9(4):284–90. https://doi.org/10.1159/000529906.
21. Riddel C, Rashid R, Thomas V. Ungual and periungual human papillomavirus-associated squamous cell carcinoma: a review. J Am Acad Dermatol. 2011;64(6):1147–53. https://doi.org/10.1016/j.jaad.2010.02.057.
22. Sanchez-Carpintero I, Serrano-Pardo R, Enguita AB, Feito M, Ruiz-Rodriguez R. Unique presentation of squamous cell carcinoma with longitudinal melanonychia. Dermatol Ther. 2020;33(6):e14087. https://doi.org/10.1111/dth.14087.
23. García-Lozano JA, Salerni G, Cardenas-de la Garza JA, Perez MR, Schreiber FG. Longitudinal melanonychia as the only sign of in situ squamous cell carcinoma. Dermatol Pract Concept. 2023;13(1):e2023062. https://doi.org/10.5826/dpc.1301a62.
24. Gatica-Torres M, Arguello-Guerra L, Manuel Ruiz-Matta J, Dominguez-Cherit J. Subungual pigmented squamous cell carcinoma presenting as a grey longitudinal melanonychia in a young patient. BMJ Case Rep. 2016;2016:bcr2016215390. https://doi.org/10.1136/bcr-2016-215390.
25. Lallas A, Korecka K, Apalla Z, et al. Seven plus one steps to assess pigmented nail bands (melanonychia striata longitudinalis). Dermatol Pract Concept. 2023;13(4):e2023204. https://doi.org/10.5826/dpc.1304a204.

26. Lee J, Shin DM, Oh SJ, Park JH, Lee D. A retrospective study of nail squamous cell carcinoma at a single tertiary center: a relationship between longitudinal melanonychia and the depth of invasion. J Am Acad Dermatol. 2022;87(5):1123–5. https://doi.org/10.1016/j.jaad.2022.01.044.
27. Nojima K, Namiki T, Hanafusa T, Miura K, Yokozeki H. Pigmented squamous cell carcinoma of the right thumb: longitudinal melanonychia and dermoscopic features. Eur J Dermatol. 2017;27(5):561–3. https://doi.org/10.1684/ejd.2017.3122.
28. Serret CA, Wang S, Marsch A, Hernandez C. Pigmented squamous cell carcinoma presenting as longitudinal melanonychia in a transplant recipient. Cutis. 2018;101(5):375–7.
29. Stetsenko GY, McFarlane RJ, Chien AJ, et al. Subungual Bowen disease in a patient with epidermodysplasia verruciformis presenting clinically as longitudinal melanonychia. Am J Dermatopathol. 2008;30(6):582–5. https://doi.org/10.1097/DAD.0b013e31817e6f0d.
30. Williams NM, Obayomi AO, Diaz-Perez JA, Morrison BW. Monodactylous longitudinal melanonychia: a sign of Bowen's disease in skin of color. Skin Appendage Disord. 2021;7(4):306–10. https://doi.org/10.1159/000514221.
31. Teysseire S, Dalle S, Duru G, et al. Dermoscopic features of subungual squamous cell carcinoma: a study of 44 cases. Dermatology. 2017;233(2–3):184–91. https://doi.org/10.1159/000479059.
32. Lesort C, Debarbieux S, Duru G, Dalle S, Poulhalon N, Thomas L. Dermoscopic features of onychomatricoma: a study of 34 cases. Dermatology. 2015;231(2):177–83. https://doi.org/10.1159/000431315.
33. Carlioz V, Perier-Muzet M, Debarbieux S, et al. Intraoperative dermoscopy features of subungual squamous cell carcinoma: a study of 53 cases. Clin Exp Dermatol. 2021;46(1):82–8. https://doi.org/10.1111/ced.14345.
34. Young LC, Tuxen AJ, Goodman G. Mohs' micrographic surgery as treatment for squamous dysplasia of the nail unit. Australas J Dermatol. 2012;53(2):123–7. https://doi.org/10.1111/j.1440-0960.2011.00813.x.
35. Dalle S, Depape L, Phan A, Balme B, Ronger-Savle S, Thomas L. Squamous cell carcinoma of the nail apparatus: clinicopathological study of 35 cases. Br J Dermatol. 2007;156(5):871–4. https://doi.org/10.1111/j.1365-2133.2006.07744.x.
36. Saito T, Uchi H, Moroi Y, Kiryu H, Furue M. Subungual Bowen disease revealed by longitudinal melanonychia. J Am Acad Dermatol. 2012;67(5):e240–1. https://doi.org/10.1016/j.jaad.2012.03.031.

Metastasis to the Nail Unit

19

Kaya L. Curtis and Shari R. Lipner

19.1 Description of Disease

Metastases to the nail unit/distal phalanx are rare. Lung cancer is the most frequent primary origin of malignancy [1, 2]. Prognosis is poor, with a mean survival time of 3.4 months after diagnosis in Curtis et al.'s systematic review [1].

19.2 Epidemiology

In Curtis et al.'s systematic review [1], there were 224 cases reported in PubMed 1900–2021. The mean age at diagnosis was 58 years, and 65.6% of patients were male. Though race was not reported in the majority of cases (79%), the most commonly represented races were 15.2% White, 3.6% African American, and 1.3% Asian.

19.3 Risk Factors

In Curtis et al.'s systematic review [1], the most common primary origin of malignancy was the lungs (38%), genitourinary tract organs (18.8%, of which the kidneys represented 57.6%), and gastrointestinal organs (17%, of which the esophagus represented 34.2%). The most common histology of primary malignancy was squamous cell carcinoma (29.9%) and adenocarcinoma (17.4%). In this systematic review, there was no preceding diagnosis of visceral malignancy prior to nail dystrophy presentation in 31.7% of cases. A predilection for male patients is likely reflective of lung cancer epidemiology (higher incidence in males vs. females). Overrepresentation of lung cancer in metastases to the nail unit/distal phalanx is hypothesized to be due to direct lung cancer cell entry into the systemic circulation via the left heart with subsequent dissemination to acral areas [3]. In contrast, cancer cells in other visceral malignancies are initially filtered by the lungs and liver [3].

S. R. Lipner, *Atlas of Nail Disorders Across All Skin Colors*,
https://doi.org/10.1007/978-3-031-74272-9_19

19.4 Clinical Features

Metastases to the nail unit/distal phalanx most frequently involved the fingernail(s) (80.4%) in Curtis et al.'s systematic review [1]. The thumb is the most commonly involved digit (21.4%), followed by the fourth finger (17.6%). Of the toenails, the great toenail was most frequently affected (9.4%). There is no predilection for laterality. On physical examination, there may be swelling (37.1%), erythema (26%), ulceration (13%), distal digit discoloration (10.7%), and nail plate changes (e.g., detachment, elevation) (11.2%). Subungual hematomas and dilated vessels may be present on dermoscopy. Patients reported a history of trauma in around a tenth of cases. The most common symptom was pain and/or tenderness (69.6%). There was a history of bleeding in 6.7% of cases. Metastases to the nail unit frequently mimic other nail conditions; the most common differential diagnosis in Curtis et al.'s systematic review was infection (38.4%), followed by gout (1.8%) and pyogenic granuloma (1.8%).

19.5 Clinical Features in Skin of Color

Distinct clinical presentations of metastases to the nail unit in skin of color have not been characterized due to their rarity. Erythema and hyperpigmentation of the surrounding skin may be more subtle in darker skin tones. Dermoscopy may aid in visualization. Physiologic longitudinal melanonychia may be present in patients with skin of color.

19.6 Requirements for Diagnosis

X-ray of the involved digit aids in diagnosis and frequently demonstrates distal phalanx destruction and soft tissue swelling (94.6% and 21%, respectively) [1]. Ultrasound may also be conducted to assess for vascularization [4]. Biopsy with histopathological confirmation is required for definitive diagnosis. For patients without a preceding diagnosis of visceral malignancy, a thorough workup for the primary origin of malignancy and other metastases is crucial.

19.7 Cases

Figures 19.1, 19.2, 19.3, 19.4, 19.5, 19.6, 19.7, and 19.8 demonstrate the presentation of metastases to the nail unit in a clinical setting.

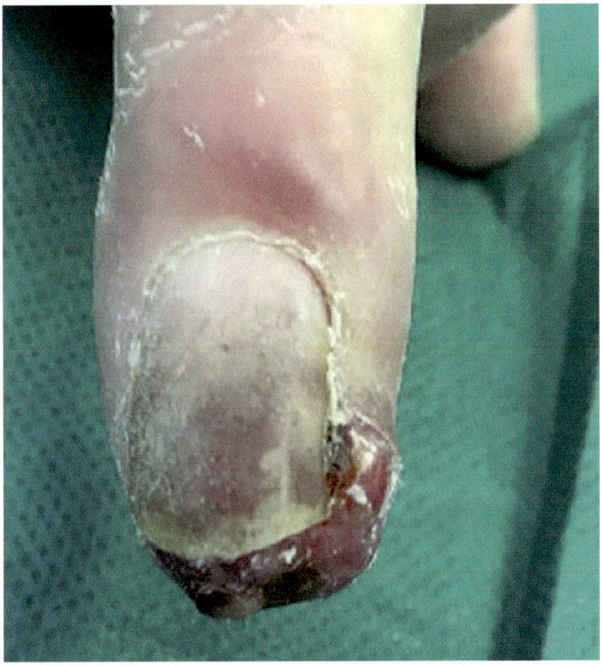

Fig. 19.1 72-Year-old male, Fitzpatrick type I, metastasis to the nail unit, with subungual metastatic lung adenocarcinoma with erythematous-violaceous, subungual plaque involving the third finger of the right hand. The primary origin of malignancy is lung adenocarcinoma (*from* Lora et al. [5]; *with permission*)

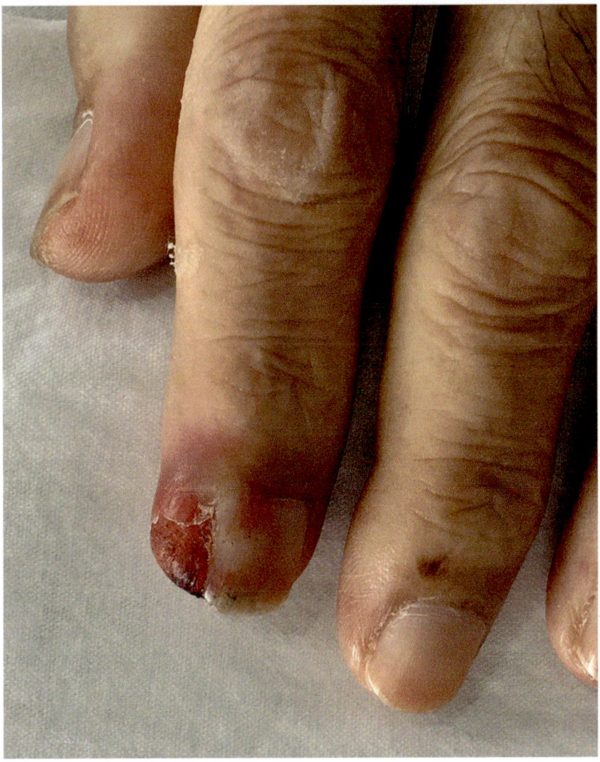

Fig. 19.2 61-Year-old male, Fitzpatrick type II, metastasis to the nail unit, with the appearance of the nail change. The primary origin of malignancy is tongue squamous cell carcinoma (*from* Aiempanakit et al. [6]; *with permission*)

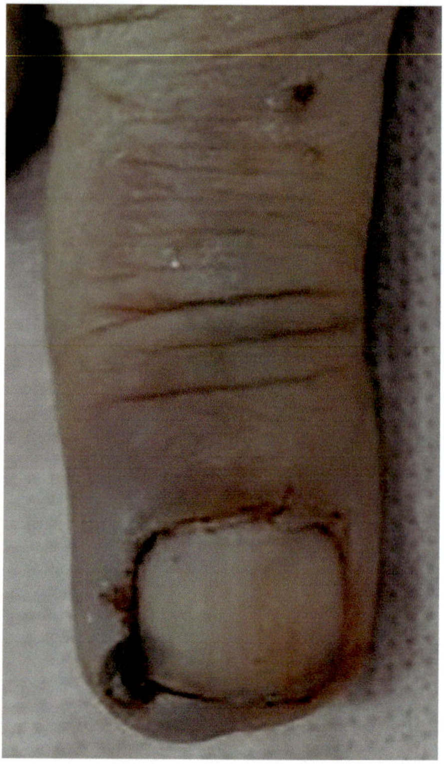

Fig. 19.3 80-Year-old male, Fitzpatrick type II, metastasis to the nail unit, with localized bluish swelling around the lateral nail fold with a crust over the edge of the nail, mimicking paronychia. The primary origin of malignancy is rectal adenocarcinoma (*from* Ko et al. [7]; *with permission*)

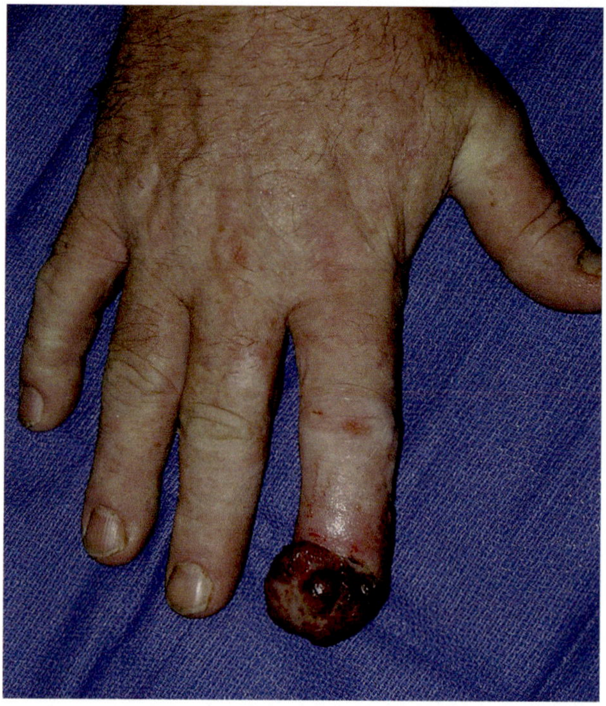

Fig. 19.4 55-Year-old male, Fitzpatrick type II, metastasis to the nail unit, with right index finger lesion. Anteroposterior view. The primary origin of malignancy is pulmonary squamous cell carcinoma (*from* Madjidi et al. [8]; *with permission*)

Fig. 19.5 84-Year-old male, Fitzpatrick type III, metastasis to the nail unit, with swelling and hemorrhaging at the distal part of the right thumb. The primary origin of malignancy is follicular-type adenocarcinoma of the thyroid gland (*from* Huri et al. [9]; CC-BY 3.0, https://creativecommons.org/licenses/by/3.0)

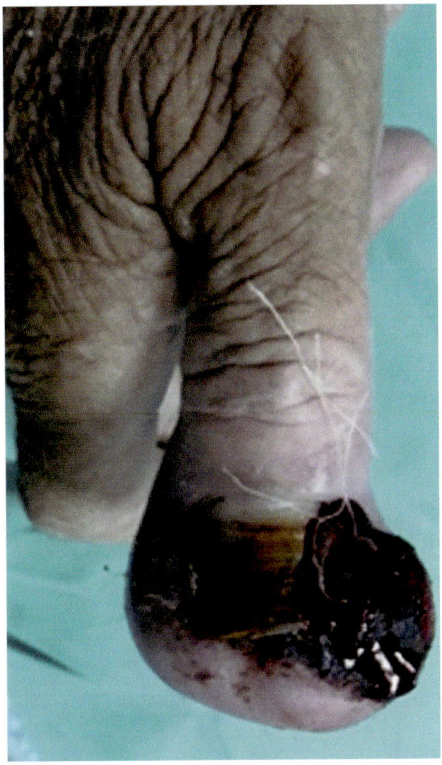

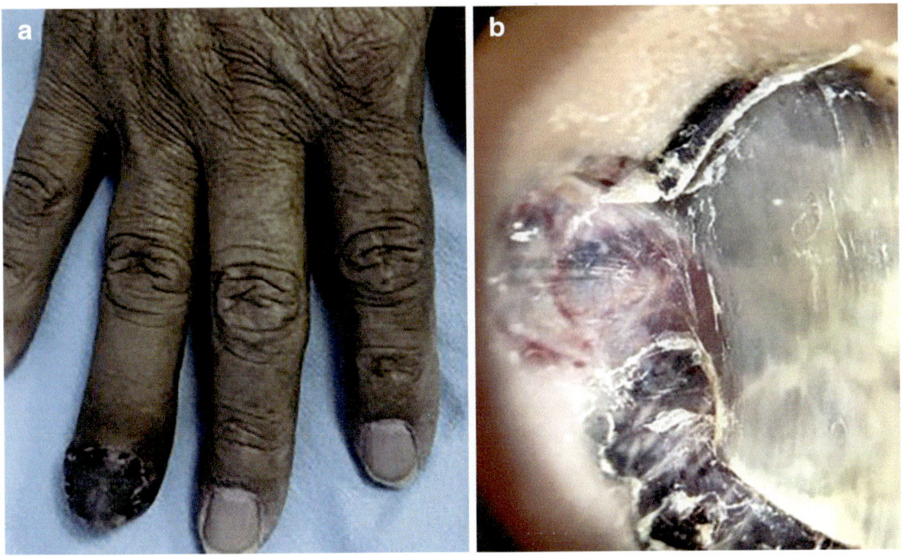

Fig. 19.6 (**a**) 66-Year-old male, Fitzpatrick type III, metastasis to the nail unit, with a painful enlargement on the nail plate of the fourth right finger, with violaceous discoloration, without destroying the nail plate. The primary origin of malignancy is adenocarcinoma of the prostate. (**b**) 66-year-old male, Fitzpatrick type IV, metastasis to the nail unit, with onychoscopy showing non-melanocytic black pigmentation of the nail bed, with hematomas and vascular-like nodules, as well as dilated blood vessels. The nail plate was unremarkable (*from* García-Galaviz et al. [10]; *with permission*)

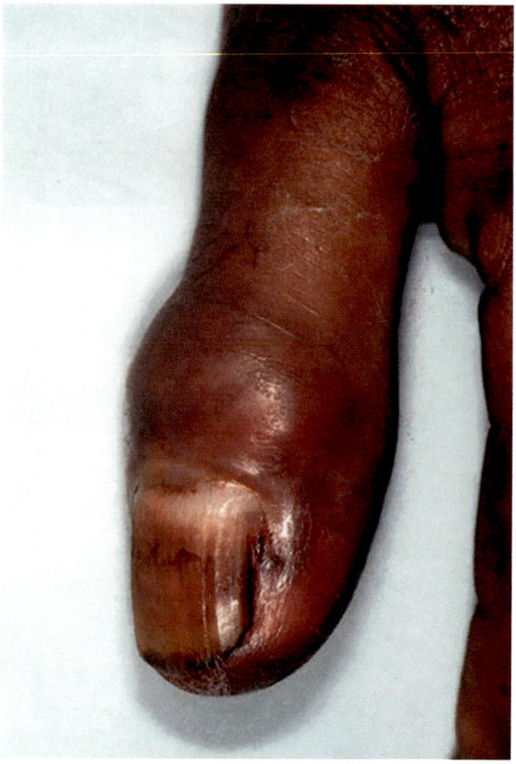

Fig. 19.7 56-Year-old male, Fitzpatrick type IV, metastasis to the nail unit, with inflammation of the distal phalanx of the thumb. The primary origin of malignancy is squamous cell esophageal carcinoma (*from* Aguiar Bujanda et al. [11]; *with permission*)

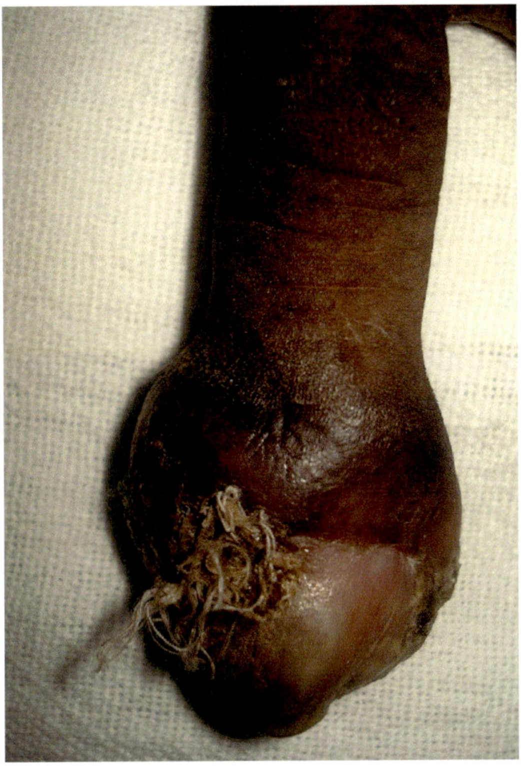

Fig. 19.8 76-Year-old male, Fitzpatrick type V, metastasis to the nail unit, with digital metastasis as globular swelling on the tip of the right little finger. The primary origin of malignancy is well-differentiated adenocarcinoma of the colon (*from* Anoop et al. [12]; *with permission*)

References

1. Curtis KL, Lipner SR. Metastases to the nail unit and distal phalanx: a systematic review. Arch Dermatol Res. 2023;315(3):347–58.
2. Cohen PR. Metastatic tumors to the nail unit: subungual metastases. Dermatologic Surg. 2001;27(3):280–93.
3. Stomeo D, Tulli A, Ziranu A, Perisano C, De Santis V, Maccauro G. Acrometastasis: a literature review. Eur Rev Med Pharmacol Sci. 2015;19(15):2906–15.
4. Feito-Sancho L, Rubio-Flores C, Lorido-Cortés MM, Vazquez-Contreras G, Santa-Cruz Martín A, Prats-Caelles I. Cutaneous metastasis of a sarcomatoid-rhabdoid renal tumor to a distal phalanx. Int J Dermatol. 2024;63(2):207–9.
5. Lora V, Haneke E, Scarabello A, Morrone A, Cota C. Subungual metastasis: expanding the spectrum. J Eur Acad Dermatol Venereol. 2019;33(8):e282–4.
6. Aiempanakit K. Digital metastasis of tongue squamous cell carcinoma. JAAD Case Rep. 2018;4(2):200–2.
7. Ko JH, Young A, Wang KH. Paronychia-like digital cutaneous metastasis. Br J Dermatol. 2014;171(3):663–5.
8. Madjidi A, Cole P, Laucirica R. Digital acrometastasis: a rare initial sign of occult pulmonary squamous cell carcinoma. J Plast Reconstr Aesthet Surg. 2009;62(10):e365–7.
9. Huri G. An atypical metastasis of follicular-type adenocarcinoma of the thyroid gland to thumb. Case Rep Orthop. 2011;2011:735789.

10. García-Galaviz R, Domínguez-Cherit J, Caro-Sánchez C, Salazar-Rojas E. Subungual metastasis of an adenocarcinoma of the prostate in a finger. Skin Appendage Disord. 2018;5(1):46–9.
11. Aguiar Bujanda D, Bohn Sarmiento U, Aguiar Morales J. Some unusual paraneoplastic syndromes. Case 1. Metastatic squamous cell esophageal cancer to the thumb. J Clin Oncol. 2003;21(13):2620.
12. Anoop TM, George S, Divya KP, Jabbar PK. Metastatic phalangeal osteolysis as an initial presentation of carcinoma colon. Am J Surg. 2010;200(5):e61–3.

Part V

Traumatic Nail Disorders

Onychotillomania 20

Rachel C. Hill and Shari R. Lipner

20.1 Description of Disease

Onychotillomania, also known as "nail picking," describes self-induced trauma to the fingernails or toenails and periungual skin using one's own fingers or other tools, including knives, scissors, or toothpicks, and is classified as a body-focused repetitive behavior [1–3]. Patients with onychotillomania may pick or excessively manicure their nails, resulting in onychodystrophy and other complications, including paronychia [3]. Onychotillomania is commonly seen in clinical practice, but prevalence estimates vary widely, suggesting that it is underreported. In a cross-sectional survey-based study by Pacan et al. examining the prevalence of onychotillomania and onychophagia in 339 Polish medical students, the estimated prevalence of onychotillomania was 0.9% [1, 4], In a cross-sectional survey study of 181 graduate students by Wu et al., 46.4% of respondents (84/181) reported nail picking [5].

20.2 Epidemiology

20.2.1 Sex

Previous studies have not supported a sex predilection of onychotillomania. In Pacan et al.'s cross-sectional study of 339 Polish medical students, onychotillomania was reported in three students, including two female students and one male student [4]. In Wu et al.'s cross-sectional survey study of 181 graduate students, the male-to-female ratio of respondents with onychotillomania was 38:57 [5]. In a retrospective study of 63 patients with onychophagia and/or onychotillomania by Chen et al. including 16 patients with only onychotillomania, 50% of the onychotillomania cohort was female ($n = 8$) [6].

S. R. Lipner, *Atlas of Nail Disorders Across All Skin Colors*,
https://doi.org/10.1007/978-3-031-74272-9_20

20.2.2 Age

Patients of all ages can be affected by onychotillomania [7], however, large studies have not been in patients with a wide age range, and onychotillomania may be underreported in adults. In Pacan et al.'s cross-sectional study of medical students, the mean age of onychotillomania onset was 8.6 years old and ranged from 6 to 10 years. The average duration of the disease was 14 years and ranged from 12 to 17 years [4]. In Wu et al.'s cross-sectional survey study of 181 graduate students ages 18–45 years old, the median age of disease onset in the onychotillomania cohort was 10 years (range 1–37 years) [5]. In Chen et al.'s retrospective study of 63 patients with onychophagia and/or onychotillomania, including 16 patients with only onychotillomania, the average age of the onychotillomania cohort was 34 years old (standard deviation 20.61 years) [6]. The rate of nail biting decreases as age increases, and such habits may be instead replaced by nail picking, which patients may consider a more socially acceptable alternative behavior [8].

20.3 Risk Factors

Psychiatric comorbidities, including depression, obsessive-compulsive disorder, specific phobia, delusional disorders, and suicidal ideation, are reported in patients with onychotillomania [4, 9–12]. In Wu et al.'s cross-sectional survey study of 181 graduate students, 33.8% (32/181) of students who reported nail picking were previously diagnosed with a psychiatric disorder [5]. To date, these associations have only been reported in case reports and survey studies and require larger cohort studies to adequately characterize the relationship and temporality of onychotillomania and psychiatric disease [11].

Onychotillomania is a clinical feature of Smith-Magenis syndrome, a neurodevelopmental syndrome that develops due to a heterozygous deletion at chromosome 17p11.2 that includes the *RAI1* gene. The syndrome is characterized by coarse facial features, developmental delay and cognitive impairment, behavioral abnormalities, and childhood-onset obesity [13]. The behavioral phenotype of Smith-Magenis syndrome includes maladaptive and self-injurious behaviors that become recognizable at age 18 months or older. In addition to self-biting and skin picking, individuals with Smith-Magenis syndrome may pull at their fingernails and/or toenails [1, 13].

Nail picking is also associated with Lesch-Nyhan syndrome, a rare, X-linked recessive disorder caused by a deficiency of hypoxanthine-guanine phosphoribosyltransferase which leads to an accumulation of uric acid. The syndrome is characterized by gout, neurological symptoms including lack of muscle control with involuntary writhing, developmental disabilities, and self-mutilating behaviors, including onychotillomania and lip and finger biting [1, 14].

Onychotillomania is also associated with forkhead box protein 1 (FOXP1) syndrome, a neurodevelopmental disorder caused by mutations in the FOXP1 gene that is associated with intellectual disability and dysmorphic features. The prevalence of body-focused repetitive behaviors among individuals with FOXP1 is high, with an estimated 29.7% prevalence of onychotillomania in this population [15].

20.4 Clinical Features

Onychotillomania presents with a broad spectrum of clinical appearances due to the spectrum and severity of picking mechanisms [11]. Both fingernails and toenails may be involved, although fingernails are more commonly affected [1]. Notably, nail dystrophy may be asymmetric and bizarre appearing, with nail plate abnormalities present in some nails and absent in others [16]. Generalized onychodystrophy may occur, with other clinical features including transverse grooves, thinning or thickening, macrolunula, nail plate atrophy, pitting, and brittleness [2, 8, 11]. The periungual skin and nail matrix may also be traumatized, leading to nail plate ridging with or without accompanying nail fold erythema and erosions [8]. Due to repetitive trauma to the proximal and lateral nail folds, acute or chronic paronychia may occur. In severe cases, onychotillomania may lead to anonychia, absence of fingernails and toenails, or secondary, superimposed infections, including bacterial cellulitis [11, 17].

Longitudinal melanonychia (LM) has also been described as a clinical feature of onychotillomania. A case series including six patients affected by onychotillomania described LM in all cases, likely due to activation of melanocytes in the nail matrix because of repetitive trauma [18]. In one case, a pause in the repetitive trauma resulted in the lightening of the LM [18].

Onychoscopy may be used to support the diagnosis of onychotillomania. In a retrospective study of 36 patients with onychotillomania by Maddy et al., scales (n = 34, 94.4%), absence of the nail plate (n = 30, 83.3%), wavy lines in the nail plate (n = 25, 69.4%), hemorrhages (n = 23, 63.9%), crusts (n = 22, 61.1%), and nail plate pigmentation (n = 17, 47.2%) were the most common onychoscopic features of the disease [19]. Melanonychia was also present in four cases (11.1%) [19]. In Chen et al.'s retrospective study of 63 patients with onychophagia and/or onychotillomania, including 16 patients with only onychotillomania, the most common onychoscopic features of the nail plate included washboard-like nails (n = 9, 56.3%), Beau's lines (n = 8, 50%), and lamellar onychoschizia (n = 6, 37.5%), of the subungual area included macrolunula (n = 5, 31.3%), splinter hemorrhages (n = 4, 25%), and subungual hyperkeratosis (n = 4, 25%), and of the periungual area included damage to or less of the cuticle (n = 16, 100%) and erythema (n = 10, 62.5%) [6].

20.5 Clinical Features in Skin of Color

Although features of onychotillomania in skin of color patients have not been explicitly described, patients with skin of color are more likely to have physiologic melanonychia affecting the fingernails and toenails, which may make the clinical diagnosis more challenging.

20.6 Requirements for Diagnosis

Onychotillomania is a clinical diagnosis that can be made if characteristic nail plate or nail fold dystrophy, such as grooves, melanonychia, thinning, macrolunula, cuticle damage, and/or erosion, is present in conjunction with the patient-reported history of picking or manipulation of the nail unit. If the patient denies picking or is unaware of the behavior, it may be observed during history taking or clinical examination.

The differential diagnosis of onychotillomania includes onychomycosis, nail psoriasis, or nail lichen planus, and requires a high degree of clinical suspicion [19]. In rare cases in which the patient denies picking and picking is not observed in the office, a nail biopsy may be required to rule out other diagnoses. Histopathology of onychotillomania shows epithelial hyperplasia with hyperkeratosis and lack of inflammatory infiltrate [9]. Patients diagnosed with onychotillomania may also benefit from a psychiatric evaluation, as treatment of the underlying psychiatric disorder may result in regression of onychotillomania [20]. In Maddy et al.'s retrospective study of 36 patients with onychotillomania, follow-up images of 15 patients who were referred to psychiatry were examined, showing the resolution of onychodystrophy with the treatment of underlying psychiatric disorders [19].

20.7 Cases

Figures 20.1, 20.2, 20.3, 20.4, 20.5, and 20.6 demonstrate the presentation of onychotillomania in a clinical setting.

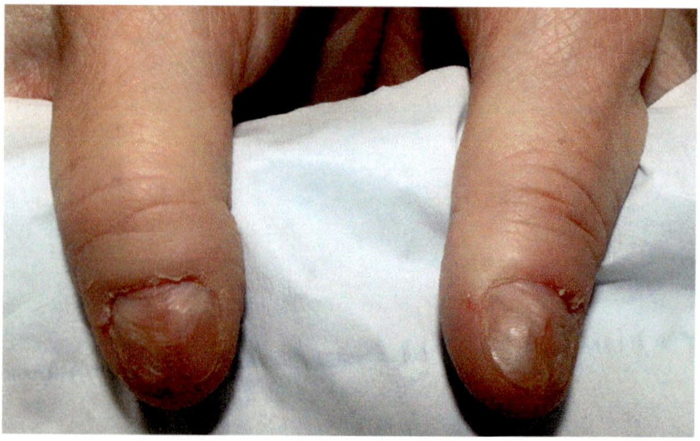

Fig. 20.1 58-Year-old female, Fitzpatrick type II, onychotillomania, with transverse grooves, missing cuticles, erosions of the nail folds, and macrolunula of the bilateral thumbnails

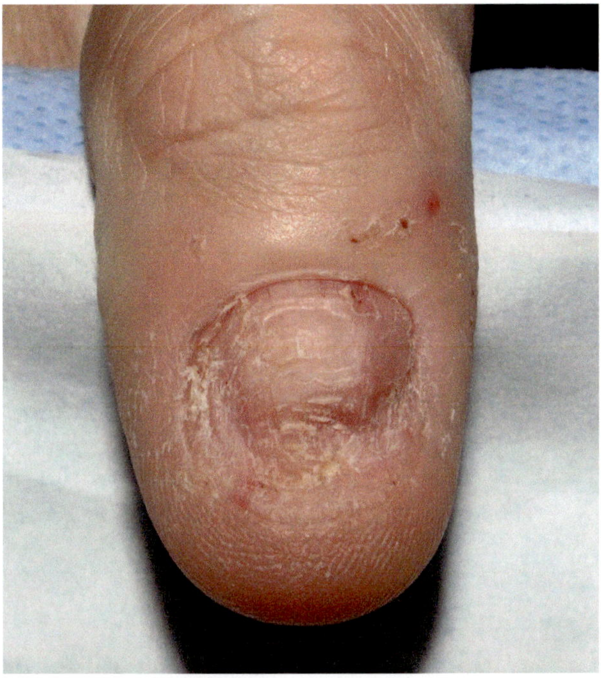

Fig. 20.2 38-Year-old female, Fitzpatrick type II, onychotillomania, with short and dystrophic right thumbnail and nail fold erosions

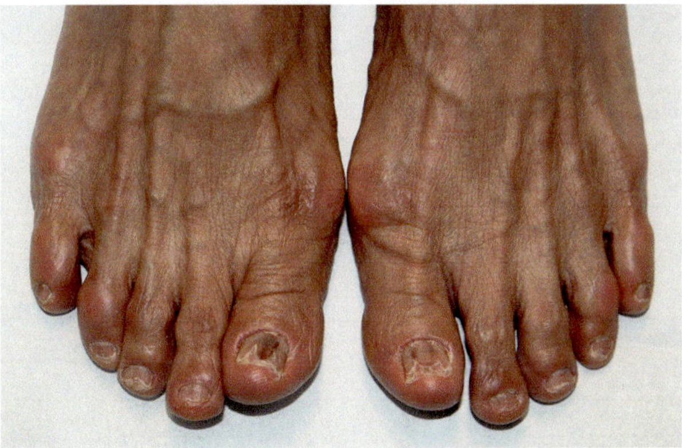

Fig. 20.3 70-Year-old female, Fitzpatrick type III, onychotillomania, with thin and shortened nail plate and missing cuticles, mainly affecting the bilateral great toenails

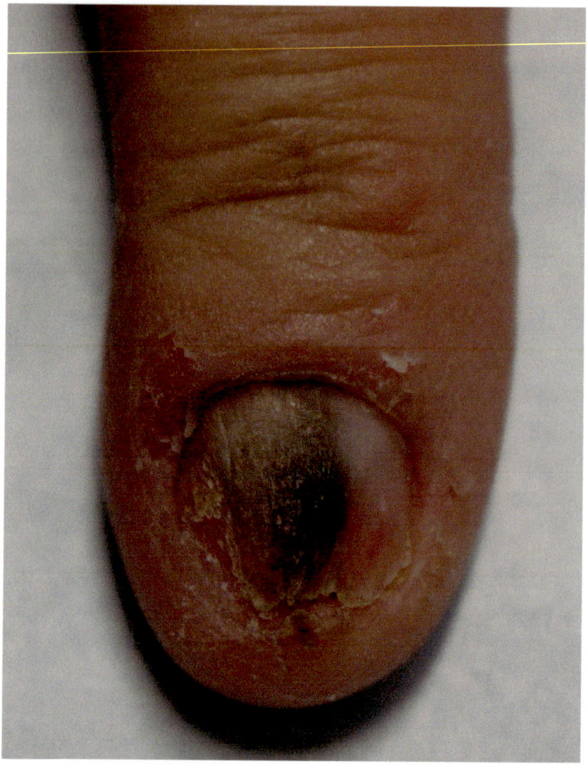

Fig. 20.4 60-Year-old male, Fitzpatrick type III, onychotillomania, with short and uneven right second fingernail accompanied by nail fold erosions and a longitudinal grey-brown band of the nail plate

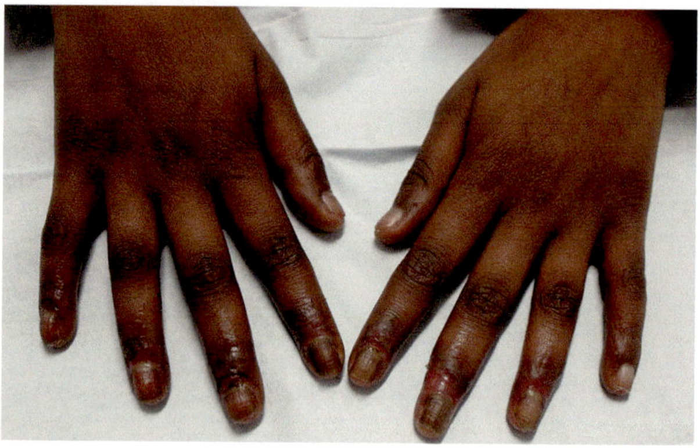

Fig. 20.5 10-Year-old female, Fitzpatrick type IV, onychotillomania, with nail fold erosions, yellowing, and thickening of all fingernails

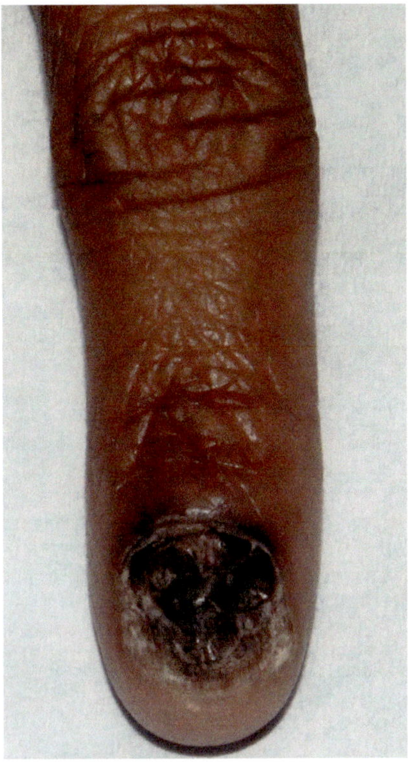

Fig. 20.6 33-Year-old female, Fitzpatrick type IV, onychotillomania, with ridges, grooves, diffuse gray-brown pigmentation, shortened nailbed, and general dystrophy of the right second fingernail

References

1. Halteh P, Scher RK, Lipner SR. Onychotillomania: diagnosis and management. Am J Clin Dermatol. 2017;18(6):763–70. https://doi.org/10.1007/s40257-017-0289-6.
2. Starace M, Cedirian S, Alessandrini A, Bruni F, Piraccini BM, Iorizzo M. Self-induced nail disorders (SINDs): what do we know so far? Ann Dermatol Venereol. 2023;150(4):253–9. https://doi.org/10.1016/j.annder.2023.05.005.
3. Sidiropoulou P, Sgouros D, Theodoropoulos K, Katoulis A, Rigopoulos D. Onychotillomania: a chameleon-like disorder: case report and review of literature. Skin Appendage Disord. 2019;5(2):104–7. https://doi.org/10.1159/000489941.
4. Pacan P, Grzesiak M, Reich A, Kantorska-Janiec M, Szepietowski JC. Onychophagia and onychotillomania: prevalence, clinical picture and comorbidities. Acta Derm Venereol. 2014;94(1):67–71. https://doi.org/10.2340/00015555-1616.
5. Wu AG, Lin K, Cooley V, Lipner SR. A cross-sectional study of onychotillomania and onychophagia in graduate students. Dermatol Ther. 2021;34(1):e14639. https://doi.org/10.1111/dth.14639.
6. Chen Y, Pradhan S, Lyu L, Xue S. Clinical and dermoscopic characteristics of onychophagia and onychotillomania: a retrospective study of 63 cases. Clin Exp Dermatol. 2022;47(5):961–3. https://doi.org/10.1111/ced.15057.
7. Koo JY, Smith LL. Obsessive-compulsive disorders in the pediatric dermatology practice. Pediatr Dermatol. 1991;8(2):107–13. https://doi.org/10.1111/j.1525-1470.1991.tb00296.x.
8. Lee DK, Lipner SR. Update on diagnosis and management of onychophagia and onychotillomania. Int J Environ Res Public Health. 2022;19(6):3392. https://doi.org/10.3390/ijerph19063392.

9. Reese JM, Hudacek KD, Rubin AI. Onychotillomania: clinicopathologic correlations. J Cutan Pathol. 2013;40(4):419–23. https://doi.org/10.1111/cup.12098.
10. Grzesiak M, Pacan P, Reich A, Szepietowski JC. Onychotillomania in the course of depression: a case report. Acta Derm Venereol. 2014;94(6):745–6. https://doi.org/10.2340/00015555-1805.
11. Rieder EA, Tosti A. Onychotillomania: an underrecognized disorder. J Am Acad Dermatol. 2016;75(6):1245–50. https://doi.org/10.1016/j.jaad.2016.05.036.
12. Lin YC, Lin YC. Onychotillomania, major depressive disorder and suicide. Clin Exp Dermatol. 2006;31(4):597–9. https://doi.org/10.1111/j.1365-2230.2006.02143.x.
13. Smith ACM, Boyd KE, Brennan C, et al. Smith-Magenis syndrome. In: Adam MP, Feldman J, Mirzaa GM, et al., editors. GeneReviews® [Internet]. Seattle, WA: University of Washington; 2001. https://www.ncbi.nlm.nih.gov/books/NBK1310/.
14. National Institute of Neurological Disorders and Stroke. Lesch-Nyhan syndrome. https://www.ninds.nih.gov/health-information/disorders/lesch-nyhan-syndrome. Accessed 19 Mar 2024.
15. Curtis KL, Lipner SR. Supplementary material for: Body focused repetitive behaviors in patients with FOXP1 syndrome: an international cross-sectional survey-based study. Karger Publishers; 2024. https://doi.org/10.6084/m9.figshare.25232255.v1.
16. Abdo HM. Marvelous response of severe onychotillomania to treatment with local steroid injection plus topical calcipotriol/betamethasone dipropionate combination. Skin Appendage Disord. 2020;6(3):158–61. https://doi.org/10.1159/000506139.
17. Bayes A, Parker G. Onychotillomania and secondary foot cellulitis. Aust N Z J Psychiatry. 2017;51(11):1158–9. https://doi.org/10.1177/0004867417710732.
18. Baran R. Nail biting and picking as a possible cause of longitudinal melanonychia. A study of 6 cases. Dermatologica. 1990;181(2):126–8. https://doi.org/10.1159/000247900.
19. Maddy AJ, Tosti A. Dermoscopic features of onychotillomania: a study of 36 cases. J Am Acad Dermatol. 2018;79(4):702–5. https://doi.org/10.1016/j.jaad.2018.04.015.
20. Singal A, Daulatabad D. Nail tic disorders: manifestations, pathogenesis and management. Indian J Dermatol Venereol Leprol. 2017;83(1):19–26. https://doi.org/10.4103/0378-6323.184202.

Habit-Tic Deformity

21

Rachel C. Hill and Shari R. Lipner

21.1 Description of Disease

Habit-tic deformity, or "washboard nails," is a type of body-focused repetitive behavior in which an individual, consciously or subconsciously, uses a finger and/or fingernail, typically the second digit, to repeatedly rub the proximal nail fold of an adjacent fingernail, typically the thumb. This habitual behavior traumatizes the nail matrix and results in characteristic grooves in the affected nail. While some argue that median canaliform nail dystrophy (MCND) is a distinct clinical entity from habit-tic deformity due to the lack of cuticle involvement in the former, it is more likely that the two lie on a spectrum [1, 2]. Habit-tic deformity is classified as a nail tic disorder [2–4].

21.2 Epidemiology

21.2.1 Sex

While it is a very commonly observed clinical finding, the epidemiology of habit-tic deformity is understudied. No studies have suggested a sex predilection for habit-tic deformity. Both men and women are affected. In a prospective case series of eight patients with habit-tic deformity by Elmas et al., most patients were male ($n = 6$) [2]. Similarly, in a case series of five patients with MCND or habit-tic deformity by Mooney et al., four patients were male [5].

S. R. Lipner, *Atlas of Nail Disorders Across All Skin Colors*,
https://doi.org/10.1007/978-3-031-74272-9_21

21.2.2 Age

While habit-tic deformity is typically acquired in adulthood, case reports have described the condition in children as young as seven [1, 6, 7]. In the case series of five patients with MCND or habit-tic deformity by Mooney et al., patient ages ranged from nine to 62 years old, with a mean of 34.6 years and a median of 32 years [5].

21.3 Risk Factors

Several risk factors have been proposed for habit-tic deformity, although the data available to support such associations are lacking [8]. The association of habit-tic deformity with psychiatric conditions, including obsessive-compulsive disorder (OCD), remains controversial. In the prospective case series of eight patients with habit-tic deformity by Elmas et al., two patients reported a history of OCD at the time of their evaluation, while one patient was diagnosed with OCD after additional psychiatric evaluation [2]. Previous case reports have also suggested associations of habit-tic deformity with anxiety and major depression [6, 9]. A retrospective case series by Cohen suggested that patients with nail-focused body-focused repetitive behaviors, including habit-tic deformity, may be more likely to develop other body-focused repetitive behaviors, such as skin biting, and vice versa [10].

Stress is also purported to play a role in the development of nail tic disorders [3, 7–9, 11]. In a retrospective case series of two patients with alopecia areata and habit-tic deformity, both patients admitted to traumatizing their nails out of habit due to the psychosocial and emotional stress caused by chronic hair loss [4].

External trauma other than self-induced rubbing and picking may also play a role in the development of habit-tic deformity. In a single case report of an otherwise healthy late twenties male, trauma resulting from recreational guitar playing was identified as the cause of the habit-tic deformity. The nail changes resolved when the patient ceased to play guitar. As such, external trauma to the fingernails caused by activities such as playing string-based instruments should be considered [12].

21.4 Clinical Features

Habit-tic deformity has a characteristic clinical presentation that results from conscious or unconscious picking, biting, rubbing, or pushing the back of the cuticle and proximal nail fold [2]. The affected nail plate shows a longitudinal midline furrow with parallel, transverse grooves of variable width [13, 14]. The midline furrow is often yellow, grey, or brown and extends the length of the nail plate from the proximal nail fold to the distal nail edge [14, 15]. Macrolunula and altered cuticles are also typically present, the latter of which distinguishes habit-tic deformity from

MCND [16]. The cuticle may be damaged, detached, or completely absent with a lack of adhesion of the nail plate to the proximal nail fold [3, 17]. In severe cases, the lunula may be hypertrophic to the point that the nail matrix is exposed [3, 17]. Elkonyxis, which is a form of nail dystrophy consisting of a "punched-out" appearance of the nail plate beginning at the proximal nail fold, has also been described in association with habit-tic deformity [18]. Notably, when the nail-damaging behaviors cease, the nail plate will return to normal after several months [19].

The bilateral thumbnails are most frequently affected by habit-tic deformity [17]. However, other fingernails and the toenails can also be affected [7, 17]. In rare and severe instances, all fingernails may be affected [16]. Individuals typically use the second or third fingers or fingernails, or the contralateral thumb, to push back the cuticle of the affected nail, which produces the characteristic "washboard" appearance.

Due to manipulation of the nail matrix, patients with habit-tic deformity may also develop physiologic longitudinal melanonychia (LM) caused by melanocyte activation [10]. Trauma to the nails can also increase susceptibility to infection, including acute paronychia, inflammation, chronic paronychia, and periungual or subungual warts [20].

While habit-tic deformity is typically apparent on clinical examination alone, onychoscopy may be used to characterize clinical features and to identify more subtle signs of trauma, including microhemorrhage and onycholysis [2]. In the prospective case series of onyschopic features of habit-tic deformity in eight patients by Elmas et al., the most common findings were transverse grooves (100%, $n = 8$), periungual scale (100%, $n = 8$), macrolunula (87.5%, $n = 7$), longitudinal grooves (87.5%, $n = 7$), branching grooves (75%, $n = 6$), and erythematous proximal lunula (62.5%, $n = 5$) [2].

21.5 Clinical Features in Skin of Color

Distinct clinical features of habit-tic deformity in patients with skin of color have not been previously described. However, patients with darker skin tones may also have accompanying physiologic LM.

21.6 Requirements for Diagnosis

Habit-tic deformity is a clinical diagnosis that is made when the characteristic features of nail plate deformity, including a longitudinal midline furrow with parallel transverse grooves, and cuticle damage are present in addition to a history of habitual, external trauma to the nail matrix [2, 6]. In some cases, patients may be unaware of the habit, in which case onychoscopy may be used to examine subtle clinical features to support the diagnosis [2].

21.7 Cases

Figures 21.1, 21.2, 21.3, 21.4, 21.5, 21.6, and 21.7 demonstrate the presentation of habit-tic deformity in a clinical setting.

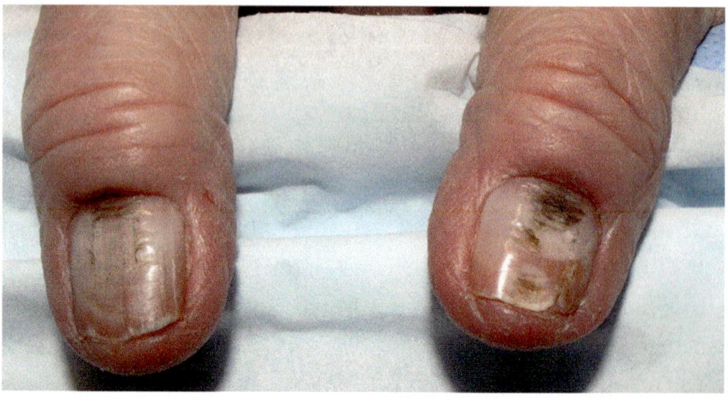

Fig. 21.1 80-Year-old female, Fitzpatrick type I, habit-tic deformity, with parallel grooves and missing cuticles of the bilateral thumbnails

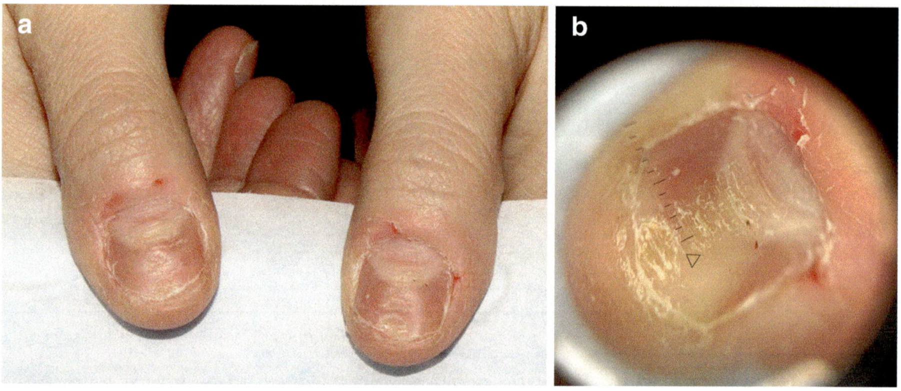

Fig. 21.2 (**a**) 39-Year-old female, Fitzpatrick type II, habit-tic deformity, with macrolunula and parallel transverse grooves of the bilateral thumbs with erosions on the nail folds reflecting complications of nail biting/picking. (**b**) These changes were also appreciated with dermoscopy

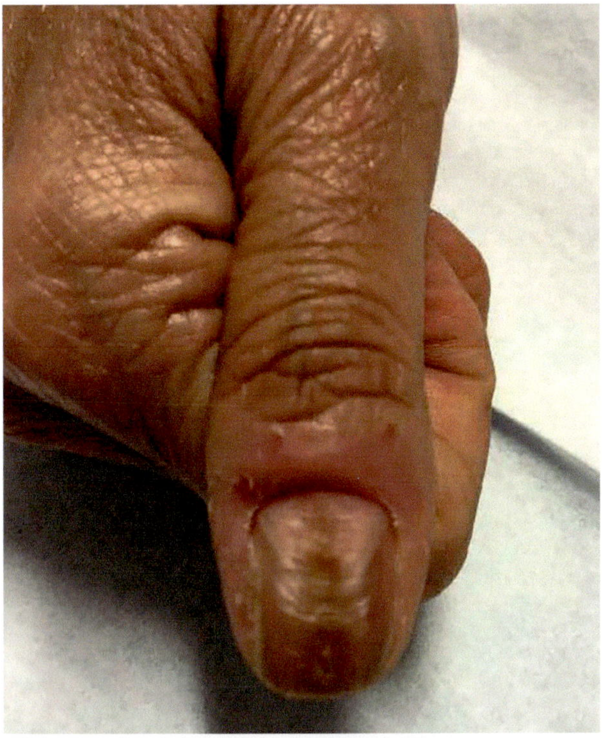

Fig. 21.3 54-Year-old female, Fitzpatrick type III, habit-tic deformity, with parallel transverse grooves, macrolunula, erythema erosions of nail folds, and missing cuticle involving the right thumbnail

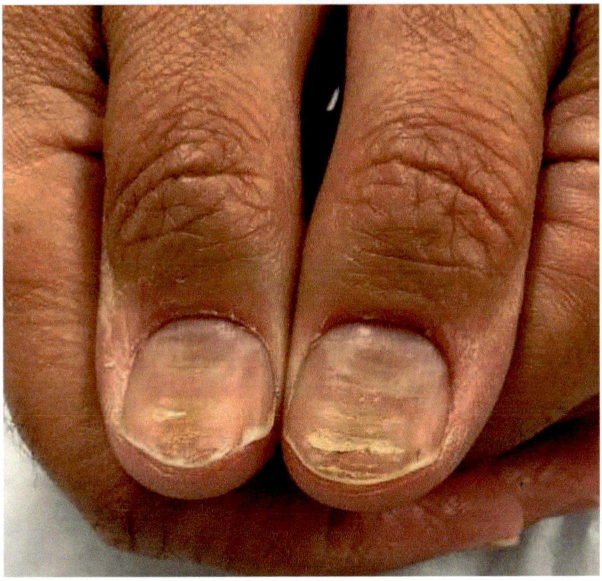

Fig. 21.4 48-Year-old male, Fitzpatrick type IV, habit-tic deformity, with parallel transverse grooves, absent cuticles, and erythema of the nail folds involving the bilateral thumbnails

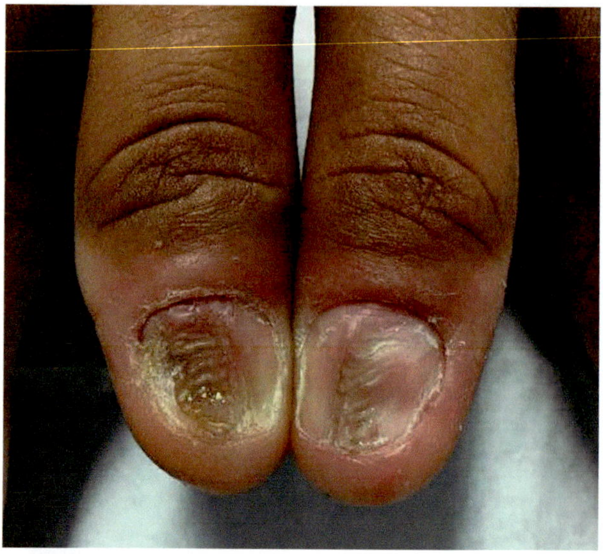

Fig. 21.5 43-Year-old male, Fitzpatrick type V, habit-tic deformity, with parallel grooves and missing cuticles involving the bilateral thumbnails

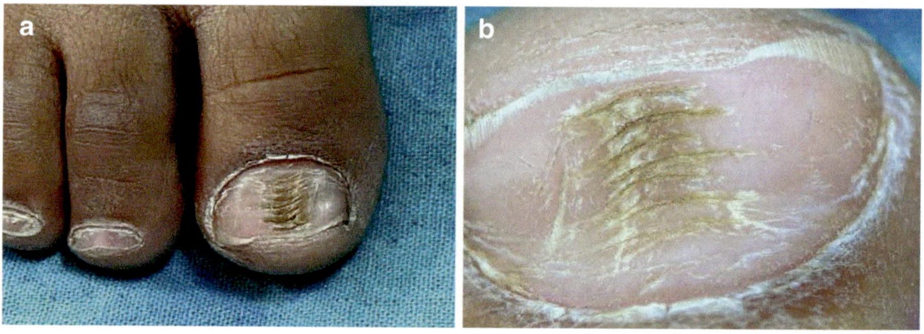

Fig. 21.6 Female patient of unknown age, Fitzpatrick type V, habit-tic deformity, with broad median longitudinal dystrophy and multiple parallel yellow-brown nail plate depressions of the right great toenail (image reused from Starace et al. with permissions)

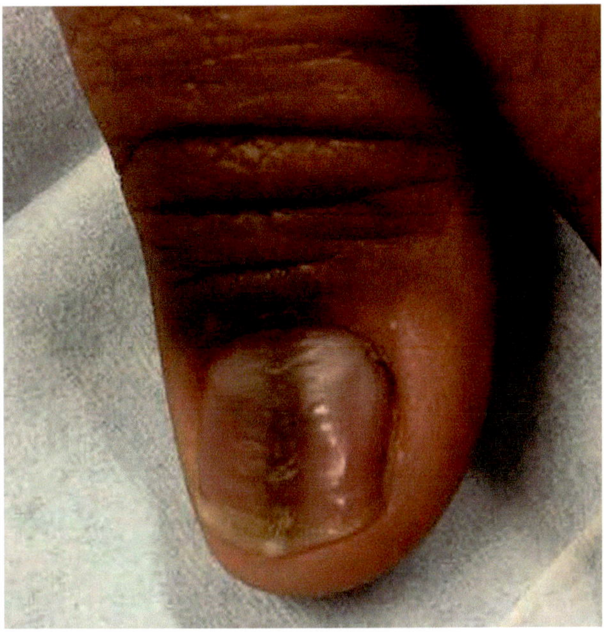

Fig. 21.7 47-Year-old woman, Fitzpatrick type V, habit-tic deformity, with light brown longitudinal band and transverse grooves involving the left thumbnail

References

1. El-Heis S, Abadie A. Habit tic nail deformity—a rare presentation in an 8 year old boy. Dermatol Online J. 2016;22(11):13030/qt16j6x5n3.
2. Elmas ÖF, Demirbaş A. Utility of dermatoscopy in the diagnosis of Habit-Tic Nail Deformity. J Cosmet Dermatol. 2021;20(2):703–4. https://doi.org/10.1111/jocd.13551.
3. Singal A, Daulatabad D. Nail tic disorders: manifestations, pathogenesis and management. Indian J Dermatol Venereol Leprol. 2017;83(1):19–26. https://doi.org/10.4103/0378-6323.184202.
4. Horne MI, Utzig JB, Rieder EA, Vincenzi C, Tosti A. Alopecia areata and habit tic deformities. Skin Appendage Disord. 2018;4(4):323–5. https://doi.org/10.1159/000486540.
5. Mooney E, Mahar P, Howard A. Median canaliform and habit-tic deformity of the nail: is there an association with macrolunulae? Australas J Dermatol. 2016;57(4):319–20. https://doi.org/10.1111/ajd.12377.
6. Perrin AJ, Lam JM. Habit-tic deformity. CMAJ. 2014;186(5):371. https://doi.org/10.1503/cmaj.121942.
7. Singal A. Habit tic deformity of bilateral thumb and toenails in a young boy: an unusual occurrence. Skin Appendage Disord. 2017;3(4):186–7. https://doi.org/10.1159/000474953.
8. Sonthalia S, Sharma P, Kapoor J, Singh P. Habit tic deformity: need for a comprehensive approach. Skin Appendage Disord. 2019;5(2):117–8. https://doi.org/10.1159/000489320.
9. Vittorio CC, Phillips KA. Treatment of habit-tic deformity with fluoxetine. Arch Dermatol. 1997;133(10):1203–4.
10. Cohen PR. Nail-associated body-focused repetitive behaviors: habit-tic nail deformity, onychophagia, and onychotillomania. Cureus. 2022;14(3):e22818. https://doi.org/10.7759/cureus.22818.
11. Kota R, Pilani A, Nair PA. Median nail dystrophy involving the thumb nail. Indian J Dermatol. 2016;61(1):120. https://doi.org/10.4103/0019-5154.174092.
12. Wu JJ. Habit tic deformity secondary to guitar playing. Dermatol Online J. 2009;15(3):16.

13. Geizhals S, Lipner SR. Clinical pearl: benzethonium chloride for habit-tic nail deformity. Cutis. 2019;104(1):81–2.
14. Griego RD, Orengo IF, Scher RK. Median nail dystrophy and habit tic deformity: are they different forms of the same disorder? Int J Dermatol. 1995;34(11):799–800. https://doi.org/10.1111/j.1365-4362.1995.tb04402.x.
15. Najafi S, Aronowitz P, Thompson GR III. The habit tic: onychotillomania. J Gen Intern Med. 2015;30(2):264. https://doi.org/10.1007/s11606-014-2991-x.
16. Jimenez-Cauhe J, Fernandez-Gonzalez P. Visual dermatology: a rare case of habit-tic deformity in all fingernails. J Cutan Med Surg. 2020;24(6):637. https://doi.org/10.1177/1203475420931777.
17. Starace M, Cedirian S, Alessandrini A, Bruni F, Piraccini BM, Iorizzo M. Self-induced nail disorders (SINDs): what do we know so far? Ann Dermatol Venereol. 2023;150(4):253–9. https://doi.org/10.1016/j.annder.2023.05.005.
18. Kim M, Jung HY, Kang JH, Cho BK, Park HJ. Elkonyxis associated with habit-tic deformity: two case reports. J Dermatol. 2014;41(8):772–3. https://doi.org/10.1111/1346-8138.12515.
19. Lipner SR. Habit tic nail deformity. J Cutan Med Surg. 2018;22(2):222. https://doi.org/10.1177/1203475417733468.
20. Tosti A, Piraccini BM. Warts of the nail unit: surgical and nonsurgical approaches. Dermatologic Surg. 2001;27(3):235–9.

Onychophagia

22

Rachel C. Hill and Shari R. Lipner

22.1 Description of Disease

Onychophagia describes chronic, habitual nail biting [1] and is classified as a body-focused repetitive behavior (BFRB) [2]. Biting may involve the nail plate, nail bed, nail matrix, and periungual skin [3] with varying clinical presentations dictated by the extent and severity of biting [4]. It is estimated that onychophagia affects between 20% and 30% of the general population [4–10]. Due to its association with psychiatric comorbidities, negative social implications, and embarrassment, onychophagia is often underrecognized in clinical practice, which may impact prevalence estimates [4, 11].

22.2 Epidemiology

22.2.1 Sex

The sex predilection of onychophagia is not well studied [5, 12–14]. In a cross-sectional survey-based study of nail biting among 362 physicians, 328 (93.0%) respondents were female, of whom 82/328 (25.0%) reported a nail-biting history, compared with 4/25 males (16.0%) ($P > 0.05$) [12]. In a cross-sectional survey study by Winebrake et al., including 281 participants administered at an outpatient pediatric clinic in New York, USA, 55 respondents were female (53%), and 49 respondents were male (47%) [5]. In a cross-sectional survey study of 181 graduate students ages 18–45 years old with onychophagia or onychotillomania at a medical school in New York, USA, by Wu et al., including 98 students with past or present onychophagia, the male-to-female ratio of students with onychophagia was 34:48 [15].

S. R. Lipner, *Atlas of Nail Disorders Across All Skin Colors*,
https://doi.org/10.1007/978-3-031-74272-9_22

22.2.2 Age

Although onychophagia can occur at any age, it is particularly prevalent in the pediatric population, with an estimated prevalence of 45% in children between the ages of 10 and the onset of puberty [4, 8, 10]. In Winebrake et al.'s cross-sectional survey-based study including 281 pediatric participants, 104 patients reported past or present nail biting behaviors that lasted ≥1 month (37%), with the age of onset at a median age of five years old, with a range of 1–13 years old [5]. As age increases, the prevalence of nail biting decreases, likely due to a lack of social acceptance of the behavior and feelings of shame [4, 8, 10]. However, nail biting may be replaced by nail picking [4]. Likewise, nail biting habits may be underreported by adult patients due to reluctance to admit to the behavior. In adults, nail biting may function as a means of stress relief [16].

22.3 Risk Factors

As with other BFRBs, onychophagia is associated with psychiatric disorders [17]. In Winebrake et al.'s cross-sectional survey-based study of 281 pediatric participants, subjects who reported nail biting were more often diagnosed with a psychiatric comorbidity compared to those who did not report nail biting (19/104, 18% vs. 11/177, 6%, $P < 0.01$) [5]. In the cross-sectional survey study of 181 graduate students with onychophagia or onychotillomania by Wu et al., including 98 students with past or present onychophagia, 34 students (34.7%) reported having a psychiatric disorder, most commonly anxiety, depression, and obsessive-compulsive disorder (21.0%, 21.0%, and 5.1%, respectively) [15].

Onychophagia may be exacerbated by stress. In a cross-sectional survey study evaluating onychophagia using the perceived stress scale (PSS) and European health impact scale among 3475 university and high school students, the PSS score was significantly higher among university students who reported onychophagia (median PSS 29.0) vs. those who did not (median PSS 28.0, $P < 0.001$). University students who reported nail biting also reported a lower quality of life score on the European health impact scale vs. those who did not bite (median 26.0 vs. 28.0, $P < 0.001$) [18]. In Wu et al.'s cross-sectional survey-based study of 181 graduate students, 98 of 181 total participants (54.1%) reported past or present nail biting, with stress reported as the top reason for biting in 33.2% of respondents [15].

Notably, onychophagia affects children who have family members with nail biting habits, which may be due to a genetic component or through learned behaviors at home [4]. In a cross-sectional survey study of 743 parents with school-aged children in Iran, including 166 children with a parent that reported nail biting, 13.2% of children bit their nails and had a parent with a similar habit ($n = 22$), while 22.9% had a sibling with a similar habit ($n = 38$) [10]. Similarly, in Winebrake et al.'s cross-sectional survey-based study of 281 pediatric participants, 65 of 101 respondents with a nail biting history (63%) reported that they had family members who also bit their nails [5].

22.4 Clinical Features

Both the fingernails and toenails can be affected by onychophagia, although toenails are rarely affected [5, 19]. In Winebrake et al.'s cross-sectional survey-based study of 281 pediatric participants, the majority of patients reported fingernail biting vs. fingernail and toenail biting (92/104, 88% vs. 12/104, 12%, respectively). The ratio of fingernail and toenail biters to only fingernail biters in this study was greater among patients with co-diagnosis of a psychiatric disorder vs. those without (0.36 vs. 0.09, $P = 0.07$) [5]. The clinical features of onychophagia are dictated by the extent of biting, and whether it is confined to the nail plate, or if it also extends to the periungual skin, nail bed, and/or nail matrix. Clinical features of onychophagia include abnormally short nails with uneven edges accompanied by erythematous or ragged cuticles with or without splinter hemorrhages [6]. If nail matrix damage is involved, Beau's lines and other textural abnormalities to the nail plate may occur [16]. Longitudinal melanonychia may also develop due to melanocytic activation resulting from damage to the nail matrix [16, 20]. In a retrospective study of 53 patients with onychophagia, 48 patients (90.6%) had only fingernail involvement vs. five patients (9.4%), with both fingernail and toenail involvement. In this study, the six most common clinical features of onychophagia included short nails with a ragged distal border ($n = 53$, 100%), a patchy or rough area of the surrounding skin ($n = 27$, 50.9%), linear and pinpoint hemorrhage ($n = 17$, 32.1%), longitudinal melanonychia ($n = 16$, 30.2%), transverse grooves ($n = 15$, 28.3%), and brittleness ($n = 15$, 28.3%) [11].

The complications of onychophagia can range from mild to severe. Chronic nail biting can lead to permanent shortening of the nail plate [4]. Periungual and subungual verruca vulgaris have been reported secondary to onychophagia [21, 22]. Acute paronychia may occur due to the transfer of bacteria from the mouth to the digit [4], which in rare case reports has been associated with osteomyelitis with bacterial spread from periungual skin to bone [6, 23, 24]. Chronic paronychia may ensue due to long-standing inflammation and cuticle loss [4]. Dental complications have also been reported, including abscess and crowding or rotation of the incisors, among others [4, 6, 25, 26].

Onychoscopy is a useful adjunct to aid in diagnosing onychophagia. In a retrospective study of 63 patients with onychophagia and/or onychotillomania, including 25 patients with only onychophagia, patients with onychophagia vs. onychotillomania more often had lamellar onychoschizia ($P < 0.01$), saw-toothed nail fringe ($P = 0.01$), shortening of the nail plate ($P = 0.01$), and subungual hyperkeratosis ($P < 0.02$) on onychoscopic exam [27].

22.5 Clinical Features in Skin of Color

Although features of onychophagia in the skin of color patients have not been explicitly described, patients with skin of color are more likely than lighter-skinned patients to have physiologic melanonychia affecting the fingernails and toenails, which may complicate the clinical diagnosis.

22.6 Requirements for Diagnosis

Onychophagia is a clinical diagnosis that is made when characteristic clinical features are present, including a shortened nail plate with a jagged and uneven edge, accompanied by a history of nail biting behaviors [6]. However, due to the similarities between the clinical appearance of onychophagia and other dermatologic conditions, including nail psoriasis and nail lichen planus [17], and a reluctance to admit to the habit by some patients [6, 17], a high index of clinical suspicion is required to clinch the diagnosis. Patients may benefit from psychiatric evaluation if the habit is severe [4, 19, 27, 28].

22.7 Cases

Figures 22.1, 22.2, 22.3, 22.4, and 22.5 demonstrate the presentation of onychophagia in a clinical setting.

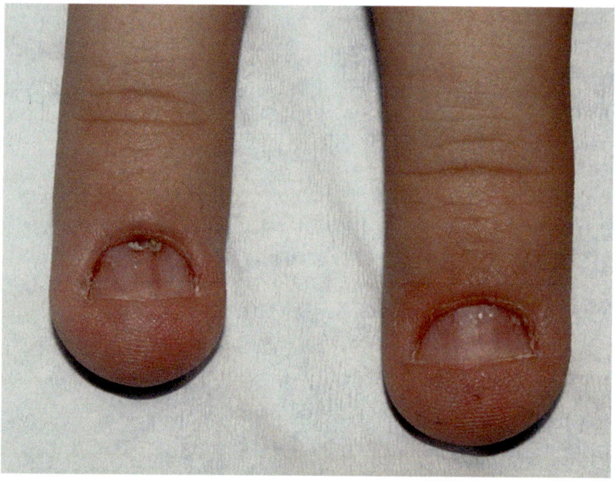

Fig. 22.1 15-Year-old male, Fitzpatrick type II, onychophagia, with short nail plates affecting the left second and third fingernails

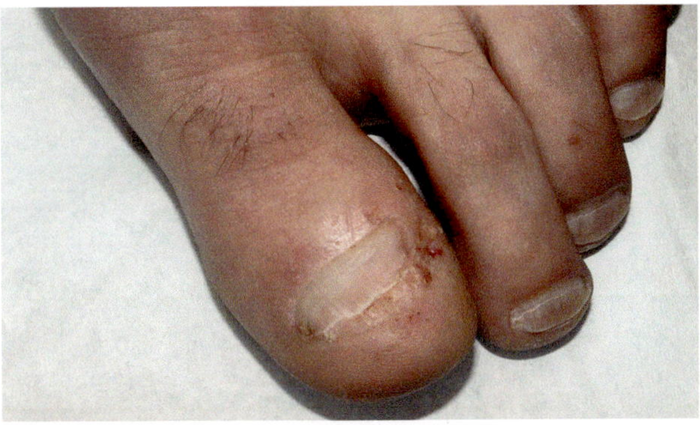

Fig. 22.2 56-Year-old male, Fitzpatrick type II, onychophagia, with short and dystrophic left great toenail accompanied by medial nail fold erosions

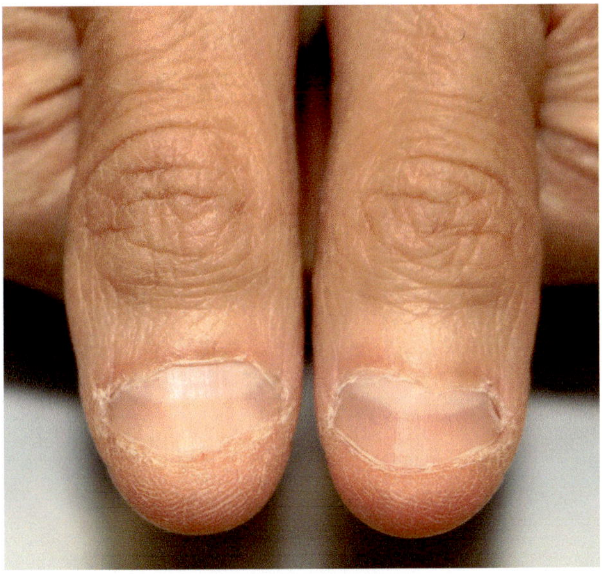

Fig. 22.3 41-Year-old male, Fitzpatrick type II, onychophagia, with short nail plates involving the bilateral thumbnails

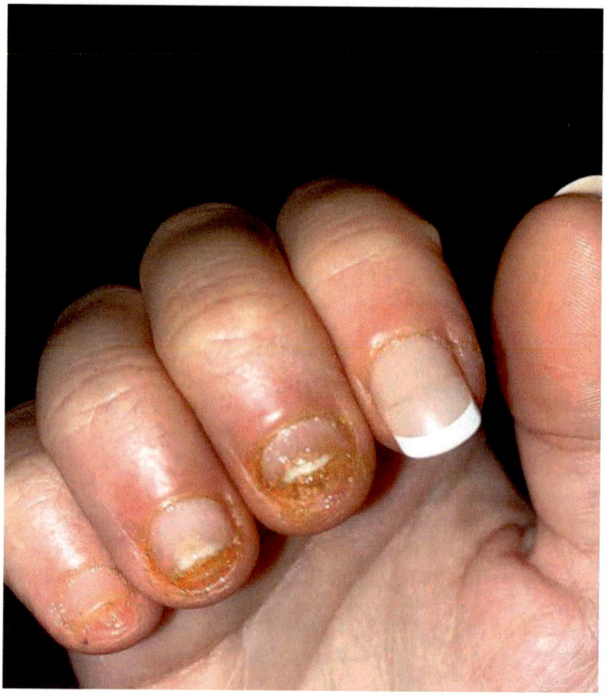

Fig. 22.4 41-Year-old female, Fitzpatrick type III, onychophagia complicated by acute paronychia The right third-fifth fingernails are short with onycholysis. There is purulent discharge. The patient had been applying acrylic nails

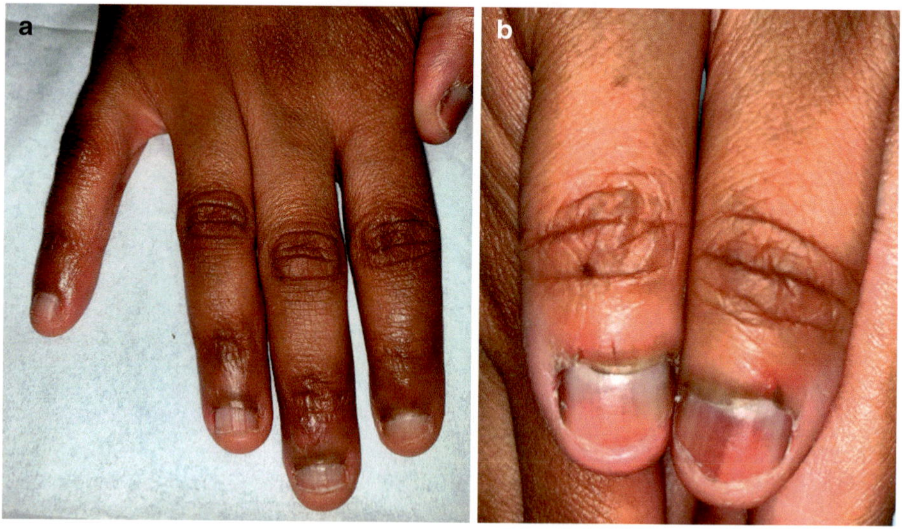

Fig. 22.5 (**a**) 45-Year-old female, Fitzpatrick type IV, onychophagia, with short, uneven nail plates affecting all fingernails of the right hand. (**b**) Bilateral thumbnails with gray longitudinal bands and erythema and erosions of the proximal and lateral nail folds

References

1. Ha EL, Magid M. Psychopharmacology in dermatology: five common disorders. Clin Dermatol. 2023;41(1):112–20. https://doi.org/10.1016/j.clindermatol.2023.03.010.
2. Gu L, Pathoulas JT, Widge AS, Idnani A, Lipner SR. Exacerbation of onychophagia and onychotillomania during the COVID-19 pandemic: a survey-based study. Int J Dermatol. 2022;61(11):e412–4. https://doi.org/10.1111/ijd.16395.
3. Cohen PR. Nail-associated body-focused repetitive behaviors: habit-tic nail deformity, onychophagia, and onychotillomania. Cureus. 2022;14(3):e22818. https://doi.org/10.7759/cureus.22818.
4. Lee DK, Lipner SR. Update on diagnosis and management of onychophagia and onychotillomania. Int J Environ Res Public Health. 2022;19(6):3392. https://doi.org/10.3390/ijerph19063392.
5. Winebrake JP, Grover K, Halteh P, Lipner SR. Pediatric onychophagia: a survey-based study of prevalence, etiologies, and co-morbidities. Am J Clin Dermatol. 2018;19(6):887–91. https://doi.org/10.1007/s40257-018-0386-1.
6. Halteh P, Scher RK, Lipner SR. Onychophagia: a nail-biting conundrum for physicians. J Dermatol Treat. 2017;28(2):166–72. https://doi.org/10.1080/09546634.2016.1200711.
7. Garde JB, Suryavanshi RK, Jawale BA, Deshmukh V, Dadhe DP, Suryavanshi MK. An epidemiological study to know the prevalence of deleterious oral habits among 6 to 12 year old children. J Int Oral Health. 2014;6(1):39–43.
8. Foster LG. Nervous habits and stereotyped behaviors in preschool children. J Am Acad Child Adolesc Psychiatry. 1998;37(7):711–7. https://doi.org/10.1097/00004583-199807000-00010.
9. Shetty SR, Munshi AK. Oral habits in children—a prevalence study. J Indian Soc Pedod Prev Dent. 1998;16(2):61–6.
10. Ghanizadeh A, Shekoohi H. Prevalence of nail biting and its association with mental health in a community sample of children. BMC Res Notes. 2011;4:116. https://doi.org/10.1186/1756-0500-4-116.
11. Shin JO, Roh D, Son JH, et al. Onychophagia: detailed clinical characteristics. Int J Dermatol. 2022;61(3):331–6. https://doi.org/10.1111/ijd.15861.
12. Lesinskiene S, Pociute K, Dervinyte-Bongarzoni A, Kinciniene O. Onychophagia as a clinical symptom: a pilot study of physicians and literature review. Sci Prog. 2021;104(4):00368504211050288. https://doi.org/10.1177/00368504211050288.
13. Gür K, Erol S, İncir N. The effectiveness of a nail-biting prevention program among primary school students. J Spec Pediatr Nurs. 2018;23(3):e12219. https://doi.org/10.1111/jspn.12219.
14. Selles RR, La Buissonnière Ariza V, McBride NM, Dammann J, Whiteside S, Storch EA. Initial psychometrics, outcomes, and correlates of the Repetitive Body Focused Behavior Scale: examination in a sample of youth with anxiety and/or obsessive-compulsive disorder. Compr Psychiatry. 2018;81:10–7. https://doi.org/10.1016/j.comppsych.2017.11.001.
15. Wu AG, Lin K, Cooley V, Lipner SR. A cross-sectional study of onychotillomania and onychophagia in graduate students. Dermatol Ther. 2021;34(1):e14639. https://doi.org/10.1111/dth.14639.
16. Starace M, Cedirian S, Alessandrini A, Bruni F, Piraccini BM, Iorizzo M. Self-induced nail disorders (SINDs): what do we know so far? Ann Dermatol Venereol. 2023;150(4):253–9. https://doi.org/10.1016/j.annder.2023.05.005.
17. Gupta MA, Gupta AK. Self-induced dermatoses: a great imitator. Clin Dermatol. 2019;37(3):268–77. https://doi.org/10.1016/j.clindermatol.2019.01.006.
18. Erdogan HK, Arslantas D, Atay E, et al. Prevalence of onychophagia and its relation to stress and quality of life. Acta Dermatovenerol Alp Pannonica Adriat. 2021;30(1):15–9.
19. Mosca M, Martin K, Hadeler E, Hong J, Brownstone N, Koo J. Review of the diagnosis and management of pediatric psychodermatologic conditions: Part I. Pediatr Dermatol. 2022;39(1):17–21. https://doi.org/10.1111/pde.14888.

20. Anolik RB, Shah K, Rubin AI. Onychophagia-induced longitudinal melanonychia. Pediatr Dermatol. 2012;29(4):488–9. https://doi.org/10.1111/j.1525-1470.2011.01496.x.
21. Sil A, Priyam P, Mondol DK. Nail biter's wart: hands that feed the mouth. J Paediatr Child Health. 2020;56(6):991. https://doi.org/10.1111/jpc.14920.
22. Patidar S. Combination treatment of periungual warts. J Cutan Aesthet Surg. 2008;1(1):23–4. https://doi.org/10.4103/0974-2077.41154.
23. Rivera JA, Aragon D, Thomas PM, et al. Bitten to the bone: a case of anxiety-induced osteomyelitis. Cureus. 2022;14(11):e31511. https://doi.org/10.7759/cureus.31511.
24. Hoof M, Cognetti DJ, McClain WD, Plucknette B. Recurrent osteomyelitis requiring surgical management secondary to nail-biting: a case report. JBJS Case Connect. 2021;11(4):e21.00346.
25. Sachan A, Chaturvedi T. Onychophagia (nail biting), anxiety, and malocclusion. Indian J Dent Res. 2012;23(5):680–2.
26. Sousa D, Pinto D, Araujo R, Rego RO, Moreira-Neto J. Gingival abscess due to an unusual nail-biting habit: a case report. J Contemp Dent Pract. 2010;11(2):085–91.
27. Chen Y, Pradhan S, Lyu L, Xue S. Clinical and dermoscopic characteristics of onychophagia and onychotillomania: a retrospective study of 63 cases. Clin Exp Dermatol. 2022;47(5):961–3. https://doi.org/10.1111/ced.15057.
28. Magid M, Mennella C, Kuhn H, Stamu-O'Brien C, Kroumpouzos G. Onychophagia and onychotillomania can be effectively managed. J Am Acad Dermatol. 2017;77(5):e143–4. https://doi.org/10.1016/j.jaad.2017.06.154.

Myxoid Cyst

23

Rachel C. Hill and Shari R. Lipner

23.1 Description of Disease

Digital myxoid cyst, also known as digital mucous cyst or myxoid pseudocyst, refers to a benign nodule that is most commonly located between the distal interphalangeal (DIP) joint and the proximal nail fold on the dorsal aspect of a finger or toe [1]. Myxoid cysts are the second most common type of benign nail growth, second to nail warts [2]. The nodule is composed of mucinous fluid resulting from degeneration of connective tissue or leakage of joint fluid from the DIP joint. Due to a lack of an epithelial lining surrounding the mucinous fluid, myxoid cysts are technically pseudocysts. The mucinous fluid flows via a one-way valve from the joint space to the pseudocyst space. Because myxoid cysts are in close proximity to the nail matrix, disruption of nail growth and onychodystrophy can occur [1].

23.2 Epidemiology

23.2.1 Sex

Myxoid cysts may be more common in adult women than in adult men, with sex ratios estimated at up to 3:1 [3, 4]. In a retrospective study of 51 patients with digital myxoid cysts across a five-year period by Lin et al., 31 patients (60.8%) identified as female, and 20 patients (39.2%) identified as male [2]. In a retrospective study of 36 consecutive patients with myxoid cysts by Kleinert et al., 27 patients (75%) identified as female and nine (25%) as male [5]. In a retrospective study of 34 patients with subungual myxoid cysts across three specialty nail clinics by de Berker et al., 22 patients (64.7%) identified as female, while 12 (35.3%) identified as male [6].

S. R. Lipner, *Atlas of Nail Disorders Across All Skin Colors*,
https://doi.org/10.1007/978-3-031-74272-9_23

23.2.2 Age

Myxoid cysts most commonly affect middle-aged individuals. In the retrospective study of 51 patients with myxoid cysts by Lin et al., the mean age was 63.2 years (range 51–79) [2]. In the retrospective study of 36 patients with myxoid cysts by Kleinert et al., the mean age was 50 years (range 35–71) [5]. In the retrospective study of 34 patients with subungual myxoid cysts by de Berker et al., the mean age was 63.5 years (range 38–83) [6].

23.2.3 Race

Previous studies have not reported on the association of myxoid cysts with race or ethnicity. Patients of all races and ethnicities are affected.

23.3 Risk Factors

In addition to sex and age, osteoarthritis is an important risk factor for the development of myoxid cysts. In the retrospective study of 51 patients with myxoid cysts by Lin et al., osteoarthritis was reported in 38 cases (74.5%), suggesting that deterioration of the joint over time leads to leakage of mucinous fluid from the joint space and accumulation near the DIP joint and proximal nail fold [2]. Lin et al. also demonstrated that nail dystrophy associated with digital myxoid cysts was more common in patients with osteoarthritis (29/38 patients, 76%) vs. those without (6/13 patients, 47%) [2]. In the retrospective study of 36 patients with myxoid cysts by Kleinert et al., 64% of patients had DIP joint osteoarthritis in the digit with the myxoid cyst [5].

Trauma may also be a risk factor for myxoid cyst development [7, 8]. In the retrospective study of 36 patients with myxoid cysts by Kleinert et al., 75% of patients under age 40 (n not stated) reported a history of trauma to the digit with the myxoid cyst [5]. Similar to osteoarthritis, trauma may result in a change in intraarticular pressure, which may promote myxoid cyst development [2].

23.4 Clinical Features

A myxoid cyst typically presents as a solitary nodule <10–15 mm in diameter, although the presence of multiple myxoid cysts in a single digit or across multiple digits has been described [2, 9, 10]. They are more frequently localized to the fingers vs. toes and most commonly present on the second and third fingers of the dominant hand [11]. In the retrospective study of 23 cases of digital myxoid cysts by Chae et al., the fingers were affected three times more often than the toes ($n = 17$, 73.9% vs. $n = 6$, 26.1%, respectively) [11]. In the retrospective study of 51 patients with 63 myxoid cysts by Lin et al., the third finger was the most common site ($n = 28$), followed by the second finger ($n = 11$) [2]. Nail dystrophy often co-occurs with myxoid cysts, with a longitudinal groove as the most common manifestation.

The depth of the longitudinal groove varies based on cyst volume [6]. In the retrospective study of 51 patients with myxoid cysts by Lin et al., nail changes were apparent in 35 patients (n = 68.6%), and the most common nail findings were a longitudinal groove (n = 20), concave longitudinal canaliform dystrophy (n = 9), and transverse lines in a "washboard" appearance (n = 5) [2].

There are three clinical subtypes of myxoid cysts, which vary by location. Type A cysts are located between the DIP and the proximal nail fold, type B is located within the proximal nail fold, and type C is located beneath the nail plate [12, 13]. Depending on the location of the cyst, nail findings may vary. In a superficially located cyst, a skin-colored nodule near the proximal nail fold may be apparent. When the cyst is in contact with the proximal nail fold, a longitudinal groove may be present [1]. Dominguez-Cherit et al. also coined the term "waves sign" for myxoid cysts that place pressure on the nail matrix, which results in a waving pattern of irregular grooves in the nail plate [12]. When the cyst is below the nail matrix, longitudinal thinning may occur [1]. Separation of the nail plate from the cuticle may also be appreciated. When a myxoid cyst is located subungually, the features of nail dystrophy may vary from those classically observed when the myxoid cyst affects the proximal nail fold. In the retrospective study of 35 cases of subungual myxoid cysts by de Berker et al., the most common clinical features included red lunula (n = 22, 62.9%), increased transverse curvature of the nail plate (n = 29, 82.9%), and ingrown lateral nail plate (n = 11, 31.4%) [6].

Dermoscopy may also be used to evaluate for the presence of myxoid cyst [9, 11]. In the retrospective study of 23 cases of digital myxoid cyst by Chae et al., vascular patterns were most often appreciated on dermoscopy (13/23 cases, 56.5%), with arborizing (n = 8, 34.8%) and dotted vessels (n = 3, 13.0%) being most common [11]. Because myxoid cysts are not solid tumors, they easily transmit light [9]. Using a dermatoscope, light can be projected from the palmar aspect of the finger through the nail unit via a technique known as "transillumination." An area near the proximal nail fold that is brighter than the surrounding skin indicates the presence of a myxoid cyst [9]. Transillumination can also be used for guidance when planning incision and drainage.

With drainage, whether via trauma or surgical manipulation, myxoid contents with jelly-like consistency are expelled, and the size of the cyst will decrease [1].

23.5 Clinical Features in Skin of Color

Although features of myxoid cysts in skin of color patients have not been explicitly described, patients with skin of color are more likely to have physiologic melanonychia affecting the fingernails and toenails.

23.6 Requirements for Diagnosis

When myxoid cysts present with classic features including a nodule between the DIP and the proximal nail fold and characteristic nail changes, such as a longitudinal groove, they can be diagnosed clinically. In equivocal cases, ultrasound (US) or magnetic resonance imaging (MRI) may be used to confirm the diagnosis. In a prospective study comparing US and MRI for the diagnosis of myxoid cyst in 11 participants, six of whom had myxoid cyst confirmed with imaging, both US and MRI showed avascularity and size measurements were similar between the two modalities (Pearson correlation coefficient = 0.91) [14]. In the retrospective study of 34 patients with subungual myxoid cysts by de Berker et al., including 20 cases in which MRI was performed, a channel indicating communication between the myxoid cyst and DIP joint was apparent on imaging in 80% of cases (16/20) [6].

23.7 Cases

Figures 23.1, 23.2, 23.3, 23.4, 23.5, 23.6, 23.7 and 23.8 demonstrate the presentation of myxoid cysts in a clinical setting.

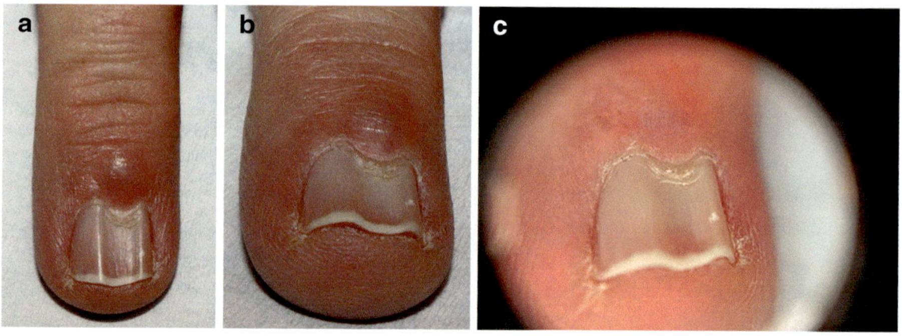

Fig. 23.1 **(a–c)** 61-Year-old male, Fitzpatrick type II, myxoid cyst, with a flesh-colored, translucent nodule localized to the right fourth fingernail proximal nail fold. A longitudinal groove in the nail plate was appreciated on physical examination and dermoscopy

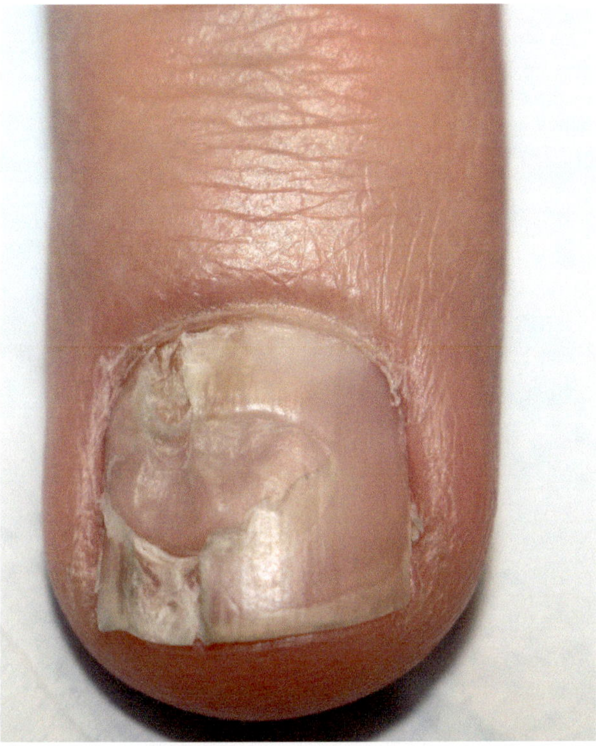

Fig. 23.2 56-Year-old male, Fitzpatrick type II, myxoid cyst, with a longitudinal groove and onychoschizia involving the right third fingernail

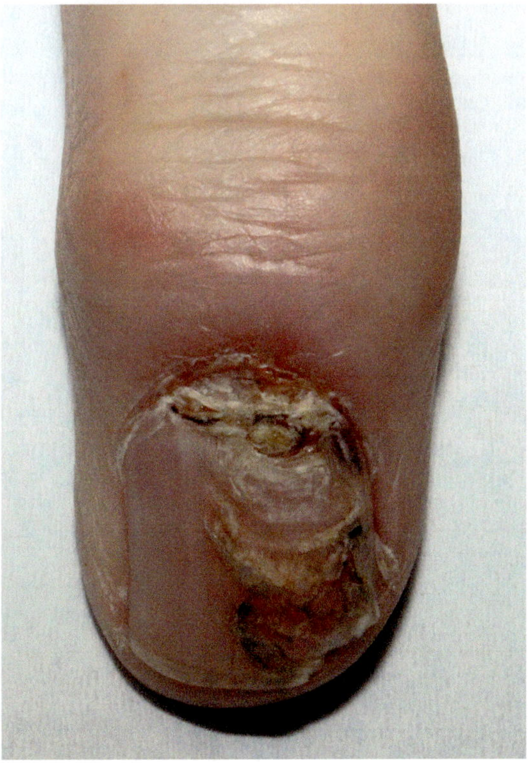

Fig. 23.3 69-Year-old male, Fitzpatrick type II, myxoid cyst, with a longitudinal groove and the “waves sign” involving the right third fingernail

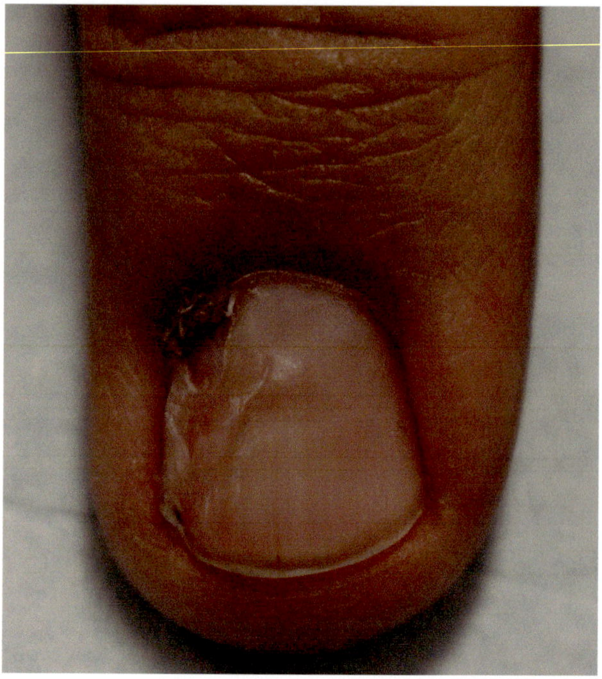

Fig. 23.4 67-Year-old male, Fitzpatrick type II, myxoid cyst, with a longitudinal groove involving the right third fingernail

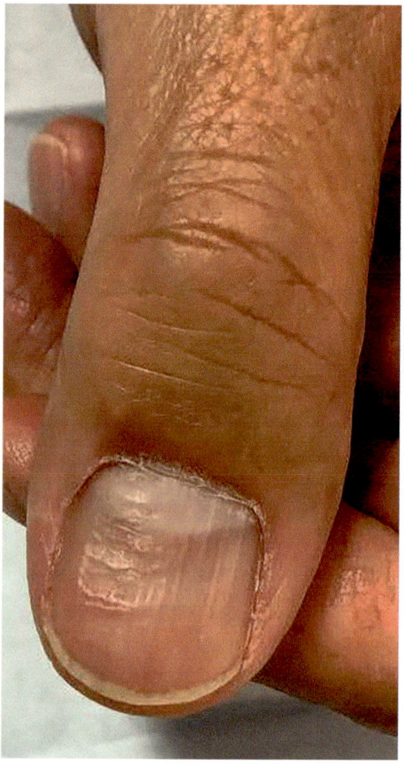

Fig. 23.5 61-Year-old male, Fitzpatrick type III, myxoid cyst, with a subtle longitudinal groove involving the left thumbnail

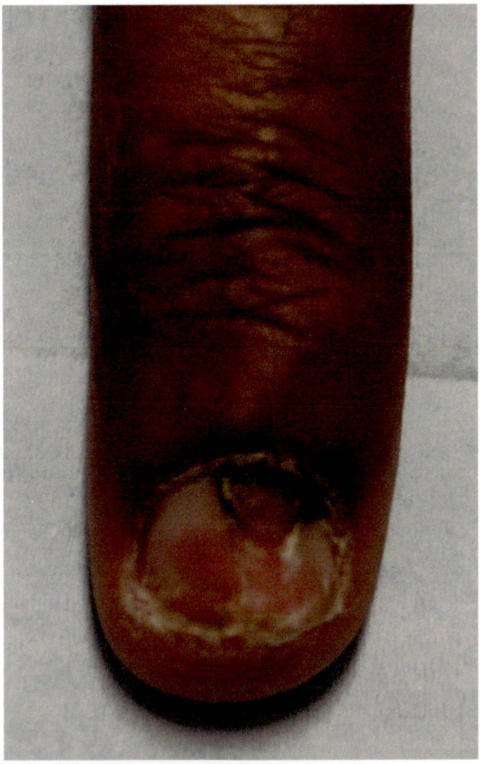

Fig. 23.6 61-Year-old male, Fitzpatrick type IV, myxoid cyst, right third fingernail with translucent nodule involving the proximal nail fold and longitudinal groove with mild green discoloration (due to *Pseudomonas aeruginosa*)

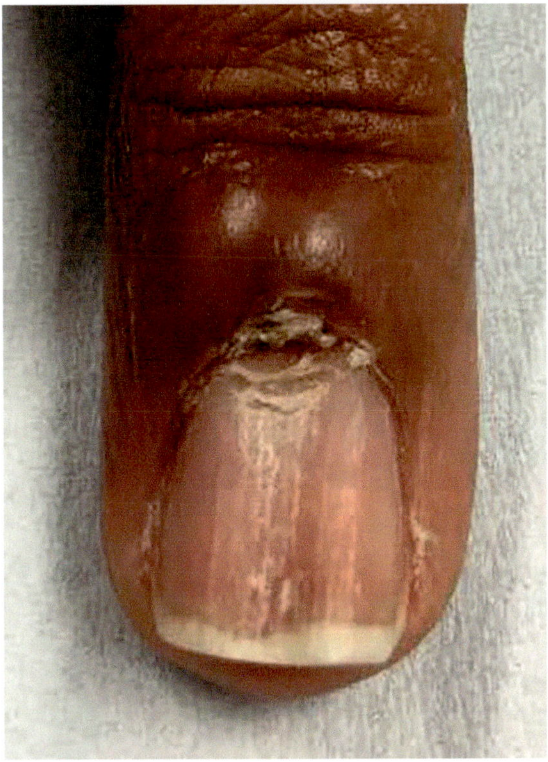

Fig. 23.7 57-Year-old female, Fitzpatrick type V, with compressible translucent nodule involving the proximal nail fold and a longitudinal groove of the right fourth fingernail

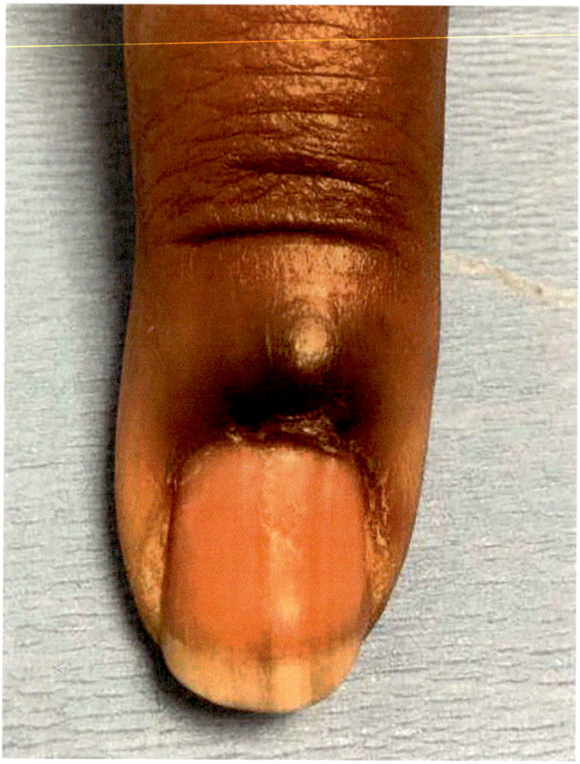

Fig. 23.8 61-Year-old female, Fitzpatrick type V, myxoid cyst, with a translucent nodule involving the proximal nail fold, accompanied by a longitudinal groove of the right third fingernail. There is hyperpigmentation of the proximal nail fold and cuticle and subtle gray longitudinal bands affecting the nail plate

References

1. Hare AQ, Rich P. Nail tumors. Dermatol Clin. 2021;39(2):281–92. https://doi.org/10.1016/j.det.2020.12.007.
2. Lin YC, Wu YH, Scher RK. Nail changes and association of osteoarthritis in digital myxoid cyst. Dermatologic Surg. 2008;34(3):364–9. https://doi.org/10.1111/j.1524-4725.2007.34070.x.
3. Monteagudo-Sánchez B, Luiña-Méndez L, Mosquera-Fernández A. Dermoscopic features of a digital myxoid cyst. Acta Dermatovenerol Croat. 2019;27(2):129–30.
4. Thornburg LE. Ganglions of the hand and wrist. J Am Acad Orthop Surg. 1999;7(4):231–8. https://doi.org/10.5435/00124635-199907000-00003.
5. Kleinert HE, Kutz JE, Fishman JH, McCraw LH. Etiology and treatment of the so-called mucous cyst of the finger. J Bone Joint Surg Am. 1972;54(7):1455–8.
6. de Berker D, Goettman S, Baran R. Subungual myxoid cysts: clinical manifestations and response to therapy. J Am Acad Dermatol. 2002;46(3):394–8. https://doi.org/10.1067/mjd.2002.119652.
7. Drapé JL, Idy-Peretti I, Goettmann S, et al. MR imaging of digital mucoid cysts. Radiology. 1996;200(2):531–6. https://doi.org/10.1148/radiology.200.2.8685352.
8. Cressey BD, Jellinek NJ. Myxoid cyst as a probable complication of nail surgery. Dermatologic Surg. 2018;44(12):1647–9. https://doi.org/10.1097/dss.0000000000001481.
9. Gupta MK, Lipner SR. Transillumination for improved diagnosis of digital myxoid cysts. Cutis. 2020;105(2):82.

10. Butler DF, Davis G, Greene JF. Multiple mucinous (myxoid) cysts of a single finger. J Am Acad Dermatol. 2005;53(5):914–6. https://doi.org/10.1016/j.jaad.2005.05.013.
11. Chae JB, Ohn J, Mun JH. Dermoscopic features of digital mucous cysts: a study of 23 cases. J Dermatol. 2017;44(11):1309–12. https://doi.org/10.1111/1346-8138.13892.
12. Domínguez-Cherit J, Rosales-Sotomayor Á. The "Waves Sign" in digital myxoid pseudocyst. Skin Appendage Disord 2024:1–3. doi: https://doi.org/10.1159/000536137.
13. Baltz JO, Telang GH, Robinson-Bostom L, Jellinek NJ. Pseudo-encapsulated digital myxoid cyst: an unusual manifestation of a common disease. Dermatologic Surg. 2021;47(3):422–4. https://doi.org/10.1097/dss.0000000000002321.
14. Dhami A, Vale SM, Richardson ML, Schachtel AK, Fleckman P. Comparing ultrasound with magnetic resonance imaging in the evaluation of subungual glomus tumors and subungual myxoid cysts. Skin Appendage Disord. 2023;9(4):262–7. https://doi.org/10.1159/000530397.

Splinter Hemorrhage

24

Rachel C. Hill and Shari R. Lipner

24.1 Description of Disease

Splinter hemorrhages are short, red, brown, and/or black longitudinal streaks that are most commonly localized to the distal one-third of the nail plate [1]. They are caused by the extravasation of blood from ruptured capillaries that are arranged longitudinally in the nail bed and were named due to their similar appearance to a wood splinter [2]. Previous studies have reported an 11–66% prevalence of splinter hemorrhages among hospitalized patients [3–5]. While splinter hemorrhages may be idiopathic, benign nail findings, they are also classically associated with serious medical conditions, including bacterial endocarditis, and can serve as an important clue to underlying disease processes [1, 2].

24.2 Epidemiology

24.2.1 Sex

Splinter hemorrhages may be more common in males [6, 7]. In a cross-sectional study of 574 consecutive patients at a city-county hospital by Kilpatrick et al., 59 patients had splinter hemorrhages, 70% of whom were male ($n = 41$) vs. 30% female ($n = 18$) ($P < 0.001$) [3]. However, certain conditions, including autoimmune or connective tissue diseases, may be more common in women, and thus, splinter hemorrhages secondary to these conditions could be more frequent in females.

S. R. Lipner, *Atlas of Nail Disorders Across All Skin Colors*,
https://doi.org/10.1007/978-3-031-74272-9_24

24.2.2 Age

Patients of all ages may develop splinter hemorrhages, and the most prevalent age groups are not well defined. Because splinter hemorrhages are associated with a variety of systemic diseases, they may be more common in older individuals. Likewise, older adults may be more susceptible to trauma since mobility declines with age. In a cross-sectional study of 220 patients in geriatric wards by Young et al. (mean age 82, range 66–98), the prevalence of splinter hemorrhages was 16%, and they were more frequent in patients using walking aids [5].

24.2.3 Race

Splinter hemorrhages may affect patients of all races and ethnicities [6]. In the cross-sectional study of 574 patients by Kilpatrick et al., including 59 patients with splinter hemorrhages, Black or African American patients were more likely to have splinter hemorrhages compared to White patients (59% vs. 41%, respectively, $P < 0.05$), although this could be attributable to the study population being from a city-county hospital, which served patients who mostly worked in labor-heavy occupations [3].

24.3 Risk Factors

24.3.1 Trauma

Trauma is the most common cause of splinter hemorrhages, either from a single event or from repetitive microtrauma to the nails [6]. Trauma may be due to physical activity, including sports or exercise, gardening, manual labor, or the use of instruments. Nail care practices, including excessive manicuring or the use of acrylic nails, can also induce trauma leading to splinter hemorrhages [8].

24.3.2 Common Medical and Dermatologic Conditions Associated with Splinter Hemorrhages (Non-Comprehensive)

Nail Psoriasis: Splinter hemorrhages are a common feature of nail psoriasis. In a systematic review including 11 studies and 723 cases of nail psoriasis, splinter hemorrhages were reported in 54% of cases ($n = 408$) [9]. In a retrospective study of 87 patients with isolated nail psoriasis, 28% of patients ($n = 24$) had splinter hemorrhages on physical examination [10]. In a prospective study of dermoscopic findings in 35 patients with severe nail psoriasis, 94.3% ($n = 33$) of patients had splinter hemorrhages on dermoscopy [11].

Other Dermatoses: Dermatologic conditions other than psoriasis that are associated with splinter hemorrhages include lichen planus and Darier disease [12, 13]. In a retrospective study of 11 patients with 79 nails affected by nail lichen planus, 35.4% ($n = 28$) had splinter hemorrhages [12].

Primary Nail conditions: Splinter hemorrhages are associated with onychomycosis and benign nail tumors, including onychopapilloma, glomus tumors, and onychomatricoma [6, 14–16]. In a retrospective study of 63 patients with splinter hemorrhages, 11.1% of patients presented with onychomycosis as a suspected cause ($n = 7$) [17]. In a retrospective study of dermoscopic findings in 32 cases of subungual glomus tumors, splinter hemorrhages were appreciated in 21.9% ($n = 7$) of cases [15]. In a retrospective study of 17 biopsy-confirmed cases of onychopapilloma, 11.7% exhibited elongated or distal, 1–2 mm splinter hemorrhages on clinical examination ($n = 2$) [16]. In a retrospective study of 34 cases of onychomatricoma in 33 patients, splinter hemorrhages were appreciated in 81.8% of patients ($n = 27$) [18].

Systemic Infectious Disease: Splinter hemorrhages were first reported in association with infective endocarditis by Sir Thomas Horder in 1920 [19, 20]. In a retrospective case-control study of 44 patients with infective endocarditis and 36 controls, splinter hemorrhages were more common in the infective endocarditis group vs. controls (6 vs. 0, $P = 0.04$) [21]. Other classic features of infective endocarditis, which may be seen in conjunction with splinter hemorrhages, include Janeway lesions, Osler nodes, and Roth spots [20–22]. Other infectious diseases, such as COVID-19, are also associated with splinter hemorrhages. In a retrospective study of 174 patients diagnosed with COVID-19 infection over a 100-day period and 57 healthy controls, splinter hemorrhage was the most common nail finding that was observed in 13.9% of patients [23].

Connective Tissue Disease: Splinter hemorrhages may be a sign of connective tissue disease, including systemic lupus erythematosus (SLE), systemic sclerosis (SS), and/or dermatomyositis, among others [24]. In a case-control study of 190 patients with SLE ($n = 56$), rheumatoid arthritis ($n = 47$), primary Sjogren's syndrome ($n = 35$), SS ($n = 39$), and dermatomyositis/polymyositis ($n = 13$), splinter hemorrhages were more common in patients with SLE, SS, and dermatomyositis/polymyositis compared to controls (all $P < 0.05$) [25]. In a retrospective study of 48 patients with SS ($n = 17$), SLE ($n = 16$), and dermatomyositis ($n = 15$), including 44 patients with nail findings, 13.6% ($n = 6$) had splinter hemorrhages [24].

Renal Disorders: Patients with chronic renal failure on or off dialysis may be at increased risk for splinter hemorrhages [26]. In a longitudinal cohort study of 20 patients who underwent hemodialysis for ≥ two years, 20% of patients developed splinter hemorrhages ($n = 4$), which is likely higher than the prevalence in the general population [27]. In a cross-sectional study of 102 patients undergoing hemodialysis, nail changes were appreciated in 67 patients, of whom 11 (11%) had splinter hemorrhages [28]. The pathogenesis of splinter hemorrhage in these patients may be capillary fragility and dysfunction of thrombocytes [29].

Medications: The use of kinase inhibitors, nitrofurantoin, tetracycline antibiotics, and terbinafine have been reported by patients with splinter hemorrhages [1, 30, 31].

Multikinase inhibitors, including sorafenib and sunitinib, cause painless splinter hemorrhages within 1–2 weeks of treatment in 60–70% of patients [30, 32].

Traumatic: Splinter hemorrhages may occur without a known, underlying etiology in healthy patients and in the elderly [1, 5, 6]. In such cases, trauma is the most likely cause, whether due to nail biting or picking, excessive manicuring, use of a walking aid, or stubbing the finger or toe [2, 5, 8].

24.4 Clinical Features

Clinically, splinter hemorrhages appear as one to three millimeter red-brown longitudinal streaks under the nail plate [6, 33]. When a splinter hemorrhage first occurs, it may appear as a dark purple color, but will become brown and/or black over time [6]. Splinter hemorrhages are non-blanchable when pressure is applied [6, 33]. As the nail grows, splinter hemorrhages typically move distally, but will appear stationary if the blood attaches to the nail bed instead of the nail plate [1, 33]. When splinter hemorrhages are secondary to trauma, they are typically distal and black in color, compared to splinter hemorrhages secondary to systemic disease, which are more often proximal and appear red [1]. Although splinter hemorrhages are typically painless, they may be painful in cases of bacterial endocarditis [34]. Splinter hemorrhages may be accompanied by other nail changes, such as onycholysis and Beau's lines [6]. In rare cases, splinter hemorrhages may be painful, especially when associated with systemic disease or other diseases of the nail, including nail psoriasis, lichen planus, and primary nail tumors [35]. However, cases of recurrent and painful splinter hemorrhages have also been reported in healthy individuals [36].

Splinter hemorrhages more often affect the fingernails vs. toenails, especially the thumb and second fingernails in patients who work in manual labor [1, 6, 33]. When splinter hemorrhages occur in multiple fingernails at once, the potential for an underlying, systemic disease should be considered [1, 6, 7].

24.5 Clinical Features in Skin of Color

In patients with skin of color, splinter hemorrhages secondary to trauma are more likely to be accompanied by benign longitudinal melanonychia caused by concurrent activation of melanocytes in the nail matrix. The presence of benign longitudinal melanonychia may camouflage splinter hemorrhages, making them more difficult to visualize on physical examination.

24.6 Requirements for Diagnosis

Splinter hemorrhage is a clinical diagnosis typically made on physical examination alone. Dermoscopy, particularly contact dermoscopy with ultrasound gel, may aid in the diagnosis, and may more clearly identify very small splinter hemorrhages [1].

In equivocal cases, a nail clipping with diaminobenzidine staining can confirm the presence of blood [37]. Importantly, when splinter hemorrhages are found on physical examination, a medical history is required to rule out systemic causes. History should be elicited to identify the history of dermatoses, nail changes, joint pain, heart disease, or possible trauma from nail care practices, physical activity, or manual occupations. If a non-idiopathic etiology is suspected, a diagnostic workup for autoimmune, infectious, thromboembolic, or drug-induced causes should be pursued [1, 6]. In cases of suspected nail psoriasis, clippings may also be used to evaluate for increased nail plate thickness and parakeratosis [38].

24.7 Cases

Figures 24.1, 24.2, 24.3, 24.4, 24.5, 24.6, 24.7, 24.8, 24.9, 24.10 and 24.11 demonstrate the presentation of splinter hemorrhage in a clinical setting.

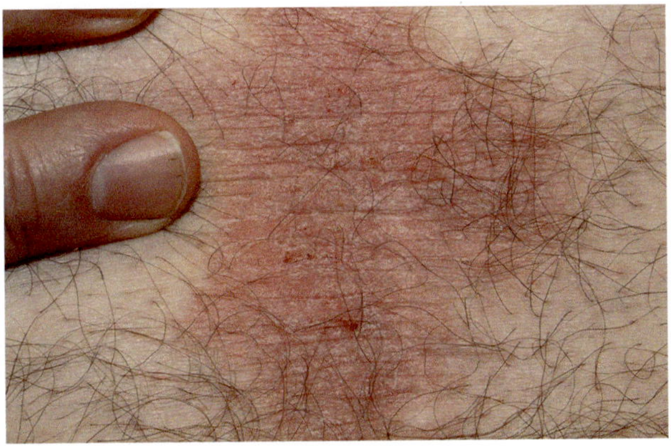

Fig. 24.1 55-Year-old male, Fitzpatrick type II, splinter hemorrhages of the left third fingernail, and an erythematous plaque on the back. Etiology: psoriasis

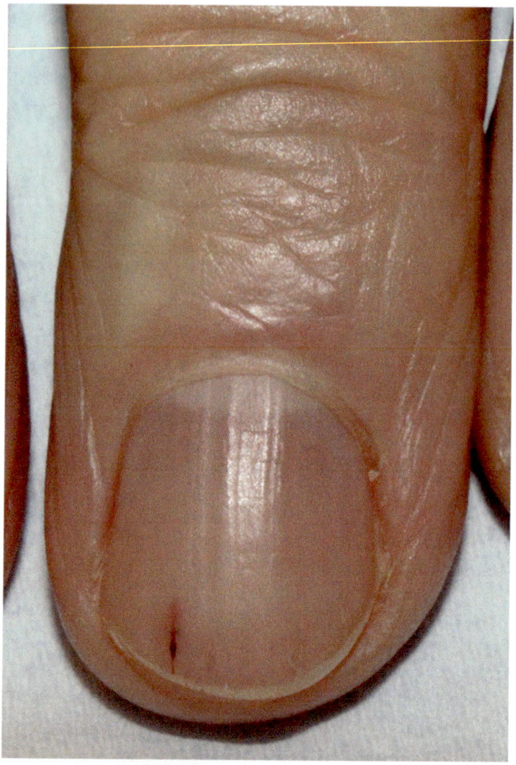

Fig. 24.2 71-Year-old female, Fitzpatrick type II, splinter hemorrhage, demonstrated by short longitudinal red lines on the distal edge of the left third fingernail. Etiology: idiopathic

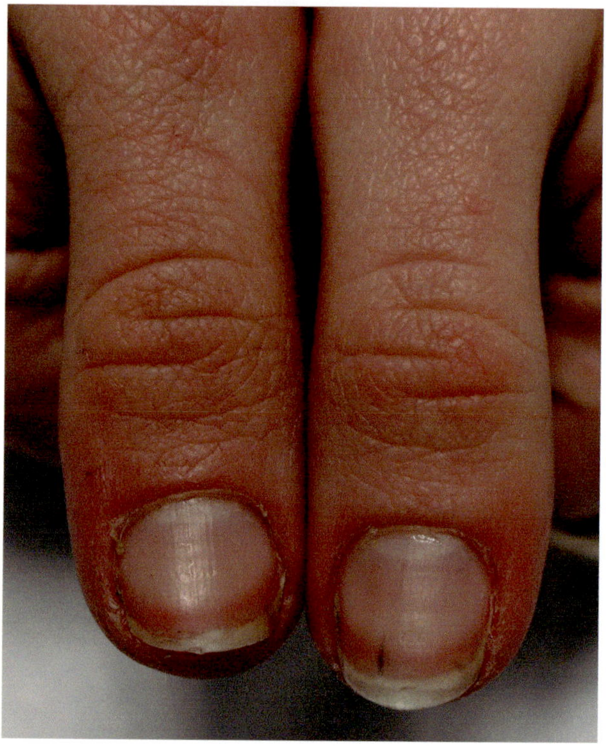

Fig. 24.3 19-Year-old female, Fitzpatrick type II, splinter hemorrhage, with short black line involving the left thumbnail. Etiology: idiopathic or traumatic

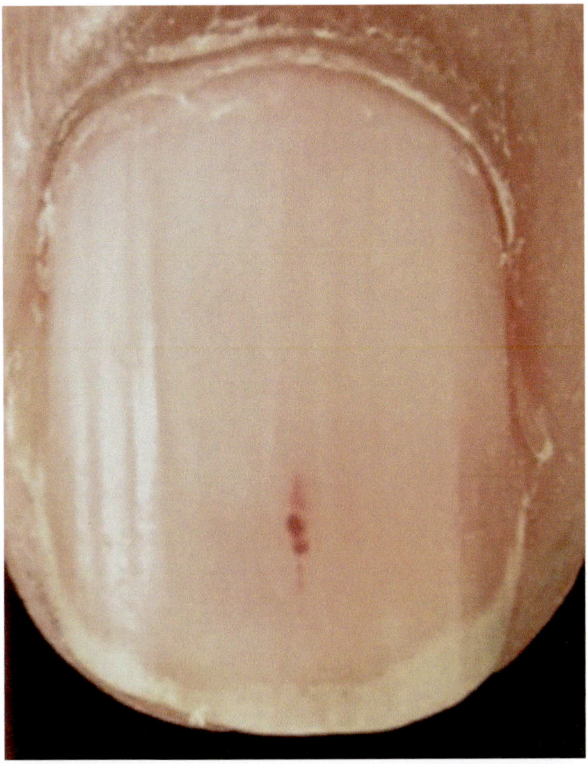

Fig. 24.4 43-Year-old female, unknown Fitzpatrick type, splinter hemorrhage, associated with fever and dyspnea. Etiology: endocarditis (*from* Haber et al. [1]; *with permission*)

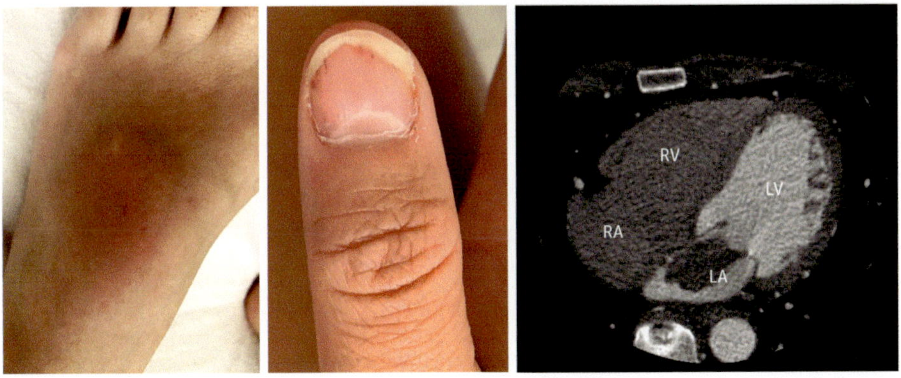

Fig. 24.5 40-Year-old female, Fitzpatrick type II, splinter hemorrhage (center panel), with an erythematous patch on the left dorsal foot (left panel). The patient also presented with petechial macules on the palms and soles. Neurologic examination revealed a right-sided internuclear ophthalmoplegia and transthoracic echocardiography demonstrated a mobile left atrial mass, which was also supported by cardiac computed tomography angiography (right panel). Etiology: Left atrial myxoma (*from* Zhang et al. [39]; *with permission*)

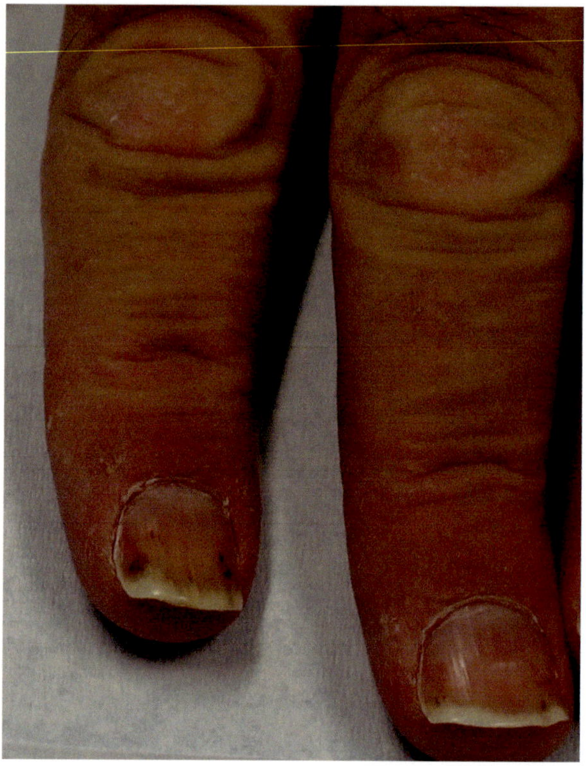

Fig. 24.6 63-Year-old male, Fitzpatrick type III, splinter hemorrhages, with thickening and onycholysis of the fingernails. Etiology: nail psoriasis

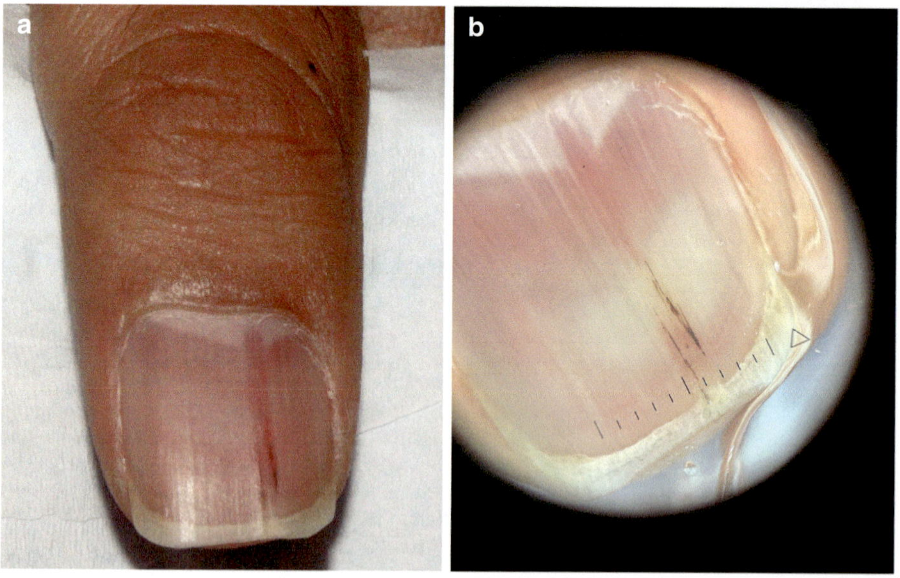

Fig. 24.7 (**a**) 37-Year-old male, Fitzpatrick type III, splinter hemorrhage, left thumbnail with longitudinal erythronychia, and subungual, hyperkeratotic papule at the hyponychium. (**b**) The splinter hemorrhages are enhanced using contact dermoscopy. Etiology: onychopapilloma

Fig. 24.8 28-Year-old female, Fitzpatrick type IV, splinter hemorrhage, with mild onycholysis of the right thumbnail. Etiology: nail psoriasis

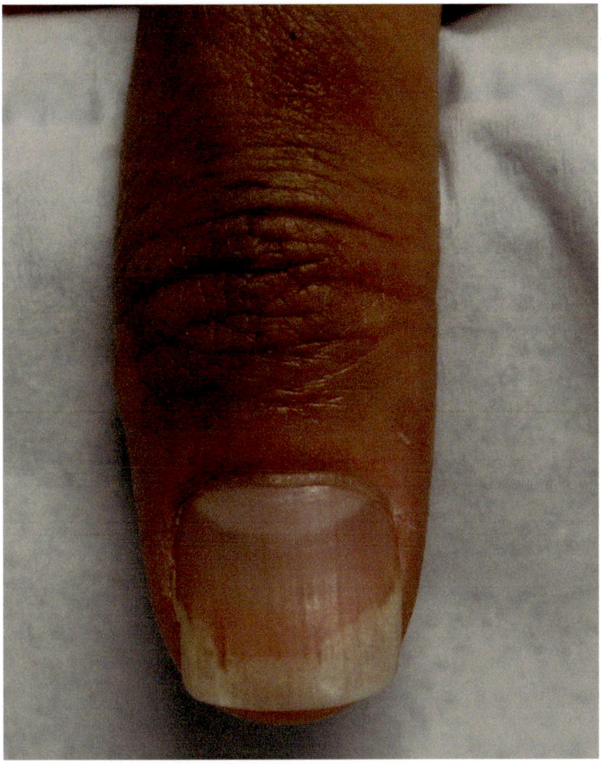

Fig. 24.9 34-Year-old male, Fitzpatrick type V, splinter hemorrhage, with involvement of the left second fingernail. Etiology: psoriasis

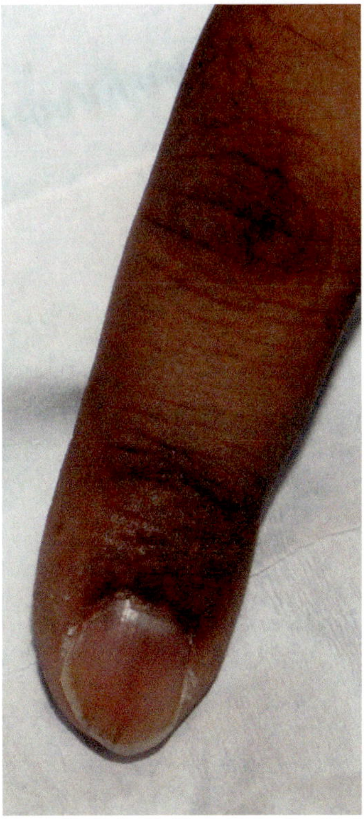

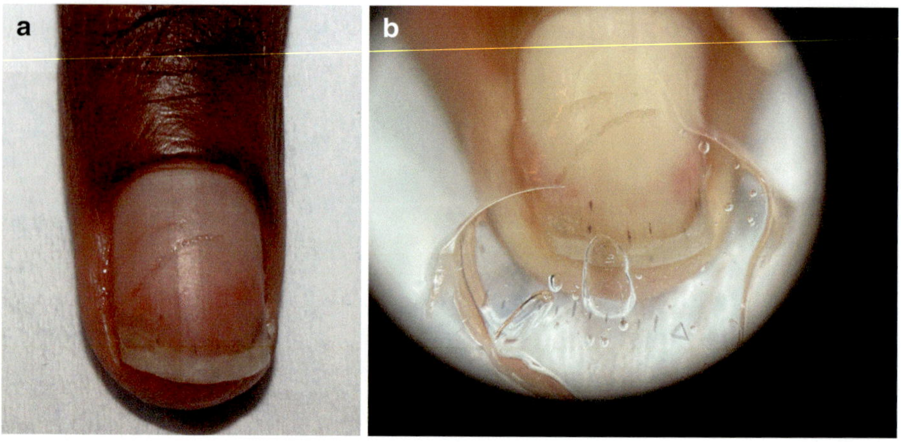

Fig. 24.10 (**a**) 23-Year-old female, Fitzpatrick type VI, splinter hemorrhage, with distal onycholysis of the left third fingernail. (**b**) The splinter hemorrhages are better appreciated with contact dermoscopy. Etiology: nail psoriasis

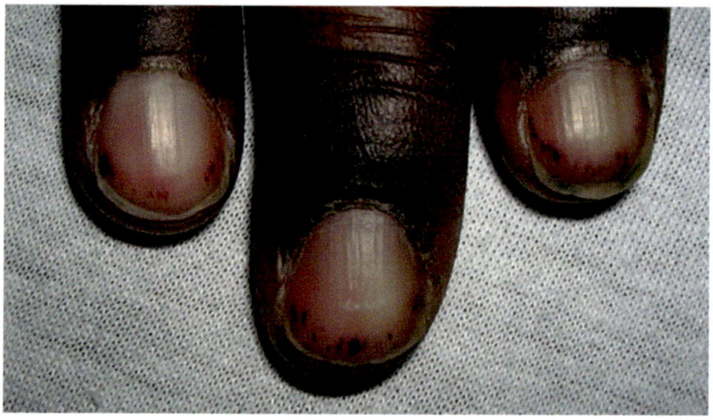

Fig. 24.11 28-Year-old female, Fitzpatrick type VI, splinter hemorrhage, who presented to the hospital suffering from headache and blurred vision. Etiology: nonbacterial thrombotic endocarditis caused by metastatic pancreatic exocrine cancer (*from* Chunhamaneewat et al. [40]; *with permission*)

References

1. Haber R, Khoury R, Kechichian E, Tomb R. Splinter hemorrhages of the nails: a systematic review of clinical features and associated conditions. Int J Dermatol. 2016;55(12):1304–10. https://doi.org/10.1111/ijd.13347.
2. Grugan BM, Dyer SP. Splinter hemorrhage. J Emerg Med. 2022;63(2):304–5. https://doi.org/10.1016/j.jemermed.2022.05.021.
3. Kilpatrick ZM, Greenberg PA, Sanford JP. Splinter hemorrhages—their clinical significance. Arch Intern Med. 1965;115:730–5. https://doi.org/10.1001/archinte.1960.03860180102019.
4. Gross NJ, Tall R. Clinical significance of splinter haemorrhages. Br Med J. 1963;2(5371):1496–8. https://doi.org/10.1136/bmj.2.5371.1496.
5. Young J, Mulley G. Splinter haemorrhages in the elderly. Age Ageing. 1987;16(2):101–4. https://doi.org/10.1093/ageing/16.2.101.
6. Saladi RN, Persaud AN, Rudikoff D, Cohen SR. Idiopathic splinter hemorrhages. J Am Acad Dermatol. 2004;50(2):289–92. https://doi.org/10.1016/j.jaad.2003.07.012.

7. Monk BE. The prevalence of splinter haemorrhages. Br J Dermatol. 1980;103(2):183–5. https://doi.org/10.1111/j.1365-2133.1980.tb06588.x.
8. Tyagi M, Singal A. Nail cosmetics: what a dermatologist should know! Indian J Dermatol Venereol Leprol 2023:1–8. doi: https://doi.org/10.25259/ijdvl_77_2023.
9. Rachadi H, Chiheb S. Dermoscopic features of nail psoriasis: a systematic review. Int J Dermatol. 2024; https://doi.org/10.1111/ijd.17138.
10. Chang MJ, Lee D, Desai AD, Lipner SR. The untold burden of isolated nail psoriasis: Delayed diagnosis and significant risk of psoriatic arthritis in a retrospective study at an academic center. J Am Acad Dermatol. 2023;88(5):1192–4. https://doi.org/10.1016/j.jaad.2022.12.031.
11. Yorulmaz A, Aksoy GG. Dermoscopic features of nail psoriasis: revisited. Skin Appendage Disord. 2022;8(5):389–98. https://doi.org/10.1159/000524109.
12. Nakamura R, Broce AA, Palencia DP, Ortiz NI, Leverone A. Dermatoscopy of nail lichen planus. Int J Dermatol. 2013;52(6):684–7. https://doi.org/10.1111/j.1365-4632.2011.05283.x.
13. Alessandrini A, Starace M, Piraccini BM. Dermoscopy in the evaluation of nail disorders. Skin Appendage Disord. 2017;3(2):70–82. https://doi.org/10.1159/000458728.
14. Wang S, Zhu J, Wang P, et al. Nail psoriasis in China: a prospective multicentre study. J Eur Acad Dermatol Venereol. 2024;38(3):549–56. https://doi.org/10.1111/jdv.19684.
15. Göktay F, Güldiken G, Altan Ferhatoğlu Z, Güneş P, Atış G, Haneke E. The role of dermoscopy in the diagnosis of subungual glomus tumors. Int J Dermatol. 2022;61(7):826–32. https://doi.org/10.1111/ijd.16042.
16. Starace M, Alessandrini A, Ferrari T, Wong V, Baraldi C, Piraccini BM. Clinical and onychoscopic features of histopathologically proven onychopapillomas and literature update. J Cutan Pathol. 2022;49(2):147–52. https://doi.org/10.1111/cup.14119.
17. Gao J, Shen C, Ko R, et al. Clinical observation and follow-up of subungual splinter hemorrhages of toenails in chinese adults. Indian J Dermatol. 2020;65(1):11–6. https://doi.org/10.4103/ijd.IJD_193_18.
18. Lesort C, Debarbieux S, Duru G, Dalle S, Poulhalon N, Thomas L. Dermoscopic features of onychomatricoma: a study of 34 cases. Dermatology. 2015;231(2):177–83. https://doi.org/10.1159/000431315.
19. Horder TJ. Infective endocarditis with an analysis of 150 cases and with special reference to the chronic form of the disease. Qj Med. 1909;2(3):289–324.
20. Silverman ME, Upshaw CB Jr. Extracardiac manifestations of infective endocarditis and their historical descriptions. Am J Cardiol. 2007;100(12):1802–7. https://doi.org/10.1016/j.amjcard.2007.07.034.
21. Ebtia M, Dewa D. Infective endocarditis revisited: clinical manifestations and echocardiographic findings of patients with infective endocarditis. J Am Coll Cardiol. 2012;59(Suppl. 13):E1894. https://doi.org/10.1016/S0735-1097(12)61895-6.
22. Lamas CC, Eykyn SJ. Suggested modifications to the Duke criteria for the clinical diagnosis of native valve and prosthetic valve endocarditis: analysis of 118 pathologically proven cases. Clin Infect Dis. 1997;25(3):713–9. https://doi.org/10.1086/513765.
23. Yanatma I, Cenk H. Evaluation of nail findings in patients with COVID-19 history and wood's lamp examination. Skin Appendage Disord. 2021;38(2):1–6. https://doi.org/10.1159/000518983.
24. Ghannem A, Zaouak A, Aydi Z, et al. Nail involvement in connective tissue diseases: an epidemiological, clinical, and dermoscopic study. Int J Dermatol. 2024; https://doi.org/10.1111/ijd.17113.
25. Tunc SE, Ertam I, Pirildar T, Turk T, Ozturk M, Doganavsargil E. Nail changes in connective tissue diseases: do nail changes provide clues for the diagnosis? J Eur Acad Dermatol Venereol. 2007;21(4):497–503. https://doi.org/10.1111/j.1468-3083.2006.02012.x.
26. Kolla PK, Desai M, Pathapati RM, et al. Cutaneous manifestations in patients with chronic kidney disease on maintenance hemodialysis. ISRN Dermatol. 2012;2012:679619. https://doi.org/10.5402/2012/679619.
27. Blum M, Aviram A. Splinter hemorrhages in patients receiving regular hemodialysis. JAMA. 1978;239(1):47.

28. Picó MR, Lugo-Somolinos A, Sánchez JL, Burgos-Calderón R. Cutaneous alterations in patients with chronic renal failure. Int J Dermatol. 1992;31(12):860–3. https://doi.org/10.1111/j.1365-4362.1992.tb03543.x.
29. Salem A, Al Mokadem S, Attwa E, Abd El Raoof S, Ebrahim HM, Faheem KT. Nail changes in chronic renal failure patients under haemodialysis. J Eur Acad Dermatol Venereol. 2008;22(11):1326–31. https://doi.org/10.1111/j.1468-3083.2008.02826.x.
30. Belloni B, Schönewolf N, Rozati S, Goldinger SM, Dummer R. Cutaneous drug eruptions associated with the use of new oncological drugs. Chem Immunol Allergy. 2012;97:191–202. https://doi.org/10.1159/000335632.
31. Acosta AS, Jafri Z, Khalil K, Kerdel F. Nitrofurantoin-induced splinter hemorrhages: a forgotten culprit. JAAD Case Rep. 2024;47:38–40. https://doi.org/10.1016/j.jdcr.2024.02.031.
32. Autier J, Escudier B, Wechsler J, Spatz A, Robert C. Prospective study of the cutaneous adverse effects of sorafenib, a novel multikinase inhibitor. Arch Dermatol. 2008;144(7):886–92. https://doi.org/10.1001/archderm.144.7.886.
33. Han MJ, Bidinger JJ, Hivnor CM, Photo quiz. Asymptomatic linear hemorrhages. Splinter hemorrhages. Am Fam Physician. 2010;81(11):1375–6.
34. Lawry M, Daniel CR. Chapter 15: Nails in systemic disease. In: Scher RK, Tosti A, Elewski BE, Daniel CR, Fleckman P, Rich P, editors. Nails. 3rd ed. W.B. Saunders; 2005. p. 147–76.
35. Hwang JK, Grover C, Iorizzo M, et al. Nail psoriasis and nail lichen planus: updates on diagnosis and management. J Am Acad Dermatol. 2024;90(3):585–96. https://doi.org/10.1016/j.jaad.2023.11.024.
36. Miller AC, Vaziri ND. Recurrent atraumatic subungual splinter hemorrhages in healthy individuals. Southern Med J. 1979;72:1418–22.
37. Stephen S, Tosti A, Rubin AI. Diagnostic applications of nail clippings. Dermatol Clin. 2015;33(2):289–301. https://doi.org/10.1016/j.det.2014.12.011.
38. Fonseca GP, Werner B, Seidel G, Staub HL. Comparative microscopic analysis of nail clippings from patients with cutaneous psoriasis and psoriatic arthritis. An Bras Dermatol. 2017;92(1):21–5. https://doi.org/10.1590/abd1806-4841.20175056.
39. Zhang M, Lipner SR. A patient with dizziness, chest pain, rash, and nail changes. JAMA. 2021;325(1):83–4. https://doi.org/10.1001/jama.2020.15176.
40. Chunhamaneewat N, Maraj S, Borate U, Figueredo VM. A 28-year-old woman with headache, blurred vision, and splinter hemorrhages. Am J Med Sci. 2009;338(6):493. https://doi.org/10.1097/MAJ.0b013e3181aa508b.

Part VI

Disorders of Nail Growth and Shape

Beau's Lines

25

Kaya L. Curtis and Shari R. Lipner

25.1 Description of Disease

Beau's lines are characterized by transverse depressions in the nail plate secondary to a temporary decrease in mitotic activity of keratinocytes in the proximal nail matrix during periods of acute or chronic stress [1, 2].

25.2 Epidemiology

There are few epidemiologic studies to date on Beau's lines. Patients of any age or gender may develop Beau's lines. In Kim et al.'s systematic review [3] of 233 Beau's lines cases, the average onset was 41.6 years. Multiple nails were affected in most patients.

25.3 Risk Factors

Risk factors for Beau's lines include medications, infections, acute systemic disease, chronic conditions, and trauma [1]. In Kim et al.'s systematic review [3] of 233 Beau's lines cases, the most common causes were medications (36.3%), particularly chemotherapeutics, followed by non-autoimmune systemic diseases (25%), trauma (12.5%), and infection (7.5%). Drug-induced Beau's lines are typically present in all 20 nails and onset is two to three weeks after beginning therapy [4]. Shorter chemotherapeutic treatment durations with higher dosages and combination regimens are more likely to result in Beau's lines [4–6]. Other associated medications include retinoids, carbamazepine, cloxacillin, dapsone, and itraconazole [7–10]. Associated infectious etiologies include diphtheria, syphilis, measles, mumps, malaria, typhoid fever, scarlet fever, COVID-19, and hand-foot-mouth disease [10–13]. Associated acute systemic diseases include sepsis, rheumatic fever, and

S. R. Lipner, *Atlas of Nail Disorders Across All Skin Colors*,
https://doi.org/10.1007/978-3-031-74272-9_25

myocardial infarction. Chronic conditions include Raynaud's disease, postpartum hyperparathyroidism, telogen effluvium, and uncontrolled diabetes mellitus. Single digit or unilateral Beau's lines are likely secondary to trauma, including nail trauma or trauma to the ipsilateral extremity [14]. The mechanism of trauma-induced Beau's lines is thought to be due to a temporary decrease in blood supply to the nail matrix [10]. Carpal tunnel syndrome and fracture-induced nerve injury is another association [15–17]. Limb immobilization from casts or splints may cause unilateral Beau's lines [7, 18, 19]. Beau's lines have been reported in association with intravenous immunoglobulin infusions [20].

25.4 Clinical Features

On physical examination, Beau's line presents with a transverse groove in the nail plate. The transverse groove generally does not span the entire nail plate width [1]. Multiple nails are involved in most cases [3]. The timing of the original insult can be dated by measuring the distance between the proximal nail fold and the transverse groove. Approximately 2–3 mm and 1 mm correspond to one month of growth for fingernails and toenails, respectively [2].

25.5 Clinical Features in Skin of Color

Distinct clinical presentations of Beau's lines in skin of color have not been characterized. Accompanying longitudinal melanonychia may be present, particularly in adult patients.

25.6 Requirements for Diagnosis

Beau's lines are a clinical diagnosis and a history of medication use, systemic disease, viral infection, or trauma may be supportive. Palpation may aid in differentiating between Beau's line (depression) and onychomadesis (complete separation).

25.7 Cases

Figures 25.1, 25.2, 25.3, 25.4, 25.5, 25.6, and 25.7 demonstrate the presentation of Beau's lines in a clinical setting.

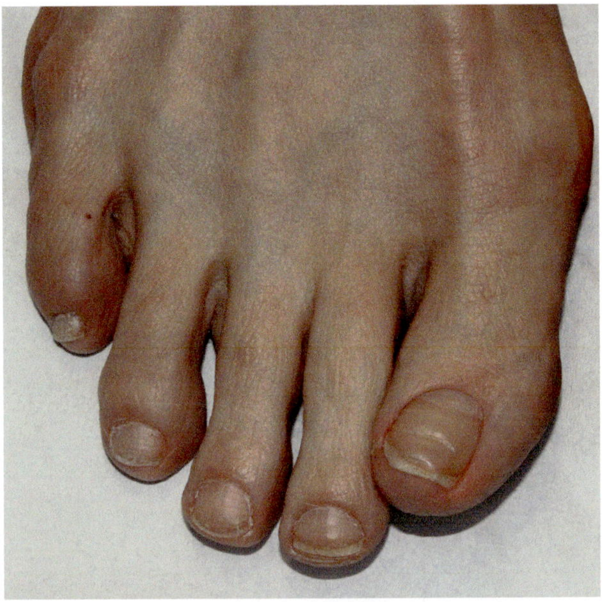

Fig. 25.1 61-Year-old female, Fitzpatrick type I, Beau's line, with transverse groove involving right great toenail

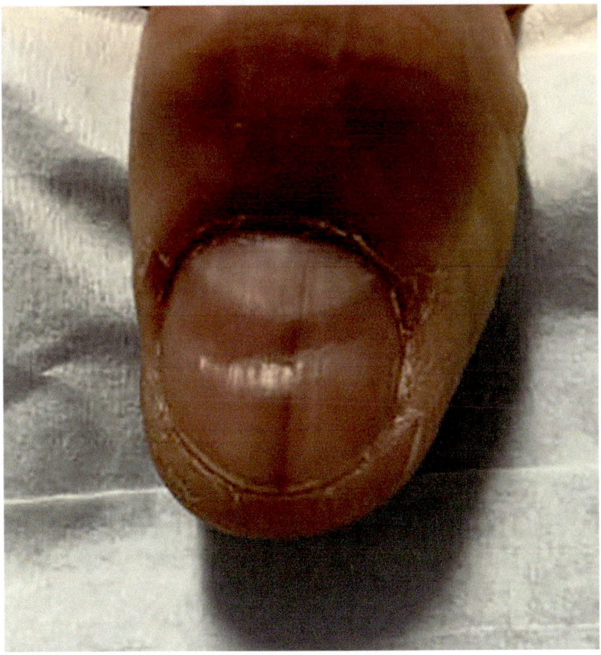

Fig. 25.2 65-Year-old female, Fitzpatrick type II, Beau's line, with transverse groove involving left thumbnail. There is also a gray-brown longitudinal band

Fig. 25.3 65-Year-old female, Fitzpatrick type III, Beau's lines, with transverse grooves involving bilateral thumbnails

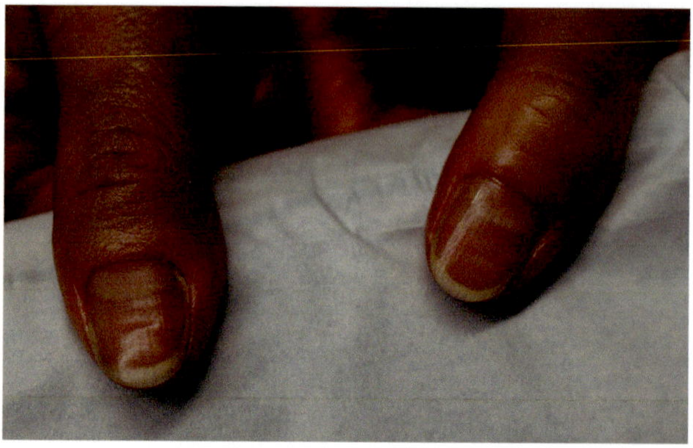

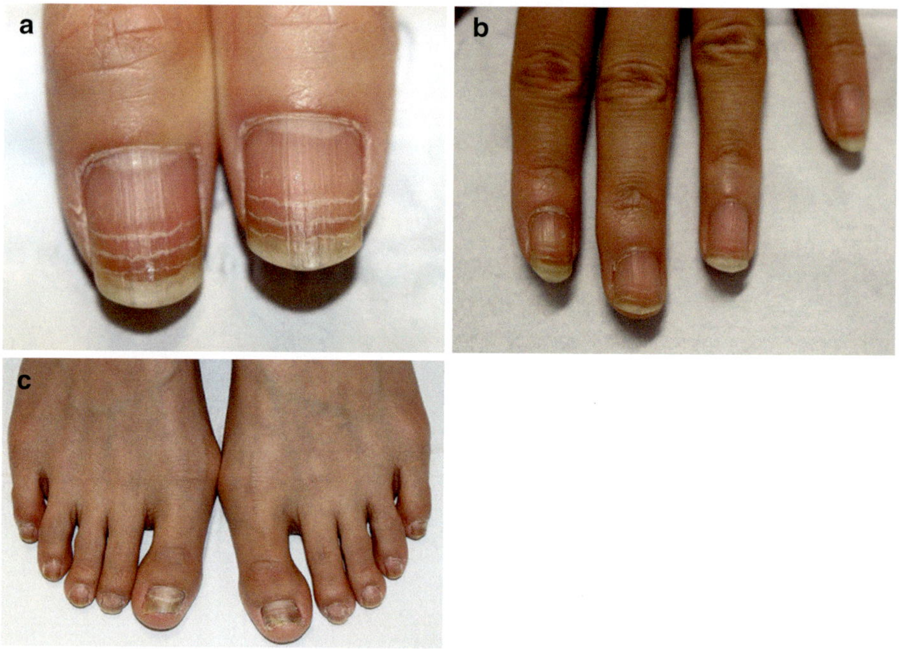

Fig. 25.4 (**a**) 33-Year-old female, Fitzpatrick type III, Beau's lines, parallel transverse grooves of the bilateral thumbnails. (**b**) 33-year-old female, Fitzpatrick type III, Beau's lines, parallel transverse grooves of the left fingernails. (**c**) 33-year-old female, Fitzpatrick type III, onychomadesis and Beau's lines, separation of the proximal and distal nail plates of the bilateral great toenails and transverse grooves of the other toenails

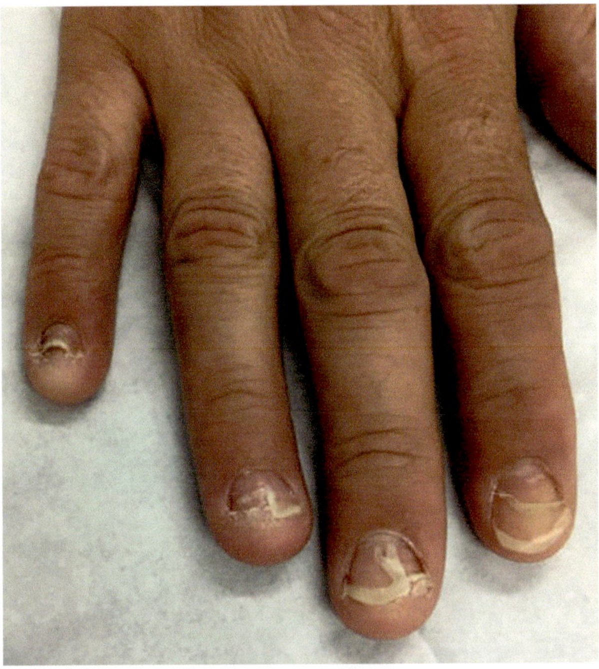

Fig. 25.5 42-Year-old female, Fitzpatrick type IV, Beau's lines, with transverse grooves involving the right fingernails following coxsackie virus infection

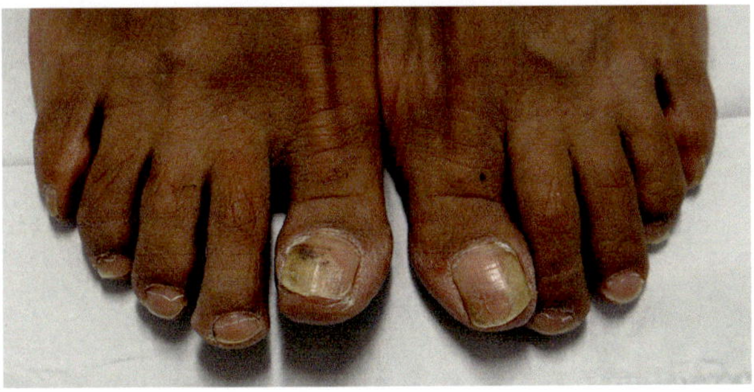

Fig. 25.6 69-Year-old female, Fitzpatrick type IV, Beau's lines, with transverse grooves involving the right second, third, and fourth toenails and left second and third toenails

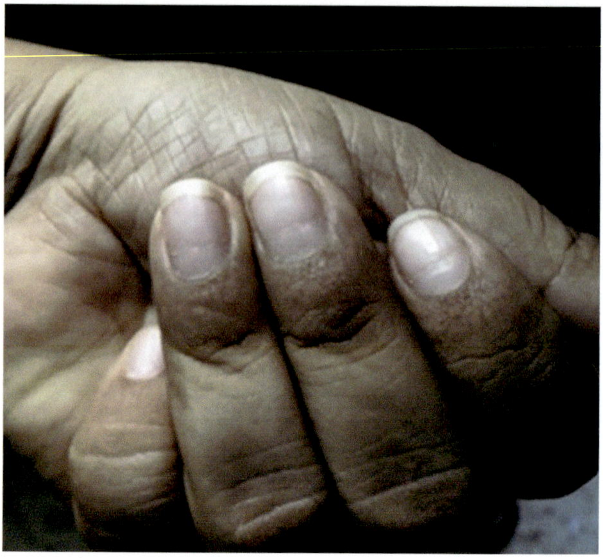

Fig. 25.7 41-Year-old female, Fitzpatrick type V, Beau's lines, with transverse grooves involving multiple fingernails associated with COVID-19 infection (*from* Deng et al. [21]; *with permission*)

References

1. Lee DK, Lipner SR. Optimal diagnosis and management of common nail disorders. Ann Med. 2022;54(1):694–712.
2. Lipner SR, Scher RK. Evaluation of nail lines: color and shape hold clues. Cleve Clin J Med. 2016;83(5):385–91.
3. Kim BR, Yu DA, Lee SR, Lim SS, Mun JH. Beau's lines and onychomadesis: a systematic review of characteristics and aetiology. Acta Derm Venereol. 2023;103:adv18251.
4. Piraccini BM, Alessandrini A. Drug-related nail disease. Clin Dermatol. 2013;31(5):618–26.
5. Ben-Dayan D, Mittelman M, Floru S, et al. Transverse nail ridgings (Beau's lines) induced by chemotherapy. Acta Haematol. 1994;91(2):89–90.
6. Park J, Li K. Images in clinical medicine. Multiple beau's lines. N Engl J Med. 2010;362(20):e63.
7. Piraccini BM, Iorizzo M, Antonucci A, et al. Drug induced nail abnormalities. Expert Opin Drug Saf. 2004;3(1):57–65.
8. Baran R. Retinoids and the nails. J Dermatol Treat. 1990;1(3):151–4.
9. Chen HH, Liao YH. Beau's lines associated with itraconazole. Acta Derm Venereol. 2002;82(5):398.
10. Avery H, Cooper HL, Karim A. Unilateral beau's lines associated with a fractured olecranon. Australas J Dermatol. 2010;51(2):145–6.
11. Ko D, Lipner SR. Concurrent beau lines, onychomadesis, and retronychia following scurvy. Cutis. 2020;105(3):146–9.
12. Chiu H-H, Liu M-T, Chung W-H, et al. The mechanism of onychomadesis (nail shedding) and beau's lines following hand-foot-mouth disease. Viruses. 2019;11(6):522.
13. Preda-Naumescu A, Penney K, Pearlman RL, Brodell RT, Daniel CR, Nahar VK. Nail manifestations in COVID-19: insight into a systemic viral disease. Skin Appendage Disord. 2021;183(6):1–6.
14. Tucker JR. Nail deformities and injuries. Prim Care. 2015;42(4):677–91.

15. Ward DJ, Hudson I, Jeffs JV. Beau's lines following hand trauma. J Hand Surg Br. 1988;13(4):411–4.
16. Tosti A, Morelli R, D'Alessandro R, et al. Carpal tunnel syndrome presenting with ischemic skin lesions, acroosteolysis, and nail changes. J Am Acad Dermatol. 1993;29(2 Pt 2):287–90.
17. Egger A, Tosti A. Carpal tunnel syndrome and associated nail changes: review and examples from the Annals of Medicine 711 author's practice. J Am Acad Dermatol. 2020;83(6):1724–9.
18. Harford RR, Cobb MW, Banner NT. Unilateral beau's lines associated with a fractured and immobilized wrist. Cutis. 1995;56(5):263–4.
19. Dawber R. The effect of immobilization on fingernail growth. Clin Exp Dermatol. 1981;6(5):533–5.
20. Conway J, Lipner SR. Beau's lines associated with IVIG infusions. J Cutan Med Surg. 2023;27(2):180.
21. Deng J, Ngo T, Zhu TH, Halverstam C. Telogen effluvium, Beau lines, and acral peeling associated with COVID-19 infection. JAAD Case Rep. 2021;13:138–40.

Onychomadesis

26

Kaya L. Curtis and Shari R. Lipner

26.1 Description of Disease

Onychomadesis refers to a complete separation of the proximal and distal nail plates due to a temporary cessation of nail growth [1–3]. An inciting trauma may result in a complete loss in the continuity of the nail matrix, resulting in a depression (Beau's line) or complete nail plate separation (onychomadesis) from the matrix [4]. As the proximal nail plate grows, the distal plate is pushed upwards and is ultimately shed [5].

26.2 Epidemiology

There are few epidemiologic studies to date on onychomadesis. Patients of any age or sex may develop onychomadesis. In Kim et al.'s systematic review [6] of 908 onychomadesis cases, the average age was 23.4 years. Patients with viral infections, including coxsackie and varicella, may be especially susceptible. During an outbreak of hand-foot-mouth disease in Taiwan, the incidence of onychomadesis following coxsackievirus A [6] infection was 37% (48/130) compared to 5% (7/145) in cases with non-coxsackie virus A6 strains [7]. In a retrospective study [8] of 88 hand-foot-mouth disease cases in a nursery outbreak in Spain, the prevalence of onychomadesis by age group was 55% (18/33) in patients 9–23 months, 30% (8/27) in patients 2–2.7 years, and 4% (1/28) in patients 2.8–3.5 years.

26.3 Risk Factors

Onychomadesis risk factors include trauma, infection, medications, acute severe disease, and autoimmune disease [4]. In a systematic review [6] of 908 onychomadesis cases, the most common etiologies were infection (36.9%), drugs

S. R. Lipner, *Atlas of Nail Disorders Across All Skin Colors*,
https://doi.org/10.1007/978-3-031-74272-9_26

(14.6%), particularly antiepileptics, and non-autoimmune systemic diseases (13.8%). The most common cause of single-digit onychomadesis is local trauma, whereas multiple-digit onychomadesis suggests a systemic etiology [2, 9]. Commonly associated medications include cytotoxic chemotherapeutics, retinoids, and antiepileptics. Associated infectious etiologies include hand-foot-mouth disease and varicella infection, more commonly in young children. Chronic paronychia is another cause. For the coxsackie virus, nail changes typically present later in the disease course and are associated with coxsackie viral serotypes A6, A10, A16, B1, and B2 [10, 11]. In a retrospective study of 11 cases of onychomadesis secondary to hand-foot-mouth disease, the average time between acute viral episodes and the onset of nail changes was 53.4 days (range: 30–96 days) [10]. Ten onychomadesis cases associated with COVID-19 have also been reported [11]. There are several hypotheses for the mechanism of viral-induced onychomadesis, including nail matrix inflammation resulting in nail plate shedding, and viral replication resulting in direct damage to the nail matrix [1, 12]. Severe acute illnesses associated with onychomadesis include Stevens-Johnson syndrome and Kawasaki disease [4, 13, 14]. Neonates who experienced intrauterine or birth trauma (e.g., breech position, maternal infection) or who have experienced candidiasis may also be at risk [15]. Associated autoimmune diseases include Guillain-Barre syndrome, alopecia areata, and pemphigus vulgaris [16–18]. Idiopathic onychomadesis is rare and is classified into familial and sporadic subtypes [19]. Onychomadesis familial patterns suggest an autosomal dominant inheritance pattern, while sporadic subtypes may be due to seasonal or random episodes of shedding [1, 20, 21]. Microtrauma is likely to play a role in sporadic idiopathic onychomadesis [19].

26.4 Clinical Features

On physical examination, there is a transverse separation of proximal and distal nail plates. Inflammation and granulation tissue of the lateral nail folds may be observed in severe cases [3]. Onychomadesis is self-limited and spontaneous regrowth of healthy nails is typically observed within 12 weeks or sooner in pediatric patients [2, 22]. In a retrospective study of 23 pediatric patients with hand-foot-mouth disease who developed cutaneous findings, 82.6% (19/23) of patients had onychomadesis. Onychomadesis was most frequently observed in the third fingernail (73.7%), followed by the thumbnail (63.2%), and fourth fingernail (52.6%).

26.5 Clinical Features in Skin of Color

Distinct clinical presentations of onychomadesis in the skin of color have not been characterized. Longitudinal melanonychia may be present, particularly in adult patients.

26.6 Requirements for Diagnosis

Onychomadesis is a clinical diagnosis and a history of viral infection, trauma, systemic disease, or medication use may be supportive. Palpation may aid in differentiating between Beau's line (depression) and onychomadesis (complete separation).

26.7 Cases

Figures 26.1, 26.2, 26.3, 26.4, 26.5, 26.6, and 26.7 demonstrate the presentation of onychomadesis in a clinical setting.

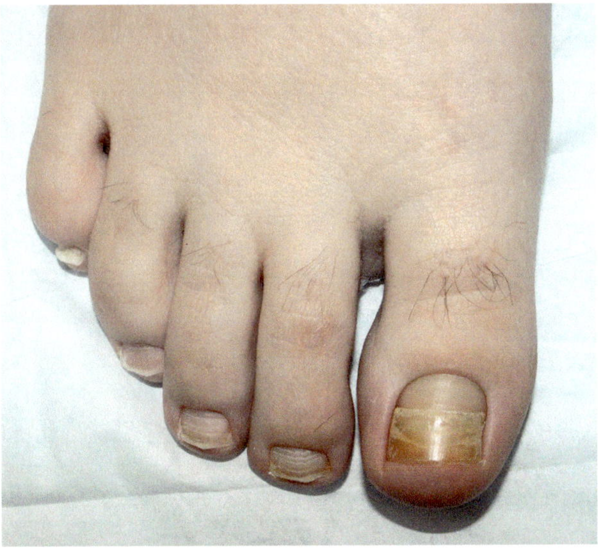

Fig. 26.1 37-Year-old female, Fitzpatrick type I, onychomadesis and Beau's lines, with separation of the proximal and distal nail plates involving the right great toenail and parallel transverse grooves of the right second and third toenails

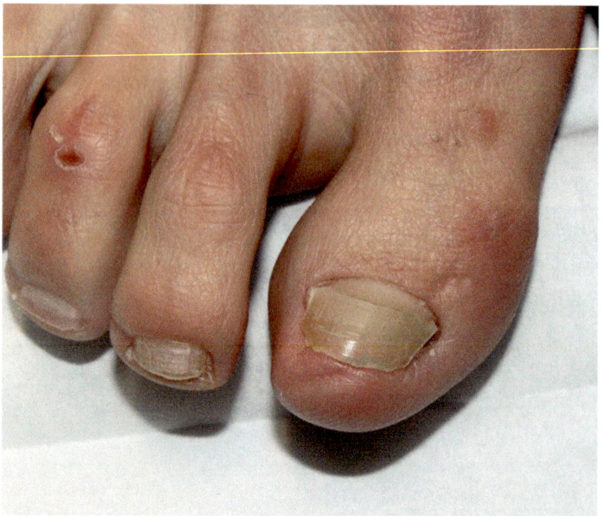

Fig. 26.2 60-Year-old female, Fitzpatrick type II, onychomadesis, with separation of the proximal and distal nail plates involving the right great toenail

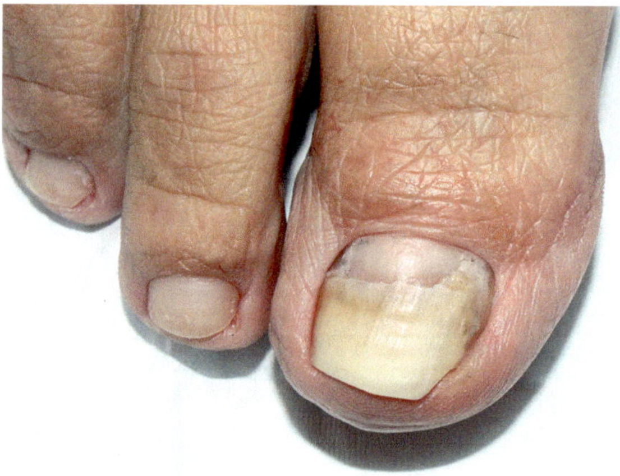

Fig. 26.3 51-Year-old female, Fitzpatrick type III, onychomadesis, with separation of the proximal and distal nail plates involving the right great toenail

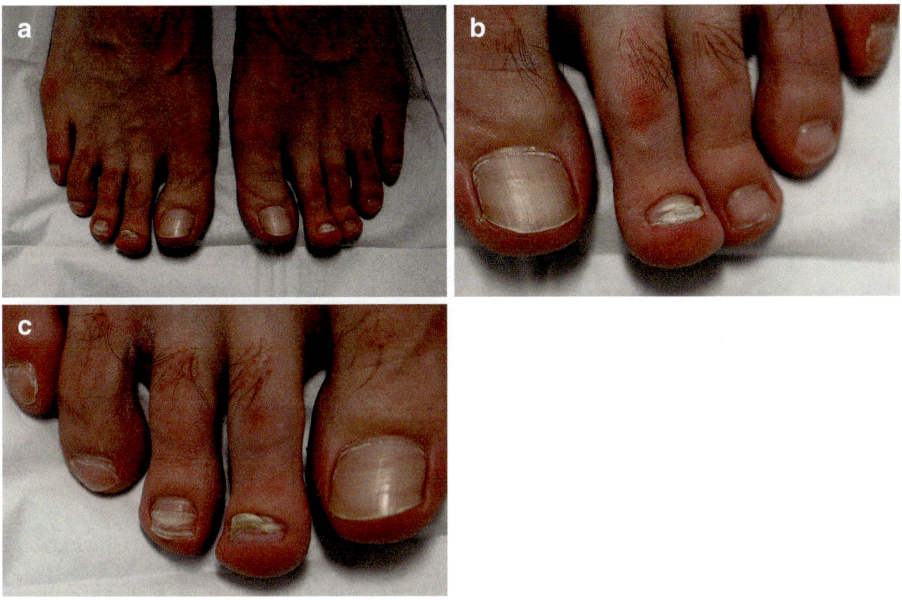

Fig. 26.4 (**a**) 40-Year-old male, Fitzpatrick type III, onychomadesis, with separation of the proximal and distal nail plates involving the right second, right third, and left second toenails. (**b**) 40-year-old male, Fitzpatrick type III, onychomadesis, with separation of the proximal and distal nail plates involving the left second toenail. (**c**) 40-year-old male, Fitzpatrick type III, onychomadesis, with separation of the proximal and distal nail plates involving the right second and third toenails

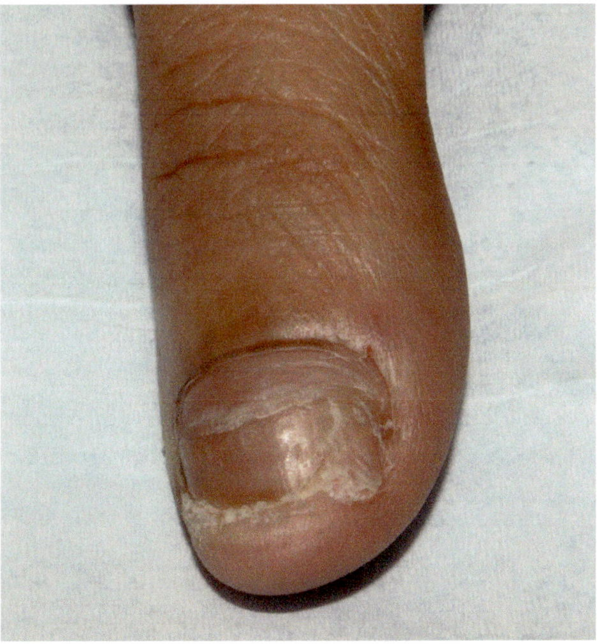

Fig. 26.5 39-Year-old female, Fitzpatrick type IV, onychomadesis, with separation of the proximal and distal nail plates involving the left thumbnail

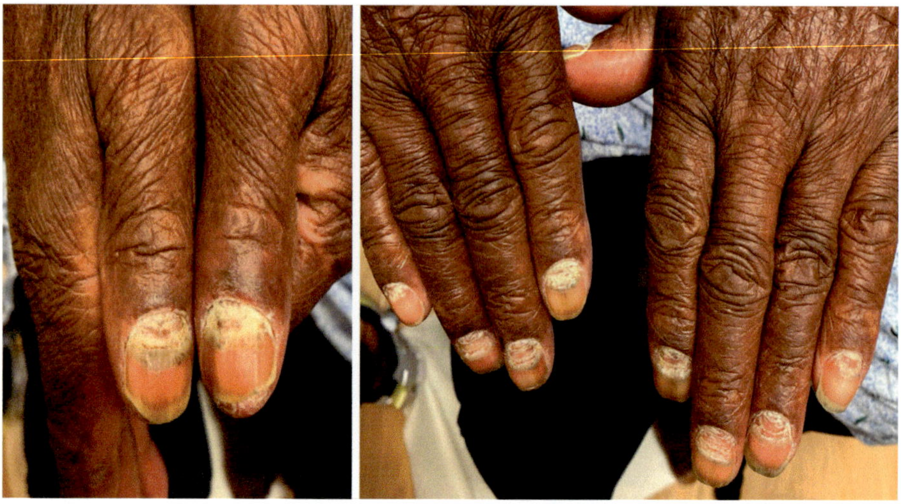

Fig. 26.6 78-year-old male, Fitzpatrick type V, onychomadesis, with separation of the proximal and distal nail plates involving multiple fingernails after starting treatment with talquetamab (*from* Narayan et al. [23]; *with permission*)

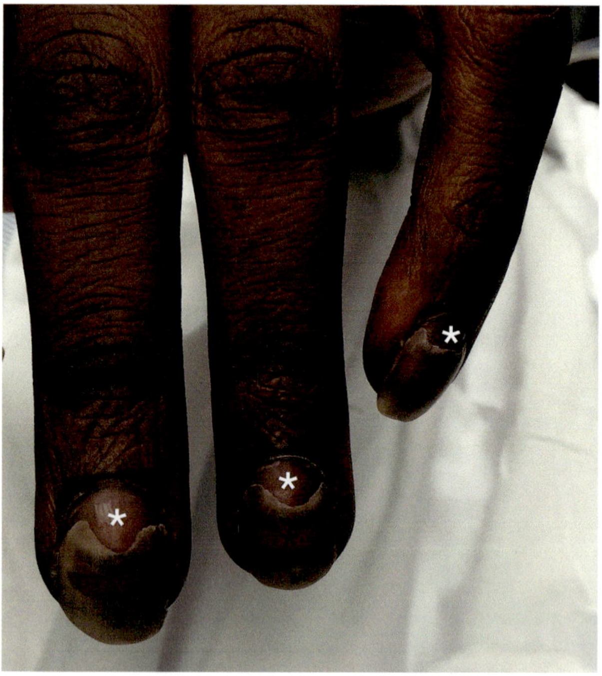

Fig. 26.7 23-Year-old male, Fitzpatrick type VI, onychomadesis, with separation of the proximal and distal nail plates involving multiple fingernails after hand, foot, and mouth disease. Examination of the patient's left hand shows the growth of new nails (white asterisk) underneath his previously healthy fingernails (black asterisk) (*from* Irving et al. [24]; *with permission*)

References

1. Lee DK, Lipner SR. Optimal diagnosis and management of common nail disorders. Ann Med. 2022;54(1):694–712.
2. Salgado F, Handler MZ, Schwartz RA. Shedding light on onychomadesis. Cutis. 2017;99(1):33–6.
3. Wortsman X, Wortsman J, Guerrero R, et al. Anatomical changes in retronychia and onychomadesis detected using ultrasound. Dermatol Surg. 2010;36(10):1615–20.
4. Hardin J, Haber RM. Onychomadesis: literature review. Br J Dermatol. 2015;172(3):592–6.
5. Braswell MA, Daniel CR, Brodell RT. Beau lines, onychomadesis, and retronychia: a unifying hypothesis. J Am Acad Dermatol. 2015;73(5):849–55.
6. Kim BR, Yu DA, Lee SR, Lim SS, Mun JH. Beau's lines and onychomadesis: a systematic review of characteristics and aetiology. Acta Derm Venereol. 2023;103:adv18251.
7. Li D, Wu Y, Xing X, Huang J, Mao A, Liu T, Rao P, Qin W, Zhang L, Feng L, Gao S, Guan X. Onychomadesis and potential association with HFMD outbreak in a kindergarten in Hubei province, China, 2017. BMC Infect Dis. 2019;19(1):995.
8. Guimbao J, Rodrigo P, Alberto MJ, Omeñaca M. Onychomadesis outbreak linked to hand, foot, and mouth disease, Spain, July 2008. Euro Surveill. 2010;15(37):19663.
9. Clark CM, Silverberg NB, Weinberg JM. What is your diagnosis? Onychomadesis following hand-foot-and-mouth disease. Cutis. 2015;95(312):319–20.
10. Chiu H-H, Liu M-T, Chung W-H, et al. The mechanism of onychomadesis (nail shedding) and beau's lines following hand-foot-mouth disease. Viruses. 2019;11(6):522.
11. Chu DH, Rubin AI. Diagnosis and management of nail disorders in children. Pediatr Clin North Am. 2014;61(2):293–308.
12. Osterback R, Vuorinen T, Linna M, et al. Coxsackievirus A6 and hand, foot, and mouth disease. Finland Emerg Infect Dis. 2009;15(9):1485–8.
13. Acharya S, Balachandran C. Onychomadesis in Stevens-Johnson syndrome. Indian J Dermatol Venereol Leprol. 1996;62(4):264–5.
14. Ciastko AR. Onychomadesis and Kawasaki disease. CMAJ. 2002;166(8):1069.
15. Patel NC, Silverman RA. Neonatal onychomadesis with candidiasis limited to affected nails. Pediatr Dermatol. 2008;25(6):641–2.
16. Mazereeuw-Hautier J, Bonafe JL. Bilateral beau's lines and pyogenic granulomas following Guillain-Barre syndrome. Dermatology. 2004;209(3):237–8.
17. LaRow JA, Mysliborski J, Rappaport IP, et al. Alopecia areata universalis in an infant. J Cutan Med Surg. 2001;5(2):131–4.
18. Habibi M, Mortazavi H, Shadianloo S, et al. Nail changes in pemphigus vulgaris. Int J Dermatol. 2008;47(11):1141–4.
19. Suchonwanit P, Nitayavardhana S. Idiopathic sporadic onychomadesis of toenails. Case Rep Dermatol Med. 2016;2016:6451327.
20. Martin S, Rudolph AH. Familial dystrophic periodic shedding of the nails. Cutis. 1980;25(6):622–3.
21. Pearson HJ, Brodell RT, Daniel Iii CR. Seasonal onychomadesis of the great toes. Skin Appendage Disord. 2018;4(3):177–9.
22. Nag SS, Dutta A, Mandal RK. Delayed cutaneous findings of hand, foot, and mouth disease. Indian Pediatr. 2016;53(1):42–4.
23. Narayan N, Williams B, Lipe B, De Benedetto A. Onychomadesis and palmoplantar keratoderma associated with talquetamab therapy for relapsed and refractory multiple myeloma. JAAD Case Rep. 2022;31:66–8.
24. Irving S, Barclay-Buchanan C. Onychomadesis: a rare sequela of hand, foot, and mouth disease. J Emerg Med. 2015;49(4):e127–8.

Retronychia

27

Kaya L. Curtis and Shari R. Lipner

27.1 Description of Disease

Retronychia refers to the proximal ingrowth of the nail into the proximal nail fold, typically resulting from trauma-induced disruption of longitudinal growth [1]. Normally, nail trauma results in the complete separation of the old nail plate from the matrix and nail bed [2]. A new nail plate subsequently grows beneath the old nail plate, advancing the old plate distally. For retronychia, an acute or repeated trauma results in partial separation of the old nail plate from the matrix and nail bed. Because the old nail plate is still partially attached, the new nail plate does not grow distally and instead grows underneath the old plate, pushing it upwards [3–5]. This process repeats, resulting in the layering of nail plates [2].

27.2 Epidemiology

Retronychia most frequently occurs in young female patients. In Pessoa et al.'s literature review [6] of 247 retronychia cases, there were 182 females (74%), 52 males (21%), and 31 patients of unknown gender, with mean age at diagnosis 31 years (range: 10–88). In Ventura et al.'s case series [2] of 20 patients, there was a female predilection of 95% (19/20), with a mean age of 28 years (range: 13–55). In Díaz et al.'s case series [7] of 9 pediatric retronychia patients (range: 0–18 years), 78% (7/9) of patients were female, suggesting that there may be a female preponderance among children and adolescents.

S. R. Lipner, *Atlas of Nail Disorders Across All Skin Colors*,
https://doi.org/10.1007/978-3-031-74272-9_27

27.3 Risk Factors

Retronychia typically results from a single acute toe trauma or repeated microtrauma [8]. Common causes of repeated microtrauma include hiking, jogging, dancing, or wearing ill-fitted shoes. Structural deformities of the feet, such as hammer toes, claw toes, or bunions, can also lead to repeated microtrauma resulting from friction between the toes and/or shoes when walking. Osteoarthritis has also been associated with retronychia [9]. In Ventura et al.'s case series [2] of 20 patients, a history of repeated trauma (particularly sports) and claw toes was present in 50% (10/20) and 45% (9/20) of patients, respectively. In Pessoa et al.'s literature review [6], 23% (57/247) had a history of acute trauma, 21% (53/247) had a history of microtrauma related to sports, and 11% (28/247) reported wearing inappropriate footwear (e.g., high heels and tight shoes). In Piraccini et al.'s case series [10] of 15 pediatric and adolescent patients, 53% (8/15) reported a history of trauma, including acute trauma, jogging, dancing, and wearing uncomfortable shoes. It remains unclear as to why retronychia is reported more often in adult patients, given the generally higher activity level of pediatric and adolescent patients, though it is hypothesized to be due to the faster rate of nail plate growth in children [10]. Adults may also accumulate more traumatic events over time.

27.4 Clinical Features

Retronychia presentation may be classified into two stages. In the early stage, there is an arrest of nail growth and xanthonychia. In the later stage, these symptoms persist but with accompanying severe paronychia and edema-induced elevation of the proximal nail fold [1, 8, 11]. Other physical examination features include onycholysis, layering, and thickening. Granulation tissue may develop between the proximal and lateral nail folds [1]. Patients universally report very slow or arrested nail growth. Patients may also complain of pain, which may be exacerbated when walking due to downward pressure from footwear [1]. There may be accompanying chronic paronychia [1]. Retronychia more commonly occurs in the toenails, in particular, the great toenail(s). In Pessoa et al.'s literature review [6] of 247 patients, there were 200 cases (80.9%) of toenail involvement, 26 cases (10.5%) of fingernail involvement, and unspecified location in 21 patients. The great toenail was involved in 92% and bilateral toenails involved in 25%. In Ventura et al.'s case series [2], 100% (20/20) of cases involved the great toenail, with bilateral toenails involved in 30% (6/20). In Piraccini et al.'s case series [10], clinical features of retronychia among 15 pediatric and adolescent patients were similar to that of adults, namely, xanthonychia, granulation tissue below the cuticle, and reported arrest of nail growth. Díaz's case series [7] of nine pediatric retronychia patients confirmed this finding, with the most common clinical signs being xanthonychia, layering, and proximal nail fold purulence.

27.5 Clinical Features in Skin of Color

Distinct clinical presentations of retronychia in the skin of color have not been characterized. Longitudinal melanonychia may be present, particularly in adult patients, in addition to classical clinical features.

27.6 Requirements for Diagnosis

Retronychia is a clinical diagnosis. A history of very slow or arrested nail growth is required for diagnosis. A history of trauma is a supportive feature. Ultrasound may aid in diagnosis, demonstrating a thickened nail plate underlying the proximal nail fold [1]; multiple superimposed nail plates confirm the diagnosis [8]. In a case-control study [12] of 43 retronychia nails and 167 normal nails, other significant ultrasound diagnostic findings included: (1) hypoechoic halo surrounding the origin of nail plate, (2) reduced distance between nail plate origin and base of distal phalanx, and (3) increased proximal nail fold thickness.

27.7 Cases

Figures 27.1, 27.2, 27.3, 27.4, 27.5, 27.6, 27.7, 27.8, 27.9, 27.10, 27.11, and 27.12 demonstrate the presentation of retronychia in a clinical setting.

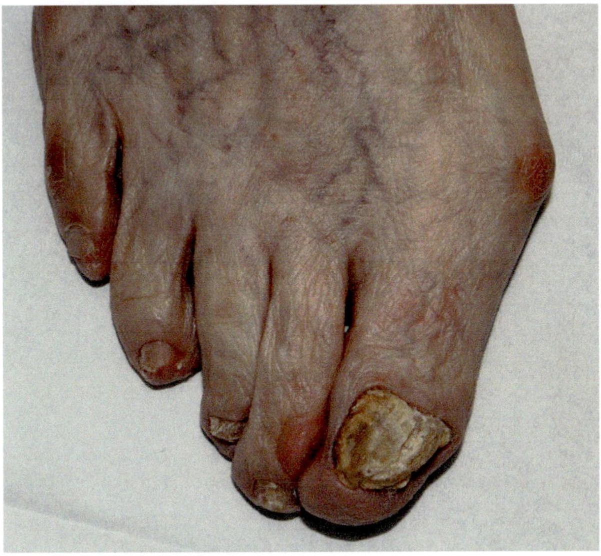

Fig. 27.1 76-Year-old female, Fitzpatrick type I, retronychia, with xanthonychia and nail thickening involving the right great toenail

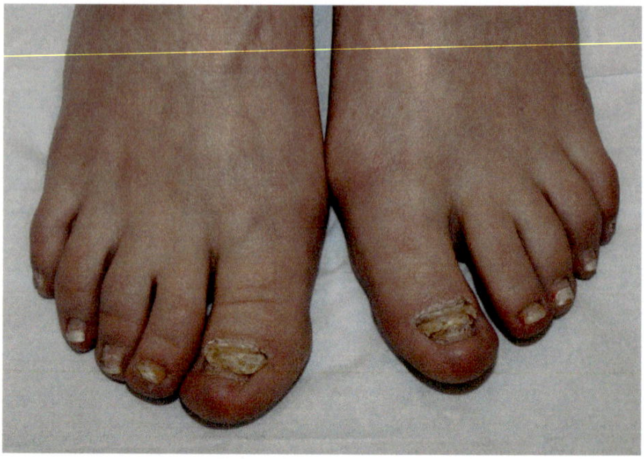

Fig. 27.2 32-Year-old female, Fitzpatrick type II, retronychia, with xanthonychia, layering, and nail thickening involving the bilateral great toenails

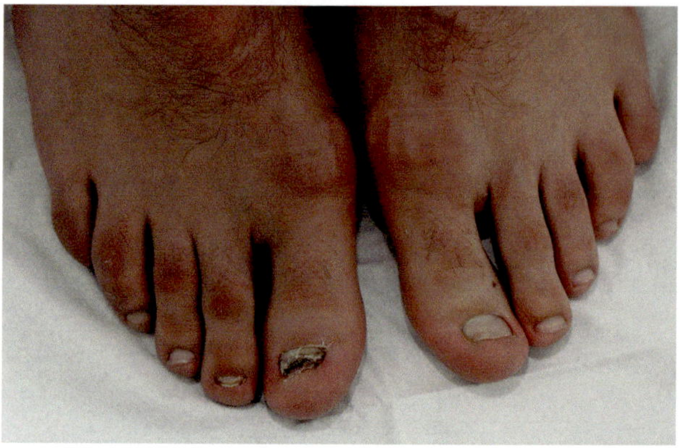

Fig. 27.3 34-Year-old male, Fitzpatrick type II, retronychia, with xanthonychia, nail thickening, and nail shortening involving the right great and second toenails

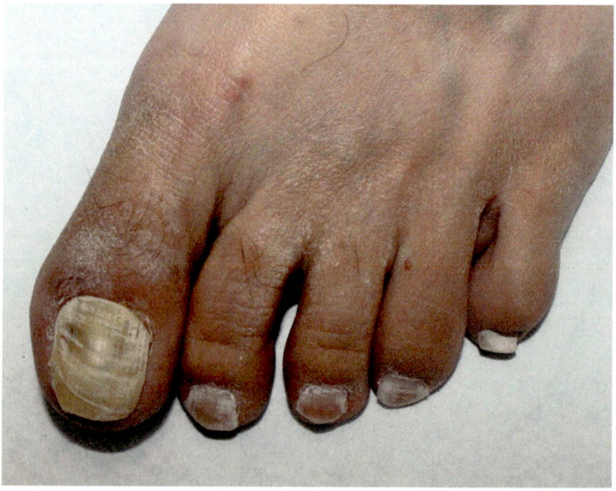

Fig. 27.4 48-Year-old male, Fitzpatrick type III, retronychia, with xanthonychia and layered nails involving the left great toenail

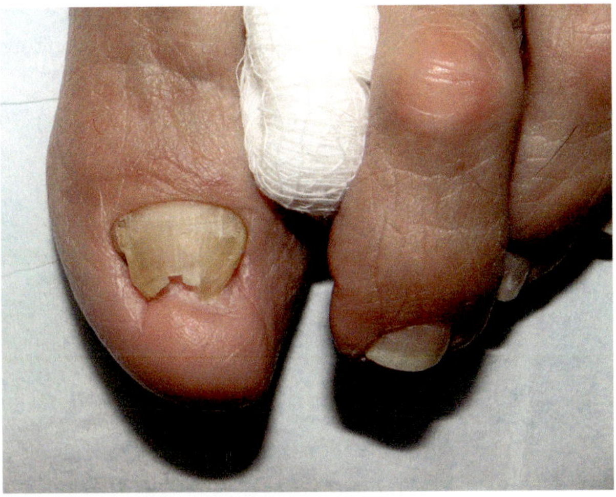

Fig. 27.5 64-Year-old female, Fitzpatrick type III, retronychia, with xanthonychia, nail thickening, and nail bed shortening involving the left great toenail

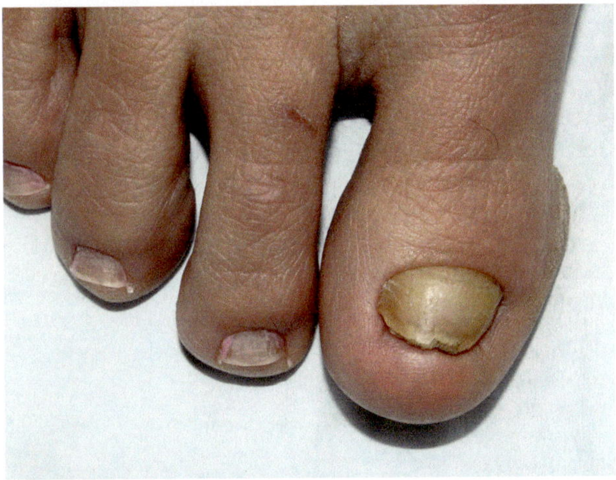

Fig. 27.6 33-Year-old female, Fitzpatrick type III, retronychia, with xanthonychia and nail thickening involving the right great toenail

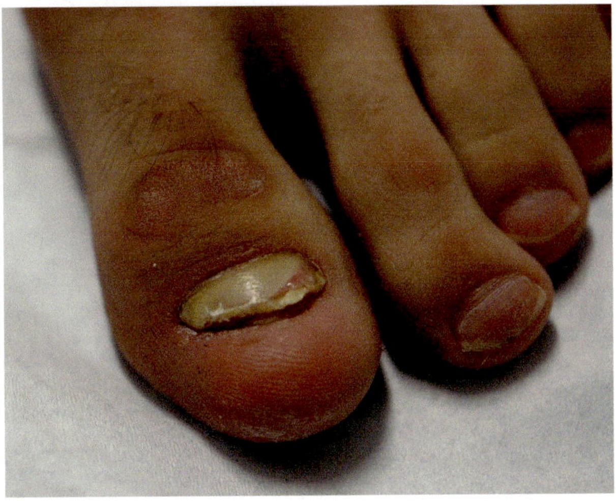

Fig. 27.7 43-Year-old male, Fitzpatrick type III, retronychia, with xanthonychia, nail thickening, and nail bed shortening involving the left great toenail

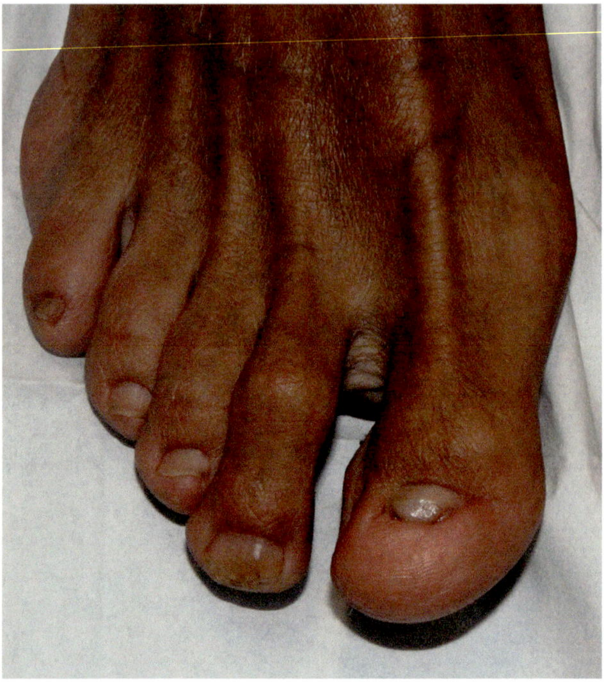

Fig. 27.8 68-Year-old male, Fitzpatrick type IV, retronychia, with nail plate thickening and nail bed shortening involving the right great toenail

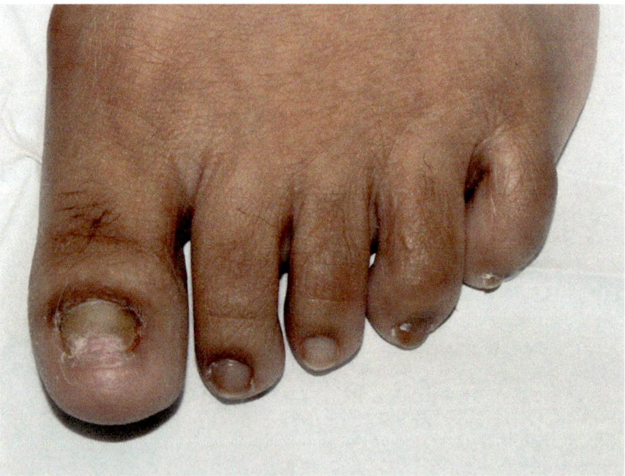

Fig. 27.9 46-Year-old female, Fitzpatrick type IV, retronychia, with nail plate thickening and nail bed shortening involving the left great toenail. There is hyperpigmentation of the proximal nail fold

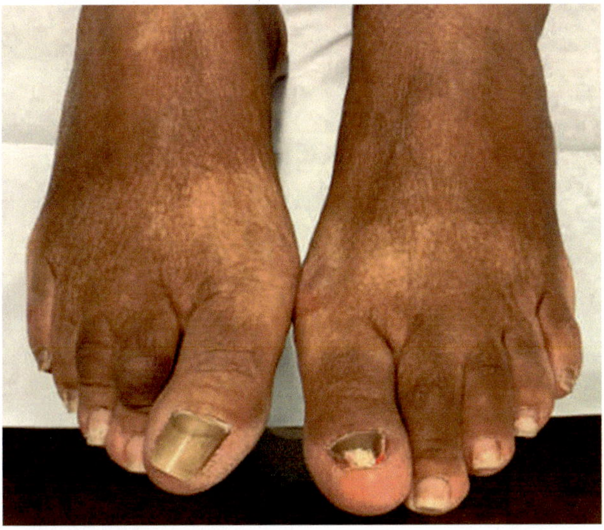

Fig. 27.10 78-Year-old female, Fitzpatrick type V, retronychia, with nail plate thickening and nail bed shortening involving the left great toenail

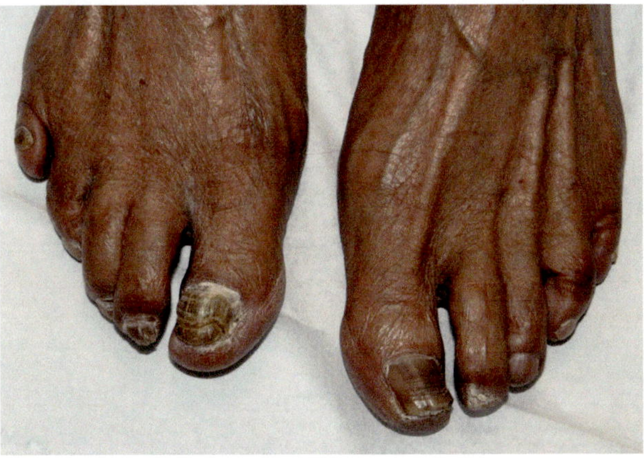

Fig. 27.11 81-Year-old female, Fitzpatrick type V, retronychia, with thickening, layering, and brown discoloration of the bilateral great toenails, with right great toenail with more severe thickening than left great toenail

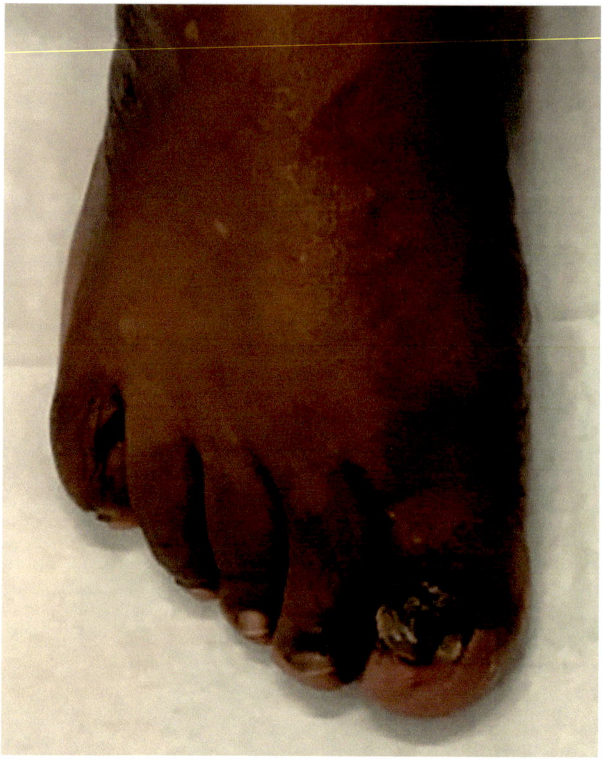

Fig. 27.12 74-Year-old female, Fitzpatrick type VI, retronychia, with thickening and brown discoloration of the right great toenail

References

1. Lee DK, Lipner SR. Optimal diagnosis and management of common nail disorders. Ann Med. 2022;54(1):694–712.
2. Ventura F, Correia O, Duarte AF, Barros AM, Haneke E. Retronychia—clinical and pathophysiological aspects. J Eur Acad Dermatol Venereol. 2016;30(1):16–9.
3. Dahdah MJ, Kibbi AG, Ghosn S. Retronychia: report of two cases. J Am Acad Dermatol. 2008;58(6):1051–3.
4. de Berker DA, Richert B, Duhard E, Piraccini BM, André J, Baran R. Retronychia: proximal ingrowing of the nail plate. J Am Acad Dermatol. 2008;58(6):978–83.
5. Baumgartner M, Haneke E. Retronychia: diagnosis and treatment. Dermatologic Surg. 2010;36(10):1610–4.
6. Pessoa E, Costa T, João AL, Lencastre A. Retronychia: a paradigm shift? Skin Appendage Disord. 2020;6(5):268–71.
7. Díaz MS, Boggio P, Calvano R, Scacchi MF, Giachetti A. Retronychia in children: a case series. Pediatr Dermatol. 2023;
8. Mello CDBF, Souza MDRE, Noriega LF, Chiacchio ND. Retronychia. An Bras Dermatol. 2018;93(5):707–11.
9. Braswell MA, Daniel CR 3rd, Brodell RT. Beau lines, onychomadesis, and retronychia: a unifying hypothesis. J Am Acad Dermatol. 2015;73(5):849–55.

10. Piraccini BM, Richert B, de Berker DA, Tengattini V, Sgubbi P, Patrizi A, Stinchi C, Savoia F. Retronychia in children, adolescents, and young adults: a case series. J Am Acad Dermatol. 2014;70(2):388–90.
11. Gerard E, Prevezas C, Doutre MS, Beylot-Barry M, Cogrel O. Risk factors, clinical variants and therapeutic outcome of retronychia: a retrospective study of 18 patients. Eur J Dermatol. 2016;26(4):377–81.
12. Fernández J, Reyes-Baraona F, Wortsman X. Ultrasonographic criteria for diagnosing unilateral and bilateral retronychia. J Ultrasound Med. 2018;37(5):1201–9.

Yellow Nail Syndrome

28

Kaya L. Curtis and Shari R. Lipner

28.1 Description of Disease

Yellow nail syndrome is characterized by a clinical triad of yellow nails, respiratory disease, and lymphedema. Impairment of lymphatic flow is frequently hypothesized as the etiology, although pathogenesis is unknown.

28.2 Epidemiology

Yellow nail syndrome is rare, with an estimated prevalence of <1/1,000,000. Cases have been reported worldwide [1]. Patients >50 years are typically affected. There may be a slight male predominance [2]. Juvenile forms affecting pediatric patients (congenital or during childhood) have been rarely reported [2]. In Piraccini et al.'s retrospective observational study [3], there were 21 patients diagnosed with yellow nail syndrome out of 15,600 patient visits to the outpatient nail clinic at the University of Bologna over a 28-year period. Overall, there were 11 male patients and 10 female patients with a mean age of 57 (range: 29–83) years [3]. In Benassaia et al.'s case series [2] of 23 yellow nail syndrome patients, there were 13 male patients and 10 female patients affected, including three pediatric patients who had yellow nails at birth or during childhood. For the remaining 20 patients, the median age at onset of yellow nail syndrome was 50.8 (range: 43–61) years [2].

28.3 Risk Factors

Yellow nail syndrome has been associated with autoimmune disease, immunodeficiency disorders, primary intestinal lymphangiectasia (Waldmann's disease), and malignancy. There have been case reports of familial forms of yellow nail

S. R. Lipner, *Atlas of Nail Disorders Across All Skin Colors*,
https://doi.org/10.1007/978-3-031-74272-9_28

syndrome, suggesting that there may be a genetic component to disease pathogenesis [4]. Titanium exposure, such as in dental or joint implants, has also been proposed as a risk factor for the development of yellow nail syndrome [5].

28.4 Clinical Features

On physical examination, nails are characterized by xanthonychia, thickening, increased transverse curvature, scleronychia, opacity, missing lunula (due to nail hyperkeratosis), missing cuticle, or onycholysis [1, 6]. Patients almost universally report a history of arrest or delay of nail growth. Patients may complain of difficulty cutting nails due to scleronychia and thickening. A complete clinical triad at presentation was reported in 27–60% of patients in a literature review of case series [1]. Common accompanying respiratory disorders include chronic sinusitis, pleural effusion, and bronchiectasia [1]. Respiratory involvement has been reported in 56–71% of patients [1]. In patients with undiagnosed respiratory disorder, reported symptoms may include chronic cough, shortness of breath, nasal drip, nasal congestion, or facial pressure [2]. Lymphedema has been reported in 29–80% of patients in a literature review [1]. Lymphedema most commonly occurs in the lower extremities, though the upper extremities and face may also be involved [2]. A bedside test for lymphedema is to pinch the skin on the dorsal side of the second toe, with a positive test being the inability to pinch the skin (Stemmer's sign) [1]. In Benassaia et al.'s case series [2] of 23 yellow nail syndrome patients, all patients had fingernail involvement, whereas only 16/23 (69.6%) had toenail involvement. In this case series, the complete clinical triad was present in only 16/23 (69.6%). The initial signs of yellow nail syndrome were chronic cough in 10/22 (45.5%), yellow nails in 6/22 (27.3%), chronic sinusitis in 4/22 (18.2%), and lymphedema in 2/22 (9.1%). In Piraccini et al.'s retrospective study [3], 15/21 (71.4%) had all nails involved, whereas 6/21 (28.6%) had only fingernail involvement. In this study, the complete clinical triad was present in only 6/21 (28.6%).

28.5 Clinical Features in Skin of Color

Yellow discoloration may be more subtle in patients with skin of color. Xanthonychia may be less apparent and may be enhanced with dermoscopy. Darker-skinned patients may have nails which have a dark greenish hue rather than the yellow coloration. Opacity and loss of lunula may be a more prominent clinical feature. Accompanying proximal nail fold erythema may be less apparent.

28.6 Requirements for Diagnosis

Yellow nail syndrome is a clinical diagnosis. Two manifestations of the clinical triad (yellow nails, respiratory disorder, lymphedema) are necessary to meet the clinical criteria for diagnosis. A history of arrest or delay of nail growth is an important diagnostic feature. A history of common comorbidities, such as malignancy and autoimmune disease, should be elicited. A family history of yellow nail syndrome may be a supportive feature. It is recommended that nail clippings are performed to rule out other causes of yellow nails, including onychomycosis. However, onychomycosis and yellow nail syndrome may present concurrently. Referral is made to pulmonology for chest imaging to assess for respiratory tract involvement. Patients with sinus symptoms are referred to otolaryngology, as sinus computed tomography may be indicated.

28.7 Cases

Figures 28.1, 28.2, 28.3, 28.4, 28.5, and 28.6 demonstrate the presentation of yellow nail syndrome in a clinical setting.

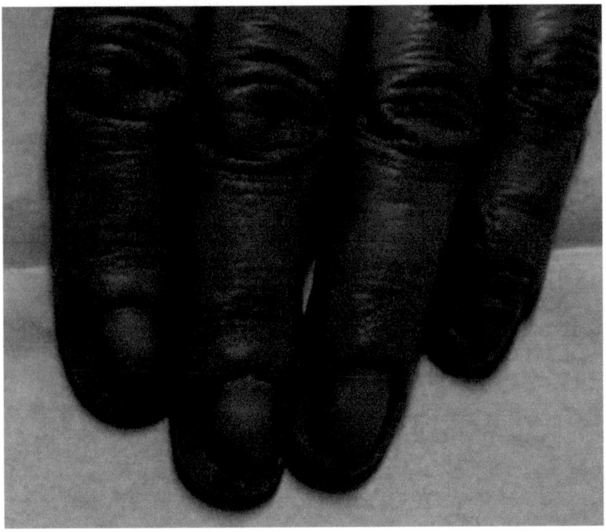

Fig. 28.1 63-Year-old female, Fitzpatrick type II, yellow nail syndrome, with xanthonychia, thickening, opacity, missing lunulae, missing cuticles, onychomadesis, proximal nail fold erythema and swelling, and increased transverse curvature of the left fingernails

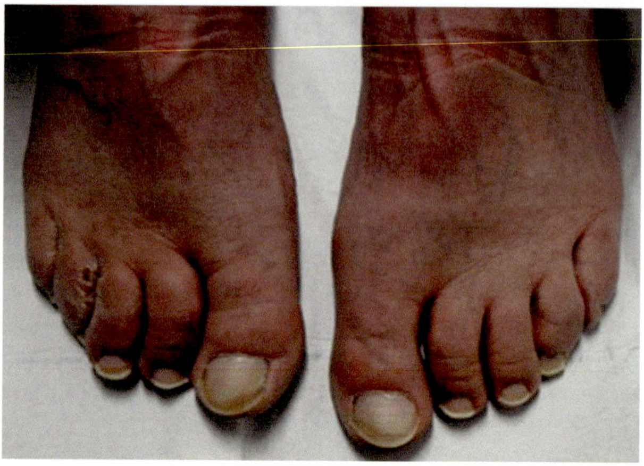

Fig. 28.2 73-Year-old male, Fitzpatrick type II, yellow nail syndrome, with xanthonychia, thickening, missing lunulae, and increased transverse curvature of the toenails. There is lymphedema of the lower extremities

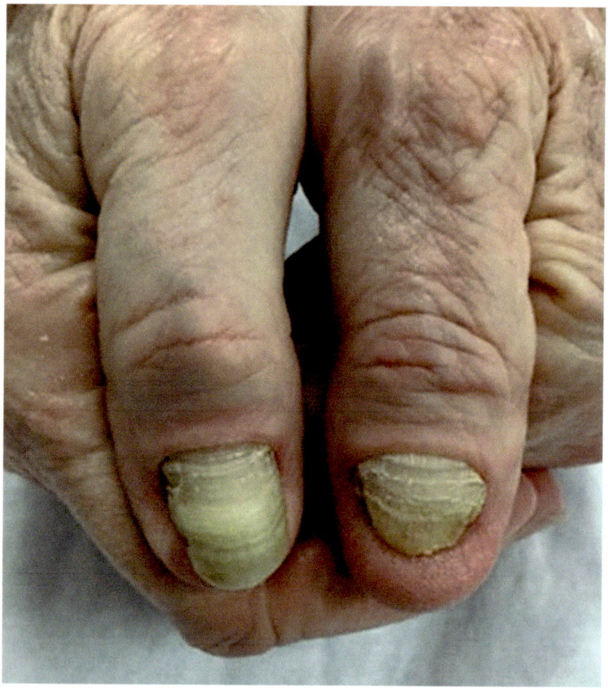

Fig. 28.3 75-Year-old male, Fitzpatrick type II, yellow nail syndrome, with xanthonychia, thickening, missing cuticles, onychomadesis, and increased transverse curvature of the bilateral thumbnails

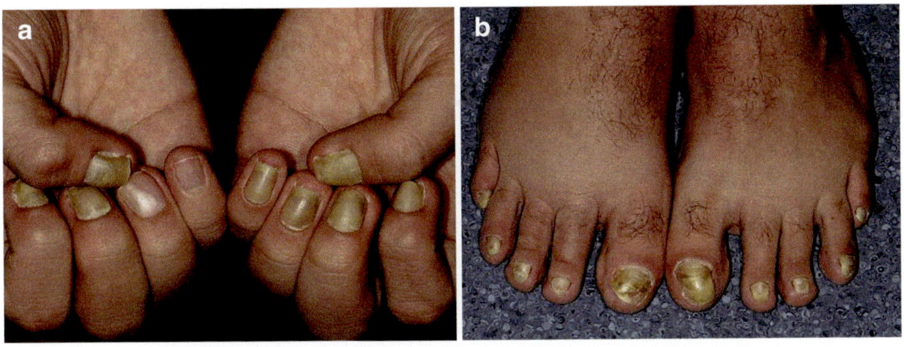

Fig. 28.4 (**a**) 14-Year-old male, Fitzpatrick type III, yellow nail syndrome, with yellow-green nail discoloration on hands. (**b**) 14-year-old male, Fitzpatrick type III, yellow nail syndrome, with yellow-green nail discoloration on feet (*from* El Alami et al. [7]; *with permission*)

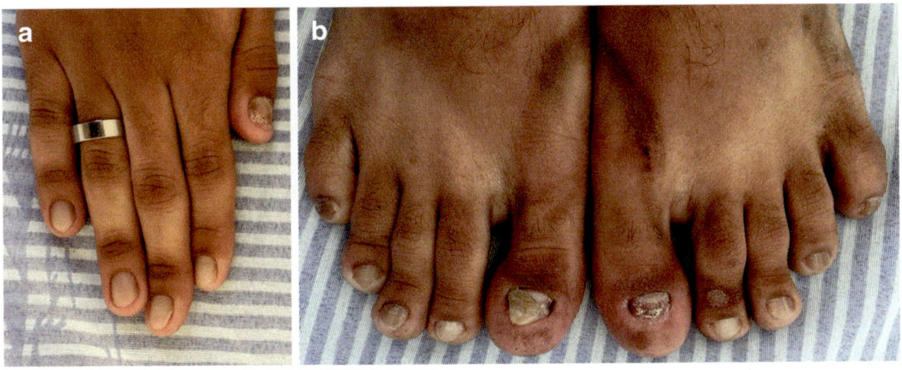

Fig. 28.5 (**a**) 21-Year-old male, Fitzpatrick type IV, yellow nail syndrome, with fingernails showing yellowish discoloration, thickening, absence of lunula and cuticle, and dystrophy of some nails. (**b**) 21-year-old male, Fitzpatrick type IV, yellow nail syndrome, with toenails showing yellowish discoloration, thickening, absence of lunula and cuticle, and dystrophy of some nails (*from* Almeida Issa et al. [8]; *with permission*)

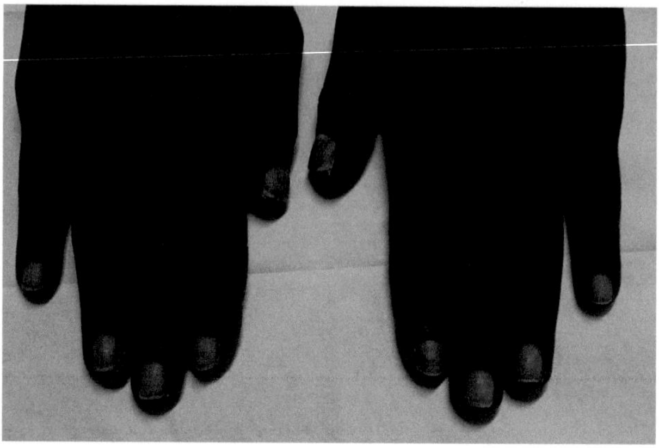

Fig. 28.6 43-Year-old male, Fitzpatrick type VI, yellow nail syndrome, with xanthonychia, increased transverse curvature, opacity, and thickening of fingernails

References

1. Vignes S, Baran R. Yellow nail syndrome: a review. Orphanet J Rare Dis. 2017;12(1):42.
2. Benassaia E, Abba S, Fourgeaud C, Mihoubi A, Vignes S. Yellow nail syndrome: analysis of 23 consecutive patients and effect of combined fluconazole-vitamin-E treatment. Dermatology. 2023.
3. Piraccini BM, Urciuoli B, Starace M, Tosti A, Balestri R. Yellow nail syndrome: clinical experience in a series of 21 patients. J Dtsch Dermatol Ges. 2014;12(2):131–7.
4. Abid N, Loukil M, Mahmoud N, Badri I, Bouzaidi K, Ghrairi H. Yellow nail syndrome: a genetic disorder? Tunis Med. 2021;99(4):475–7. English.
5. Berglund F, Carlmark B. Titanium, sinusitis, and the yellow nail syndrome. Biol Trace Elem Res. 2011;143(1):1–7.
6. Stosiek N, Peters KP, Hiller D, Riedl B, Hornstein OP. Yellow nail syndrome in a patient with mycosis fungoides. J Am Acad Dermatol. 1993;28(5 Pt 1):792–4.
7. El Alami J, Galicier L, Huynh S, Frumholtz L, Bagot M, de Masson A, Vignes S, Bouaziz JD. Congenital yellow nail syndrome presenting with eyelid lymphedema and fetal hydrops. JAAD Case Rep. 2019;5(11):1010–2.
8. Almeida Issa MC, de Oliveira BC, Vaz de Campos F, Severo Alves de Melo A, de Alencar Araripe Junior A, Pantaleão L. Yellow nail syndrome and overlap syndrome of autoimmune hepatitis and cholangitis: a rare association or an atypical presentation? Ann Dermatol Venereol. 2020;147(12):881–4.

Koilonychia

29

Rachel C. Hill and Shari R. Lipner

29.1 Description of Disease

Koilonychia, commonly known as "spoon nails," refers to flattening of the middle part of the nail plate in conjunction with upward curvature of the distal nail plate and/or lateral edges [1]. It may be caused by abnormal blood flow to the digit, nail bed hyperkeratosis leading to an abnormal shape, or a protein/amino acid deficiency state, although the pathophysiology is debated [1, 2]. Koilonychia may occur in association with primary dermatologic disease or systemic illness. Most causes of koilonychia can be classified as acquired, idiopathic, or hereditary [1].

29.2 Epidemiology

29.2.1 Sex

Sex distribution of koilonychia has not been previously described. However, some autoimmune diseases associated with koilonychia, including alopecia areata and systemic lupus erythematosus (SLE), disproportionately affect women. As such, koilonychia may be more common in women vs. men depending on the underlying etiology.

29.2.2 Age

Patients of all age groups can be affected by koilonychia, and age distribution depends on the underlying etiology. Koilonychia secondary to systemic diseases, including iron deficiency anemia and thyroid disorders, or secondary to therapies, such as hemodialysis for chronic kidney disease, more commonly affects older patients. Hereditary koilonychia affects patients of all ages. In pediatric patients, koilonychia may be idiopathic and often regresses over time [3].

S. R. Lipner, *Atlas of Nail Disorders Across All Skin Colors*,
https://doi.org/10.1007/978-3-031-74272-9_29

29.2.3 Race

Previous studies have not reported on the association of koilonychia with race or ethnicity. Patients of all races and ethnicities are affected [4].

29.3 Risk Factors

Several medical and lifestyle risk factors have been associated with koilonychia. Primary dermatologic diseases may predispose to acquired koilonychia, including inflammatory disorders such as nail psoriasis, nail lichen planus, onychomycosis, or trachyonychia [1, 5–7].

Koilonychia is classically associated with iron deficiency anemia and is reported to occur in approximately 5–6% of patients with iron deficiency anemia [1, 8–11]. Severity of iron deficiency anemia does not correlate with severity of koilonychia [1, 9]. Iron deficiency anemia may be the most common cause of koilonychia in children [1]. Other iron storage abnormalities, including hemochromatosis, have also been reported as causes of koilonychia. In a case series of 100 patients with idiopathic hemochromatosis, 49% of patients had koilonychia [12]. Koilonychia may be present in up to 50% of patients with Plummer–Vinson syndrome, characterized by a triad of iron deficiency anemia, esophageal webs, and dysphagia [1, 13]. In a case series of eight patients with Plummer–Vinson syndrome, three (37.5%) had koilonychia [1, 14].

Thyroid disorders, including both hypo- and hyperthyroidism, are also associated with koilonychia [2]. In a retrospective study of 32 patients in Iraq with koilonychia, 22 (68.8%) patients had hyperthyroidism [15].

Nutritional deficiencies in vitamin C, zinc, copper, selenium, and amino acids due to poor intake or malabsorption are also associated with koilonychia [1]. These deficiencies may occur in patients with chronic malnutrition, including children and adults living in impoverished areas, patients with alcohol use disorder, or those suffering from chronic illness that diminishes absorption capacity in the gastrointestinal tract. Likewise, patients with end-stage renal failure undergoing hemodialysis who are also at risk for nutritional deficiencies may be at increased risk for koilonychia [16].

Autoimmune conditions, including SLE and alopecia areata, have been infrequently associated with koilonychia [17, 18]. In a cross-sectional study of 197 patients with alopecia areata, koilonychia was the third most common nail change in patients with severe alopecia areata vs. mild-to-moderate alopecia areata ($P < 0.009$) after pitting and distal notching [18]. Koilonychia in SLE may accompany more common nail changes, including red lunula and nail plate thinning [19]. Raynaud's phenomenon, which may accompany autoimmune disease including SLE or scleroderma, is also a known cause of koilonychia, likely due to restricted blood flow to the digits [20].

Living at high altitude may be a risk factor for koilonychia, with prevalence estimates of koilonychia in Indian Himalayan communities ranging from 7% to 47% [21, 22]. In a cross-sectional study of 200 consecutive outpatients at a hospital in the

Himalayan region of India at an altitude of 3,840 m, 16% of patients examined had koilonychia [23]. In a cross-sectional study including 176 individuals from the Indian territory of Ladakh, a region of the Indian Himalaya, koilonychia was observed in 47.2% of subjects, perhaps due to hematologic changes that occur after spending long time periods at high altitude [21].

Occupational exposures can result in acquired koilonychia, mainly in manual labor jobs involving repeated physical trauma or exposure to motor oils or organic solvents, intricate work involving the fingers, such as coil winding, and professions with chemical exposure to the hands, including hairdressing [24–28].

Rarely, koilonychia can also be hereditary and inherited in an autosomal dominant manner with a high degree of penetrance [1, 29, 30]. Hereditary koilonychia can span multiple generations and a pedigree is used to help make the diagnosis [31]. Koilonychia may also be inherited as part of monilethrix, an autosomal dominant hair shaft disorder in which the hair shaft is fragile with a beaded appearance [32]. Other features, including keratosis pilaris and syndermatotic cataract, have been reported in conjunction with hereditary koilonychia, although only in rare case reports [33, 34]. In such cases, koilonychia occurs in the absence of iron deficiency anemia or thyroid abnormalities and can affect the fingernails, toenails, or both [1, 35, 36].

29.4 Clinical Features

On physical examination, koilonychia is characterized by concave nail dystrophy oriented laterally or transversely, in which the nail plate is centrally depressed with eversion of the lateral nail edges [1]. The nail plate may also appear thin and brittle [4]. The first, second, and third fingernails are most often affected other than in pediatric cases of hereditary congenital koilonychia, in which case fingernails and toenails may be equally affected [37]. In cases of koilonychia secondary to nail lichen planus with nail matrix involvement, there may also be longitudinal ridging, splitting, and nail plate thinning. With nail bed involvement, there may be onycholysis and nail bed hyperkeratosis [38]. When koilonychia is secondary to nail psoriasis with nail matrix involvement, pitting, leukonychia, red lunula, and crumbling may be observed. When nail psoriasis involves the nail bed onycholysis, subungual hyperkeratosis, salmon patches, and splinter hemorrhages may be seen [38].

Koilonychia should be considered in the context of other physical examination findings, review of systems, and comorbidities. In children, koilonychia present at birth or in early childhood necessitates an evaluation of family history. In patients with nail findings in addition to koilonychia, other signs and symptoms may be elicited, such as joint pain, rashes, or mucocutaneous plaques, which might suggest nail psoriasis or lichen planus as the underlying etiology. Nail clippings may also be performed to rule out onychomycosis in equivocal cases [1]. Prompt recognition of lichen planus as an etiology of koilonychia is necessary to prevent permanent scarring. If other nail findings are absent, patients can be screened for iron deficiency anemia risk factors, including family history, nutritional status and diet, and symptoms of dysphagia. When iron is replete in patients with koilonychia secondary to iron deficiency anemia, the fingernails and toenails may return to normal within 6 and 12 months of treatment, respectively [1]. In patients without risk factors for iron deficiency anemia, consider thyroid dysfunction, occupational exposures, and high-altitude living [1]. Idiopathic koilonychia may occur, in which case no underlying etiology can be elicited [1].

29.5 Clinical Features in Skin of Color

Although features of koilonychia in the skin of color patients have not been explicitly described, patients with skin of color are more likely to have physiologic melanonychia affecting the fingernails and toenails, which may accompany koilonychia upon clinical presentation.

29.6 Requirements for Diagnosis

Koilonychia is a clinical diagnosis that is made on physical examination alone. Viewing a nail with suspected koilonychia from the lateral perspective allows for a greater appreciation of the associated shape changes [1]. Simple clinical tests, such as the water-drop test, can be used to quickly assess for concavity of the nail [39]. Due to the numerous etiologies of koilonychia, an appropriate workup based on clinical features, physical examination, patient and family medical history, and occupational history can be narrowed down to specific etiologies [1, 39]. It is recommended that iron studies are performed in all patients presenting with koilonychia. A family history of koilonychia in a pediatric patient presenting with the disorder is supportive of a hereditary condition.

29.7 Cases

Figures 29.1, 29.2, 29.3, 29.4, 29.5, 29.6, 29.7, and 29.8 demonstrate the presentation of koilonychia in a clinical setting.

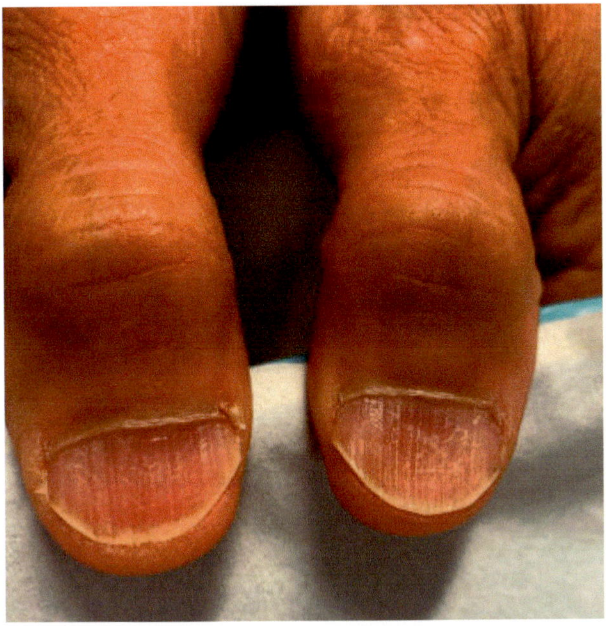

Fig. 29.1 55-Year-old male, Fitzpatrick type II, koilonychia, with involvement of the bilateral thumbnails and onychorrhexis. The patient had Crohn's disease and an iron panel, vitamin B12, folate, and thyroid function tests were all within normal limits. Etiology: unknown

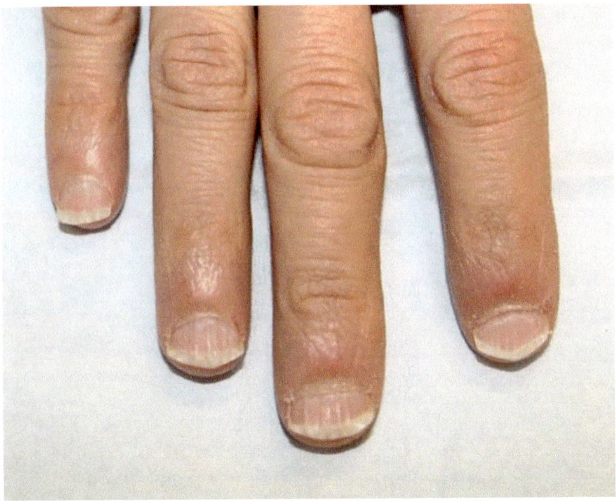

Fig. 29.2 44-Year-old male, Fitzpatrick type II, koilonychia, with onychorrhexis, onycholysis, and rapid fingernail growth involving the right 2nd–fifth fingernails. Etiology: nail psoriasis (*from* Conway et al. [5]; *with permission*)

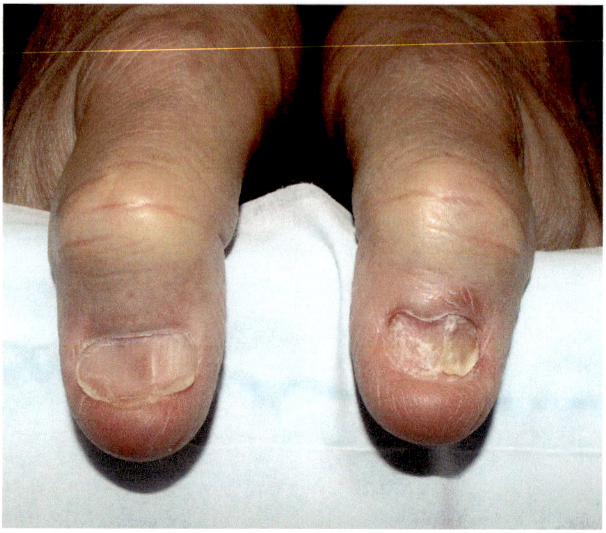

Fig. 29.3 73-Year-old male, Fitzpatrick type II, koilonychia, with nail plate atrophy and onycholysis. Etiology: lichen planus

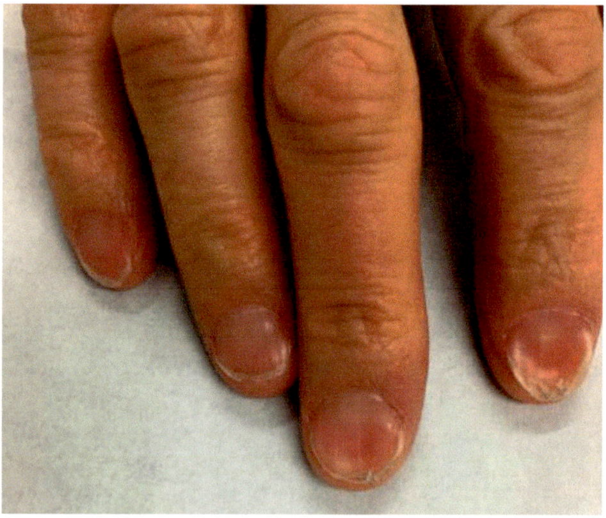

Fig. 29.4 72-Year-old female, Fitzpatrick type II, koilonychia, with onychoschizia involving all fingernails. Etiology: lichen planus

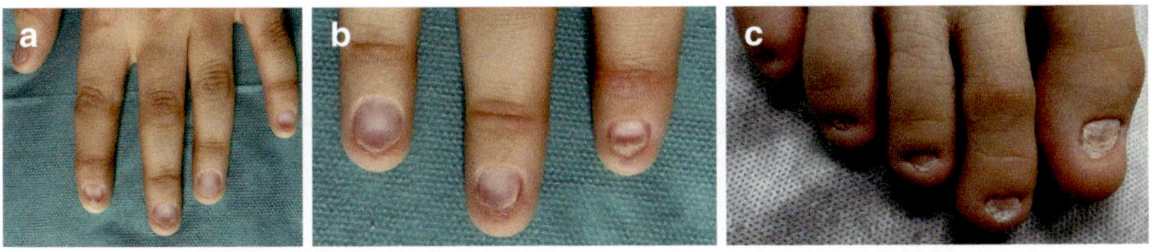

Fig. 29.5 (**a–c**), 11-Year-old male, Fitzpatrick type II–III, koilonychia, with involvement of the bilateral fingernails and toenails since early childhood. Etiology: hereditary koilonychia (*from* Callega-Algarra [30]; *with permission*)

Fig. 29.6 Adult male of unknown age, Fitzpatrick type IV, koilonychia, with distal, transverse melanonychia. Etiology: unknown. (*image used with permission from* VisualDx; www.visualdx.com)

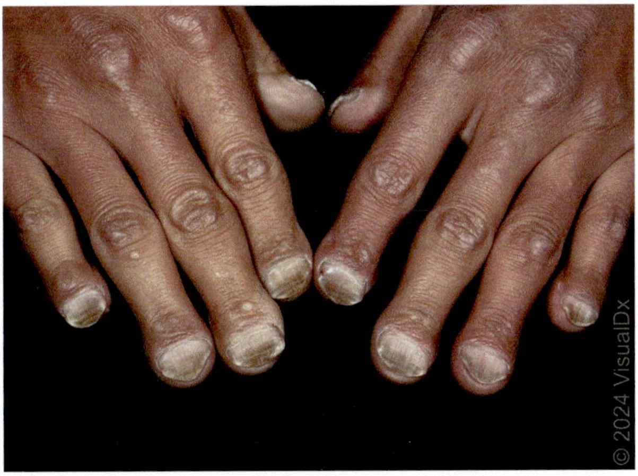

Fig. 29.7 Child of unknown sex and age, Fitzpatrick type V, koilonychia. Etiology: unknown (*image used with permission from* VisualDx; www.visualdx.com)

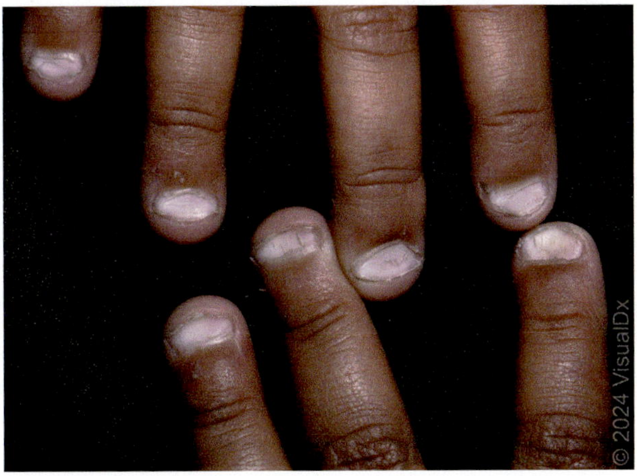

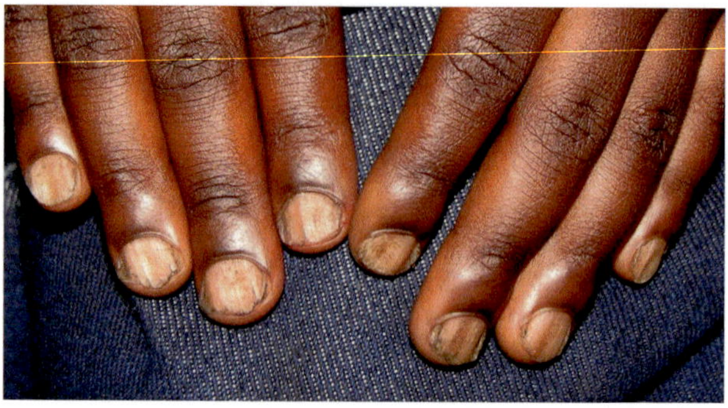

Fig. 29.8 Male of unknown age, Fitzpatrick type V, koilonychia, with bilateral fingernails affected by linear fissuring, ridging, and irregular depressions. Note the swelling of the proximal nail fold. Etiology: lichen planus (*courtesy of* Dr. Constantin E. Orfanos; *From* El-Domyati and Moftah [40]; *with permission*)

References

1. Walker J, Baran R, Vélez N, Jellinek N. Koilonychia: an update on pathophysiology, differential diagnosis and clinical relevance. J Eur Acad Dermatol Venereol. 2016;30(11):1985–91. https://doi.org/10.1111/jdv.13610.
2. Rosenberg A, Lipner SR. Nail changes associated with thyroid disease. Cutis. 2022;110(2):E8–e12. https://doi.org/10.12788/cutis.0593.
3. Starace M, Alessandrini A, Piraccini BM. Nail disorders in children. Skin Appendage Disord. 2018;4(4):217–29. https://doi.org/10.1159/000486020.
4. Rathod DG, Sonthalia S. Spoon nails. In: StatPearls. StatPearls Publishing Copyright © 2024, StatPearls Publishing LLC; 2024.
5. Conway J, Lipner SR. A case of rapid fingernail growth associated with nail psoriasis: a case report. SAGE Open Med Case Rep. 2023;11:2050313x231213149. https://doi.org/10.1177/2050313x231213149.
6. Razmi TM, Nampoothiri RV, Dogra S. Koilonychia in iron deficiency. QJM. 2018;111(4):271–2. https://doi.org/10.1093/qjmed/hcx229.
7. Starace M, Alessandrini A, Bruni F, Piraccini BM. Trachyonychia: a retrospective study of 122 patients in a period of 30 years. J Eur Acad Dermatol Venereol. 2020;34(4):880–4. https://doi.org/10.1111/jdv.16186.
8. Mangla A, Agarwal N, Yu J, Telfer M. Spooning of the nails and webbing of the esophagus: koilonychia and Plummer-Vinson syndrome. Clin Case Rep. 2015;3(12):1054–5. https://doi.org/10.1002/ccr3.419.
9. Sobolewski S, Lawrence AC, Bagshaw P. Human nails and body iron. J Clin Pathol. 1978;31(11):1068–72. https://doi.org/10.1136/jcp.31.11.1068.
10. Yamaguchi T, Shimizu K. Koilonychia in a patient with heart failure and iron deficiency anemia. Am J Med. 2022;135(10):e393–4. https://doi.org/10.1016/j.amjmed.2022.05.029.
11. Ghaffari S, Pourafkari L. Koilonychia in iron-deficiency anemia. N Engl J Med. 2018;379(9):e13. https://doi.org/10.1056/NEJMicm1802104.
12. Chevrant-Breton J, Simon M, Bourel M, Ferrand B. Cutaneous manifestations of idiopathic hemochromatosis. Study of 100 cases. Arch Dermatol. 1977;113(2):161–5.
13. Demirci F, Savaş MC, Kepkep N, et al. Plummer-Vinson syndrome and dilation therapy: a report of two cases. Turk J Gastroenterol. 2005;16(4):224–7.
14. Ogunbiyi OA, El Tahir MI. Paterson-Brown Kelly syndrome. Ann Saudi Med. 1996;16(2):130–4.

15. Al-Dabbagh TQ, Al-Abachi KG. Nutritional koilonychia in 32 Iraqi subjects. Ann Saudi Med. 2005;25(2):154–7. https://doi.org/10.5144/0256-4947.2005.154.
16. Salem A, Al Mokadem S, Attwa E, Abd El Raoof S, Ebrahim HM, Faheem KT. Nail changes in chronic renal failure patients under haemodialysis. J Eur Acad Dermatol Venereol. 2008;22(11):1326–31. https://doi.org/10.1111/j.1468-3083.2008.02826.x.
17. Litaiem N, Charfi O, Bacha T, Zeglaoui F. Koilonychia in a patient with alopecia areata. J Clin Aesthet Dermatol. 2021;14(2):42–3.
18. Shakoei S, Seifi G, Ghanami F, et al. Clinical and demographic characteristics associated with nail involvement in alopecia areata: a cross-sectional study of 197 patients. Health Sci Rep. 2024;7(4):e2020. https://doi.org/10.1002/hsr2.2020.
19. García-Patos V, Bartralot R, Ordi J, Baselga E, de Moragas JM, Castells A. Systemic lupus erythematosus presenting with red lunulae. J Am Acad Dermatol. 1997;36(5 Pt 2):834–6. https://doi.org/10.1016/s0190-9622(97)70034-3.
20. Ashrafzadeh S, Imadojemu S. Koilonychia secondary to Raynaud's phenomenon: a rare co-occurrence. JAAD Case Rep. 2021;7:117–9. https://doi.org/10.1016/j.jdcr.2020.11.021.
21. Sawhney MP. Ladakhi koilonychia. Indian J Dermatol Venereol Leprol. 2003;69(2):79–80.
22. Patial RK. High altitude koilonychia. J Assoc Physicians India. 1999;47(4):406–8.
23. Murdoch D. Koilonychia in Sherpas. Br J Dermatol. 1993;128:592–3.
24. Ancona-Alayón A. Occupational koilonychia from organic solvents. Contact Derm. 1975;1(6):367–9. https://doi.org/10.1111/j.1600-0536.1975.tb05475.x.
25. Dawber R. Occupational koilonychia. Clin Exp Dermatol. 1977;2:115–6.
26. Smith SJ, Yoder FW, Knox DW. Occupational koilonychia. Arch Dermatol. 1980;116(8):861. https://doi.org/10.1001/archderm.1980.01640320011002.
27. Alanko K, Kanerva L, Estlander T, Jolanki R, Leino T, Suhonen R. Hairdresser's koilonychia. Am J Contact Dermat. 1997;8(3):177–8. https://doi.org/10.1016/s1046-199x(97)90103-2.
28. Gupta I, Tyagi M, Dayal S, Singh J. Unilateral koilonychia secondary to chemical depilatory product. Skin Appendage Disord. 2021;7(1):25–8. https://doi.org/10.1159/000510523.
29. Prathap P, Asokan N. Familial koilonychia. Indian J Dermatol. 2010;55(4):406–7. https://doi.org/10.4103/0019-5154.74575.
30. Calleja-Algarra A, Aragón-Miguel R, Andrés-Lencina JJ, et al. Image gallery: spoon-shaped nails in an 11-year-old boy. Br J Dermatol. 2019;180(2):e34. https://doi.org/10.1111/bjd.17248.
31. Bumpers RD, Bishop ME. Familial koilonychia: a current case history. Arch Dermatol. 1980;116(7):845. https://doi.org/10.1001/archderm.1980.01640310115033.
32. Vora RV, Anjaneyan G, Mehta MJ. Monilethrix, a rare inherited hair shaft disorder in siblings. Indian Dermatol Online J. 2014;5(3):339–40. https://doi.org/10.4103/2229-5178.137795.
33. Thai KE, Sinclair RD. Keratosis pilaris and hereditary koilonychia without monilethrix. J Am Acad Dermatol. 2001;45(4):627–9. https://doi.org/10.1067/mjd.2001.116225.
34. Heidensleben E. Hereditary congenital koilonychae accompanied by syndejmatotic cataract. Acta Ophthalmol. 1960;38:1–4. https://doi.org/10.1111/j.1755-3768.1960.tb00170.x.
35. Hashizume Y, Nakamura D, Suzuki S, Endo Y. Very rare familial spoon nails (koilonychia). J Gen Fam Med. 2017;18(4):168. https://doi.org/10.1002/jgf2.32.
36. Bergeron JR, Stone OJ. Koilonychia. A report of familial spoon nails. Arch Dermatol. 1967;95(4):351–3. https://doi.org/10.1001/archderm.95.4.351.
37. Hogan GR, Jones B. The relationship of koilonychia and iron deficiency in infants. J Pediatr. 1970;77(6):1054–7. https://doi.org/10.1016/s0022-3476(70)80093-2.
38. Hwang JK, Grover C, Iorizzo M, et al. Nail psoriasis and nail lichen planus: updates on diagnosis and management. J Am Acad Dermatol. 2024;90(3):585–96. https://doi.org/10.1016/j.jaad.2023.11.024.
39. Chelidze K, Lipner SR. The water-drop test for the diagnosis of koilonychia. J Am Acad Dermatol. 2017;77(6):e157–8. https://doi.org/10.1016/j.jaad.2017.06.034.
40. El-Domyati M, Moftah NH. Nail disorders in dark skin. In: Orfanos C, Zouboulis C, Assaf C, editors. Pigmented ethnic skin and imported dermatoses. Cham, Switzerland: Springer; 2018. https://doi.org/10.1007/978-3-319-69422-1_34.

Digital Clubbing

30

Eden Axler and Shari R. Lipner

30.1 Description of Disease

Digital clubbing is characterized by an increase in the volume of the soft tissue in the nail beds, with obliteration of the angle formed between the proximal nail fold and nail bed [1]. Digital clubbing can manifest independently, as part of a secondary disease process, or as a component of hypertrophic osteoarthropathy (HOA). HOA is characterized by periostosis in long bones, joint pain, and clubbing. It may also coexist with pachydermoperiostosis, which is characterized by HOA and acromegaly [2, 3]. While the exact mechanism is not fully understood, it is thought that cytokines associated with megakaryocytes play a role in the development of clubbing. Additionally, prostaglandins, ferritin, and growth factors like vascular endothelial growth factor (VEGF), either overproduced or poorly eliminated from affected organs, may be involved in the underlying processes leading to clubbing [4]. Digital clubbing may indicate an underlying medical condition and can offer diagnostic insights during medical assessment. For example, clubbing may regress in cystic fibrosis patients who have undergone lung transplant [4].

30.2 Epidemiology

Digital clubbing is relatively rare among the general population, with prevalence rates varying depending on the underlying cause. In a prospective study, including 200 patients with Crohn's disease and 103 patients with ulcerative colitis, 38% and 15% had clubbing, respectively [5]. In a prospective study including 74 patients with primary biliary cirrhosis and 54 with other chronic liver diseases, clubbing was present in 24% of patients with primary biliary cirrhosis, 29% with HBsAg negative chronic active hepatitis, and 23% with miscellaneous liver diseases [6]. In a systematic review including 142 studies analyzing the prevalence of digital clubbing and HOA, the pooled prevalence was 33.4% (16.6–52.8), 31.3% (22.4–41.1),

S. R. Lipner, *Atlas of Nail Disorders Across All Skin Colors*,
https://doi.org/10.1007/978-3-031-74272-9_30

27% (9.4–49.5), and 22.8% (10.8–37.6) in patients with intestinal diseases, interstitial lung diseases, infective endocarditis, and hepatic diseases, respectively [7]. In children and adolescents with human immunodeficiency virus infection, hemoglobinopathies, cystic fibrosis, and tuberculosis, the pooled prevalence of digital clubbing was 29.1% (19.4–39.9), 23% (9.0–41.1), 19.5% (4.1–42.4), and 17.1% (9.5–26.5), respectively [7].

30.2.1 Common Medical Conditions Associated with Digital Clubbing (Non-Comprehensive)

Respiratory Diseases: Pulmonary pathologies that induce digital clubbing include chronic obstructive pulmonary disease (COPD), bronchiectasis, cystic fibrosis, lung abscesses, and lung cancer [8–10].

Cardiovascular Diseases: Causes of cardiovascular disease-induced digital clubbing include congenital cyanotic heart disease, infective endocarditis, and atrial myxoma [11–13].

Gastrointestinal Diseases: Implicated gastrointestinal conditions associated with digital clubbing include inflammatory bowel disease (Crohn's disease and ulcerative colitis), hereditary hemorrhagic telangiectasia, juvenile polyposis syndrome, and celiac disease [5].

Hepatic Diseases: Liver diseases associated with clubbing include hepatopulmonary syndrome, cirrhosis, alcoholic steatosis, and primary biliary cirrhosis [6, 14, 15].

Endocrine Disorders: Digital clubbing may present in endocrine disease including thyroid acropathy, a severe manifestation of Graves' disease manifesting with a triad of digital clubbing, soft tissue swelling of the hands and feet, and periosteal new bone formation [16]. Clubbing is also associated with acromegaly [17].

Neoplastic Conditions: Lung cancer and mesothelioma are two neoplasms associated with clubbing [18].

Genetic Conditions: Clubbing may be part of an inherited trait due to genetic factors rather than an underlying medical condition [19].

Miscellaneous: Clubbing may also be idiopathic, associated with laxative abuse, or associated with pregnancy [20, 21].

30.3 Risk Factors

Lifestyle choices may contribute to the risk of developing secondary medical conditions associated with digital clubbing. For instance, tobacco use is widely recognized as a significant contributor to the development of pulmonary conditions, including COPD and lung cancer, which can lead to digital clubbing secondarily.

30.4 Clinical Features

The clinical presentation of digital clubbing varies with its progression. Initially, there is periungual erythema and softening of the nail bed, accompanied by a spongy sensation with palpation. In subsequent stages there is an increase in the angle between the nail bed and proximal nail fold, exceeding 160°. As clubbing advances, there is a thickening of the distal phalanx, resulting in a bulbous appearance of the finger. This stretching of the skin over the nail bed and distal phalanx can lead to a shiny appearance of the nail and periungual skin, erythema of the nailfold, and longitudinal ridging of the nail plate. Additionally, increased vascularity may cause the nail bed to develop a lilac hue [3, 22, 23].

30.5 Clinical Features in Skin of Color

In individuals with skin of color, the findings of digital clubbing are similar to those observed in lighter-skinned individuals. However, there may be slight differences due to variations in pigmentation. For example, periungual erythema may be less apparent in individuals with darker skin tones compared to those with lighter skin.

30.6 Requirements for Diagnosis

Diagnosing digital clubbing involves both clinical observations and objective measurements. Clinically, a key diagnostic test for digital clubbing involves measuring the Lovibond angle, the angle formed between the nail plate and the proximal nail fold when viewed from the side. In clubbed nails, this angle typically exceeds 180°, whereas in normal nails the angle measures approximately 160° [3, 23, 24]. In a prospective study of four cases of digital clubbing evaluated with high-resolution magnetic resonance imaging (MRI) by Nakamura et al. [23], nail bed changes were present in all clubbed cases (soft tissue edema and hypertrophy completely involved the nail bed and were visible with contrast enhancement). The median profile angle in clubbed nails was 186° (range 179–188°) vs. 176° (range 154–179°) in normal nails ($P = 0.029$) [23].

Additionally, the Schamroth sign, loss of the diamond shape gap that forms when the dorsal surfaces of opposite nail beds and terminal phalanges are pressed together, is another diagnostic clue for digital clubbing [21, 22].

In addition to clinical measurements, diagnostic imaging including high-frequency ultrasound, point-of-care ultrasound, plain radiographs, bone scintigraphy, and high-frequency MRI can confirm the diagnosis of digital clubbing [3, 25]. After confirming the presence of clubbing, it is essential to perform a thorough clinical and physical examination to detect any underlying medical conditions. This may include assessing for respiratory, cardiovascular, gastrointestinal, or other systemic diseases associated with clubbing. In some cases, referral to pulmonology, cardiology, or gastroenterology may be warranted for further evaluation and management.

30.7 Cases

Figures 30.1, 30.2, 30.3, 30.4, 30.5, and 30.6 demonstrate the presentation of digital clubbing in a clinical setting.

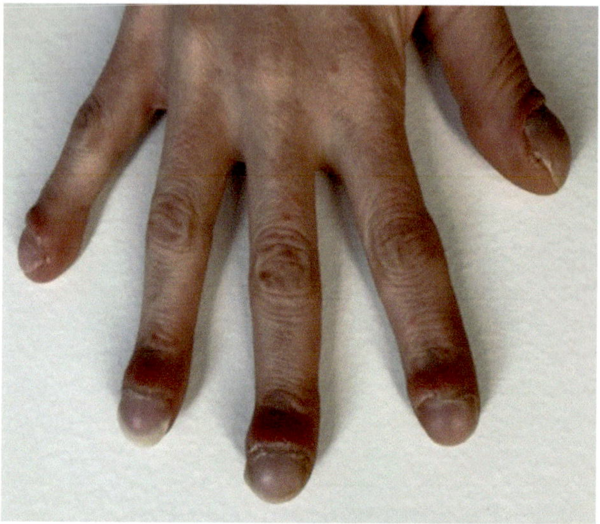

Fig. 30.1 A 36-year-old female, Fitzpatrick type II, digital clubbing in the context of laxative abuse. The digital tips are enlarged, and the nails curve around the fingertips. There is erythema of the proximal nail folds (*from* Charlton et al. [26]; CC-BY 4.0; legend modified)

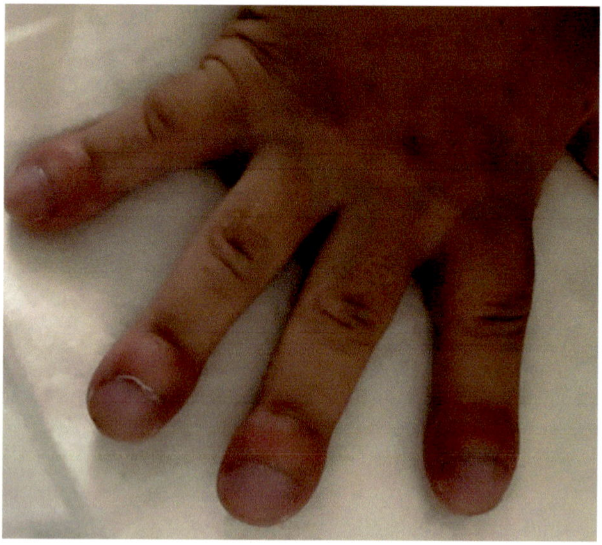

Fig. 30.2 A 4-year-old female, Fitzpatrick type II, digital clubbing in the context of hemorrhagic hereditary telangiectasia. The digital tips are enlarged with erythema of the nail folds (*from* Schultz et al. [27]; CC-BY 4.0; legend modified)

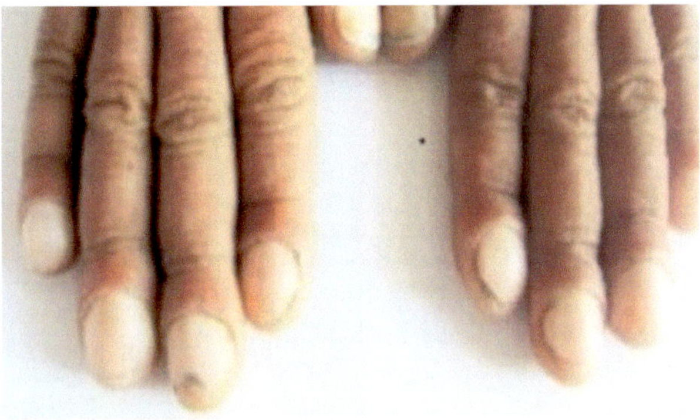

Fig. 30.3 A 35-year-old male, Fitzpatrick type III, digital clubbing in the context of pachydermoperiostosis. The digital tips are enlarged, and the nails curve around the fingertips. There is erythema of the proximal nail folds (*from* Alaya et al. [28]; CC-BY 4.0; legend modified)

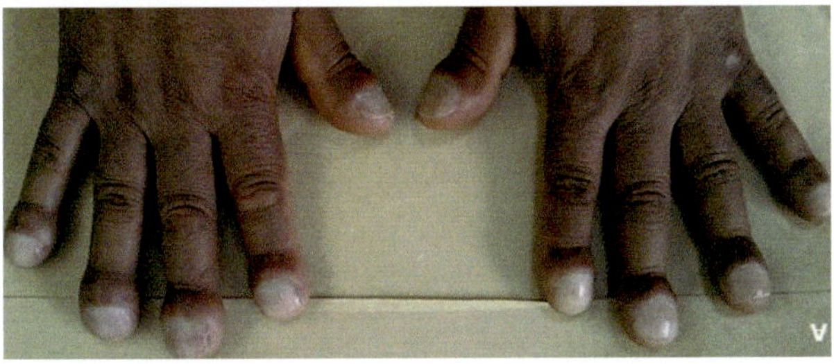

Fig. 30.4 49-year-old male, Fitzpatrick type IV, digital clubbing in the context of primary idiopathic osteoarthropathy. The digital tips are enlarged, and the nails curve around the fingertips. There is subtle hyperpigmentation of the proximal nail folds (*from* Kaffel et al. [29]; CC-BY 4.0; legend modified)

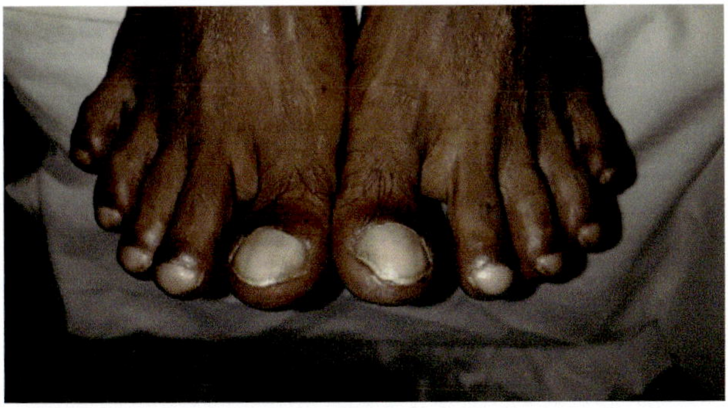

Fig. 30.5 An 18-year-old female, Fitzpatrick type V, digital clubbing in the context of a patent ductus arteriosus with pulmonary hypertension and reversal of shunt. There is bulbous swelling of the digits in the lower limbs (*from* Krishna et al. [30]; CC-BY 4.0; legend modified)

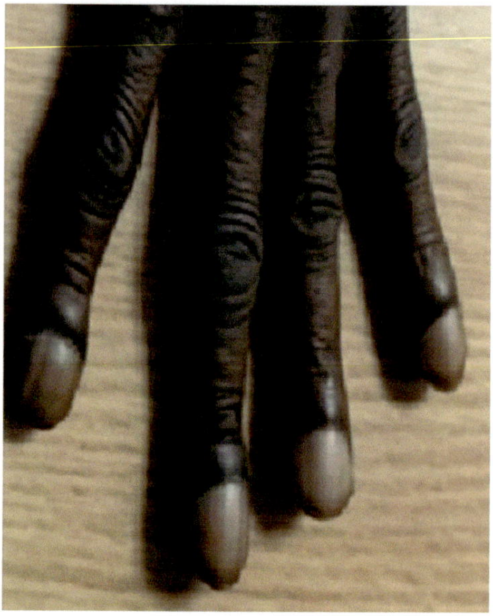

Fig. 30.6 Male patient, Fitzpatrick type VI, digital clubbing associated with alcoholic steatosis. The digital tips are enlarged. There are subtle gray-brown longitudinal bands (*from* Alnimer et al. [31]; Creative Commons Attributions License; legend modified)

References

1. Moreira AL, Porto NS, Moreira JS, Ulbrich-Kulczynski JM, Irion KL. Clubbed fingers: radiological evaluation of the nail bed thickness. Clin Anat. 2008;21(4):314–8. https://doi.org/10.1002/ca.20623.
2. Spicknall KE, Zirwas MJ, English JC 3rd. Clubbing: an update on diagnosis, differential diagnosis, pathophysiology, and clinical relevance. J Am Acad Dermatol. 2005;52(6):1020–8. https://doi.org/10.1016/j.jaad.2005.01.006.
3. McPhee SJ, Walker HK, Hall WD, Hurst JW. Clubbing. In: Clinical methods: the history, physical, and laboratory examinations. 3rd ed; 1990.
4. Augarten A, Goldman R, Laufer J, Szeinberg A, Efrati O, Barak A, Miller MS, Yahav Y. Reversal of digital clubbing after lung transplantation in cystic fibrosis patients: a clue to the pathogenesis of clubbing. Pediatr Pulmonol. 2002;34(5):378–80. https://doi.org/10.1002/ppul.10193.
5. Kitis G, Thompson H, Allan RN. Finger clubbing in inflammatory bowel disease: its prevalence and pathogenesis. Br Med J. 1979;2(6194):825–8. https://doi.org/10.1136/bmj.2.6194.825.
6. Epstein O, Dick R, Sherlock S. Prospective study of periostitis and finger clubbing in primary biliary cirrhosis and other forms of chronic liver disease. Gut. 1981;22(3):203–6. https://doi.org/10.1136/gut.22.3.203.
7. Essouma M, Nkeck JR, Agbor VN, Noubiap JJ. Epidemiology of digital clubbing and hypertrophic osteoarthropathy: a systematic review and meta-analysis. J Clin Rheumatol. 2022;28(2):104–10. https://doi.org/10.1097/rhu.0000000000001830.
8. Rasul TF, Bergholz DR, Rovinski R, Gulraiz S, Fonts E. Combined pulmonary fibrosis and emphysema and digital clubbing. Cureus. 2022;14(4):e24231. https://doi.org/10.7759/cureus.24231.

9. Nakamura CT, Ng GY, Paton JY, Keens TG, Witmer JC, Bautista-Bolduc D, Woo MS. Correlation between digital clubbing and pulmonary function in cystic fibrosis. Pediatr Pulmonol. 2002;33(5):332–8. https://doi.org/10.1002/ppul.10082.
10. Tas F, Erturk K. Digital clubbing as a first clinical presentation of pulmonary metastases in cutaneous melanoma. Postgrad Med. 2018;130(2):278–9. https://doi.org/10.1080/00325481.2018.1409050.
11. Blount SG Jr. Cyanosis: pathophysiology and differential diagnosis. Prog Cardiovasc Dis. 1971;13(6):595–605. https://doi.org/10.1016/s0033-0620(71)80005-1.
12. Moccetti F, Kaufmann BA, Tobler D. Differential clubbing and cyanosis: a pathognomonic finding in cardiology. Eur Heart J. 2014;35(21):1410. https://doi.org/10.1093/eurheartj/ehu020.
13. Ozdemir B, Sentürk T, Kaderli AA, Keçebaş M, Güllülü S, Baran I, Ozdabakoğlu O, Aydinlar A. Postoperative regression of clubbing at an unexpected rate in a patient with aortic and mitral valve replacement due to infective endocarditis. Ir J Med Sci. 2009;178(3):351–3. Epub 20081009. https://doi.org/10.1007/s11845-008-0231-2.
14. Zieliński M, Hartleb M, Sitek P, Ziora D. Dyspnoea, cyanosis and digital clubbing in a 28-year-old patient as a result of hepatopulmonary syndrome. Adv Respir Med. 2017;85(6):339–44. https://doi.org/10.5603/arm.2017.0058.
15. Gonçalo M, Pinho A, Agner T, Andersen KE, Bruze M, Diepgen T, Foti C, Giménez-Arnau A, Goossens A, Johanssen JD, Paulsen E, Svedman C, Wilkinson M, Aalto-Korte K. Allergic contact dermatitis caused by nail acrylates in Europe an EECDRG study. Contact Dermatitis. 2018;78(4):254–60. https://doi.org/10.1111/cod.12942.
16. Moule B, Grant MC, Boyle IT, May H. Thyroid acropachy. Clin Radiol. 1970;21(3):329–33. https://doi.org/10.1016/S0009-9260(70)80065-4.
17. Freeman AG. Gross digital clubbing and exophthalmic ophthalmoplegia in thyroid disorders. Lancet. 1958;2(7037):57–60. https://doi.org/10.1016/s0140-6736(58)91238-8.
18. Mondal S, Rath D, Sinha D, Lahiri D, Ghosh P, Ghosh A. Lung cancer, clubbing and hypertrophic pulmonary osteoarthropathy. QJM. 2018;111(11):825. https://doi.org/10.1093/qjmed/hcy119.
19. Lu Q, Xu Y, Zhang Z, Li S, Zhang Z. Primary hypertrophic osteoarthropathy: genetics, clinical features and management. Front Endocrinol (Lausanne). 2023;14:1235040. https://doi.org/10.3389/fendo.2023.1235040.
20. Cullen DR, Maskery PJ. Clubbing of the fingers and hypertropic osteoarthropathy in pregnancy. Lancet. 1966;2(7461):473–5. https://doi.org/10.1016/s0140-6736(66)92777-2.
21. Talley RC, Baldwin BJ, Symbas PN, Nutter DO. Right atrial myxoma. Unusual presentation with cyanosis and clubbing. Am J Med. 1970;48(2):256–60. https://doi.org/10.1016/0002-9343(70)90123-3.
22. Martínez-Lavín M. Hypertrophic osteoarthropathy. Best Pract Res Clin Rheumatol. 2020;34(3):101507. https://doi.org/10.1016/j.berh.2020.101507.
23. Nakamura J, Halliday NA, Fukuba E, Radjenovic A, Tanner SF, Emery P, McGonagle D, Tan AL. The microanatomic basis of finger clubbing—a high-resolution magnetic resonance imaging study. J Rheumatol. 2014;41(3):523–7. https://doi.org/10.3899/jrheum.130823.
24. Salerno D, Delwaide J, Detry O. Digital clubbing. Rev Med Liege. 2010;65(2):88–92.
25. Roberts C, Khodaee M. Digital clubbing as a result of metastatic lung cancer. Korean J Intern Med. 2022;37(4):883–4. https://doi.org/10.3904/kjim.2022.002.
26. Charlton OA, Dickison P, Smith SD, Roger SD. Nail clubbing in laxative abuse: case report and review of the literature. J Eat Disord. 2019;7:6. https://doi.org/10.1186/s40337-019-0236-4.
27. Schultz K, Divanovic A, Towe C, Miethke A, Wusik K, Hammill A, Brunner H. Clinicopathologic conference: a four-year-old child with digital clubbing. Arthritis Care Res (Hoboken). 2021;73(10):1379–86. https://doi.org/10.1002/acr.24428.
28. Alaya Z, Osman W. A rare cause of digital clubbing: pachydermoperiostosis. Pan Afr Med J. 2016;25:194. https://doi.org/10.11604/pamj.2016.25.194.10890.

29. Kaffel D, Riahi H. Primary idiopathic osteoarthropathy. Pan Afr Med J. 2017;28:88. https://doi.org/10.11604/pamj.2017.28.88.13295.
30. Krishna MR, Sennaiyan UN. Differential clubbing of the lower extremities. J Pediatr. 2016;175:234. https://doi.org/10.1016/j.jpeds.2016.04.082.
31. Alnimer Y, Subedi S, Dawood T, Bachuwa G. Primary idiopathic osteoarthropathy: could it be related to alcoholism? Case Rep Rheumatol. 2017;2017:2583762. https://doi.org/10.1155/2017/2583762.

Part VII

Environmental and Mechanical Nail Disorders

Brittle Nails

31

Jose W. Ricardo and Shari R. Lipner

31.1 Description of Disease

Nail brittleness (NB) is characterized by nails that are prone to splitting, flaking, and crumbling, and potentially becoming soft and inelastic [1, 2]. The nail plate (NP), which is produced in the nail matrix (NM), comprised roughly 25 layers of densely packed, completely differentiated cells called onychocytes, forming a 0.5–1 mm thick, fully keratinized structure with a smooth surface [2, 3]. The NM is localized under the proximal nail fold. NB is thought to occur due to factors that alter NP production and/or factors that damage the already formed NP [1, 2]. It may occur secondary to dermatologic and systemic diseases, nutritional deficiencies, and drug intake [2]. When none of these causes are identified, the condition is defined as idiopathic or referred to as brittle nail syndrome, which is the most common type of NB [2]. In the idiopathic form, electron microscopy shows an intrinsic or acquired defect in intracellular cement substance or the keratinous lamellae holding together onychocytes [3, 4]. Cell adhesion in the NP is facilitated by membrane-coating granules with linkage by lipids, and therefore, low lipid content in the NP contributes to the pathogenesis of NB [1, 2].

31.2 Epidemiology

31.2.1 Sex

NB affects up to 20% of the general population, with a predilection for women, who are twice as likely to be affected compared to men, in a survey-based study by Lubach et al., including 1584 randomly selected people from inpatient clinics, outpatient clinics, and nursing homes [5]. This disparity is attributed to the weaker intracellular keratinocyte bridges observed in women [1, 2].

S. R. Lipner, *Atlas of Nail Disorders Across All Skin Colors*,
https://doi.org/10.1007/978-3-031-74272-9_31

31.2.2 Age

Lubach et al's study found that NB was most prevalent in older adults, with 36% of women and 31% of men aged 60 years or older being affected [5]. In another study of fingernail plate samples including 70 healthy subjects, there was a negative correlation between NP cholesterol sulfate and age ($R = -0.59$, $P < 0.01$) in women, potentially explaining why older women are disproportionately affected by the condition [6].

31.2.3 Other Factors

NB may also occur secondary to dermatologic and systemic diseases, nutritional deficiencies, and drug intake. Normal NP formation is dependent on vascularization and inflammation [1]. Dermatoses affecting the nail apparatus, including psoriasis, lichen planus, lichen striatus, alopecia areata, eczema, and Darier disease may therefore precipitate NB [7]. Vascular disorders, including Raynaud's and peripheral artery disease, can disrupt NP production, leading to nail fragility [7]. Vitamins A–E play a role in NP strength and growth and NM circulation; consequently, severe deficiencies in these vitamins can contribute to NB [2, 7]. Similarly, the NP is rich in iron, zinc, and selenium, and low levels of these oligo elements can exacerbate NB [2]. Thyroid disorders are also associated with brittle nails [8]. In a review of eight studies, 70%, 48%, and 40% of hypothyroid patients developed NP fragility, slow growth, and thinning, respectively, whereas 9.2% of hyperthyroid patients showed brittleness [8]. Systemic medications, including chemotherapeutic agents, retinoids, or antiretrovirals may also exacerbate or cause NB [1, 2, 7].

31.3 Risk Factors

Advanced age and female sex are the most important non-modifiable risk factors for NB. Occupational and environmental risk factors play a key role in the disease pathogenesis. In an in vitro study including nail samples from ten healthy subjects exposed to frequent alternating wetting and drying cycles, electron microscopy demonstrated onychoschizia as early as 48 h [4]. Consequently, NB is prevalent in housekeepers, healthcare workers, and hairdressers [9]. Nail cosmetics and chemical agents used in manicures can disturb cell adhesion and alter keratinocyte composition of the NP [7, 10, 11]. Nail varnishes can cause NP keratin granulation, while nail polish removers, cuticle removers, and solvents can exacerbate drying of the NP [1, 2]. Repetitive trauma from typing, telephone dialing, or maintaining overly long NPs can cause fractures between onychocytes, exacerbating NB [9, 12]. Additionally, all secondary causes of NB outlined in Sect. 31.2.3 are considered risk factors for NB.

31.4 Clinical Features

Three main clinical signs have been described in NB: onychorrhexis, lamellar onychoschizia, and superficial keratin granulation [1]. Onychorrhexis is characterized by longitudinal splitting and shallow parallel furrows running through superficial NP [1]. Severity can vary from a few superficial ridges to deep furrows causing NP splitting. Pain and functional limitations due to splitting are often the reason for seeking medical advice [1]. Lamellar onychoschizia presents with horizontal exfoliation of the NP's free margin, appearing as thin layering of the NP [1]. Disruption of intercellular adhesive factors exacerbates onychoschizia [1, 3]. Superficial granulation of tissue refers to fragility and crumbling of the dorsal NP [1]. It is associated with prolonged use of nail polish and is thought to occur due to gradual granulation of keratin, leading to the formation of small white-yellow patches and striations [1].

31.5 Clinical Features in Skin of Color

The clinical features of NB in patients with skin of color have not been previously described. Melanocytic activation, a form of longitudinal melanonychia, develops from NM insult [13], and therefore, longitudinal melanonychia may be particularly prevalent in patients with NB.

31.6 Requirements for Diagnosis

The diagnosis of brittle nails is mainly based on clinical assessment. Exclusion of underlying nail conditions is helpful when the diagnosis is unclear. Histopathologic examination of nail clippings and a nail matrix/bed biopsy are instrumental in ruling out underlying onychomycosis, nail psoriasis, and nail lichen planus. Van de Kerkhof et al. proposed a semiquantitative grading system for NB that evaluates five elements: onychoschizia, transverse splitting, ridging, longitudinal splitting, and NP thickness [14]. Each element is scored on a scale from 0 to 3, resulting in a cumulative score ranging from 0 to 15, with 15 indicating the worst possible nail condition [14].

31.7 Cases

Figures 31.1, 31.2, 31.3, 31.4, 31.5, 31.6, and 31.7 depict the clinical presentation of brittle nails.

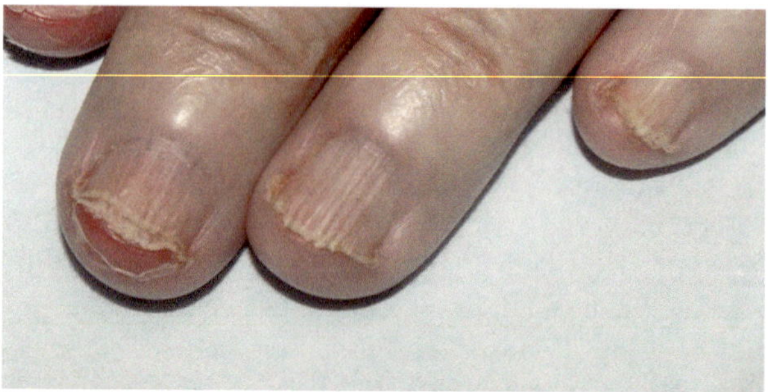

Fig. 31.1 60-Year-old female, Fitzpatrick type I, brittle nails, with severe onychorrhexis of the left third, fourth, and fifth fingernails. The third and fifth fingernails also show onychoschizia

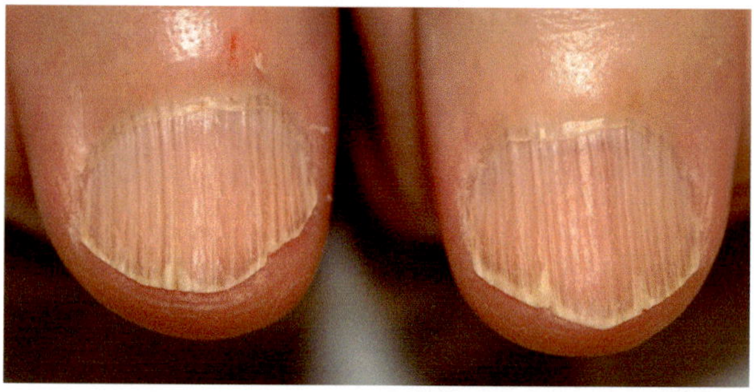

Fig. 31.2 65-Year-old female, Fitzpatrick type II, brittle nails, with severe onychorrhexis and distal longitudinal splitting of the NP affecting the left and right thumbnails

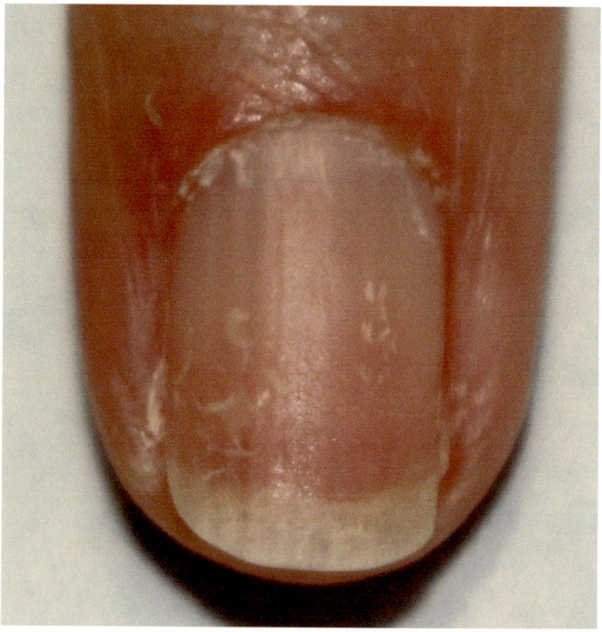

Fig. 31.3 74-Year-old female, Fitzpatrick type III, brittle nails, with superficial granulation of keratin affecting the distal half of the right fifth fingernail plate

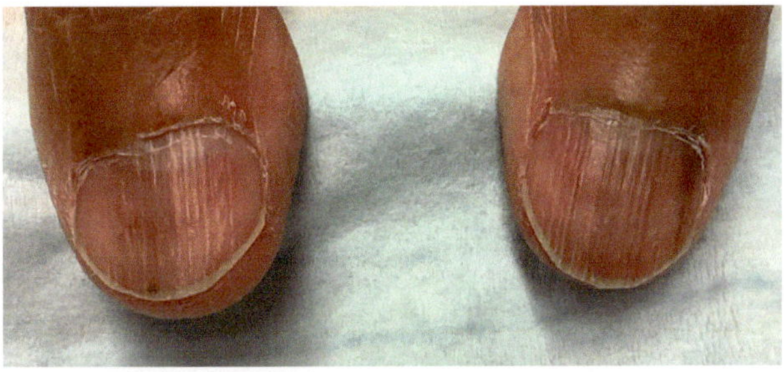

Fig. 31.4 44-Year-old male, Fitzpatrick type IV, brittle nails, with onychorrhexis and light brown to gray longitudinal bands affecting 60% of the right thumbnail and 80% of the left thumbnail

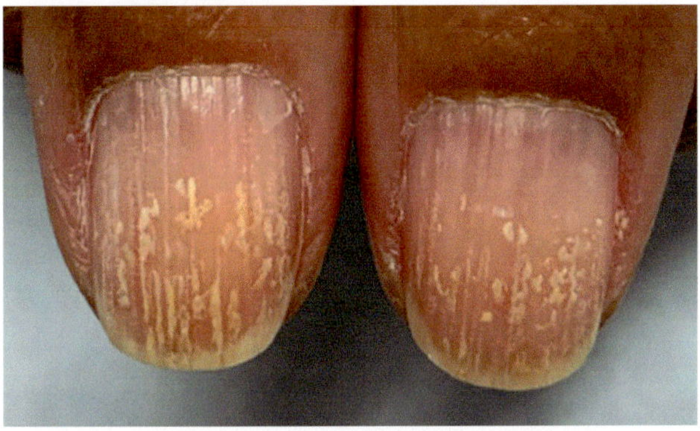

Fig. 31.5 64-Year-old female, Fitzpatrick type V, brittle nails, with onychorrhexis and superficial keratin granulation in a linear distribution on the distal halves of the right and left thumbnail plates

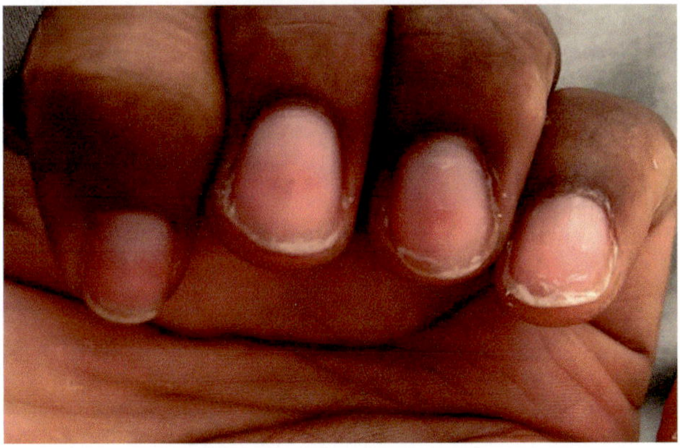

Fig. 31.6 36-Year-old female, Fitzpatrick type V, brittle nails, with onychoschizia at the free end of the right fingernails, particularly the second and third fingernails

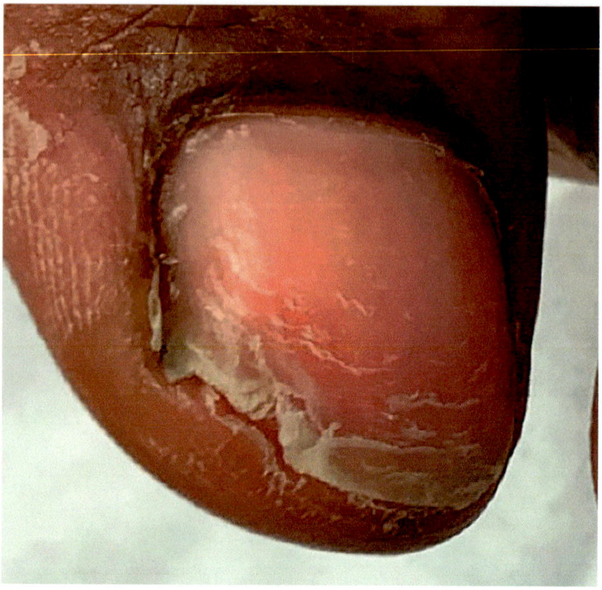

Fig. 31.7 36-Year-old female, Fitzpatrick type V, brittle nails, with lamellar splitting on the distal half and fragmentation on the right distal end of the nail plate of the left first toenail

References

1. Chessa MA, Iorizzo M, Richert B, López-Estebaranz JL, Rigopoulos D, Tosti A, Gupta AK, Di Chiacchio N, Di Chiacchio NG, Rubin AI, Baran R, Lipner SR, Daniel R, Chiheb S, Grover C, Starace M, Piraccini BM. Pathogenesis, clinical signs and treatment recommendations in brittle nails: a review. Dermatol Ther (Heidelb). 2020;10(1):15–27. https://doi.org/10.1007/s13555-019-00338-x. Epub 2019 Nov 20. Erratum in: Dermatol Ther (Heidelb). 2020 Jan 22;: PMID: 31749091; PMCID: PMC6994568
2. Iorizzo M, Pazzaglia M, Piraccini BM, Tullo S, Tosti A. Brittle nails. J Cosmet Dermatol. 2004;3(3):138–44. https://doi.org/10.1111/j.1473-2130.2004.00084.x.
3. Shelley WB, Shelley ED. Onychoschizia: scanning electron microscopy. J Am Acad Dermatol. 1984;10(4):623–7. https://doi.org/10.1016/s0190-9622(84)80268-6.
4. Wallis MS, Bowen WR, Guin JD. Pathogenesis of onychoschizia (lamellar dystrophy). J Am Acad Dermatol. 1991;24(1):44–8. https://doi.org/10.1016/0190-9622(91)70007-o.
5. Lubach D, Cohrs W, Wurzinger R. Incidence of brittle nails. Dermatologica. 1986;172(3):144–7. https://doi.org/10.1159/000249319.
6. Brosche T, Dressler S, Platt D. Age-associated changes in integral cholesterol and cholesterol sulfate concentrations in human scalp hair and finger nail clippings. Aging (Milano). 2001;13(2):131–8. https://doi.org/10.1007/BF03351535.
7. Lee DK, Lipner SR. Optimal diagnosis and management of common nail disorders. Ann Med. 2022;54(1):694–712. https://doi.org/10.1080/07853890.2022.2044511.
8. Rosenberg A, Lipner SR. Nail changes associated with thyroid disease. Cutis. 2022;110(2):E8–E12. https://doi.org/10.12788/cutis.0593.
9. Dimitris R, Ralph D. Management of simple brittle nails. Dermatol Ther. 2012;25(6):569–73. https://doi.org/10.1111/j.1529-8019.2012.01518.x.
10. Kechijian P. Nail polish removers: are they harmful? Semin Dermatol. 1991;10(1):26–8.

11. Shemer A, Daniel CR 3rd. Common nail disorders. Clin Dermatol. 2013;31(5):578–86. https://doi.org/10.1016/j.clindermatol.2013.06.015.
12. Lubach D, Beckers P. Wet working conditions increase brittleness of nails, but do not cause it. Dermatology. 1992;185(2):120–2. https://doi.org/10.1159/000247425.
13. Tosti A, Baran R, Piraccini BM, Cameli N, Fanti PA. Nail matrix nevi: a clinical and histopathologic study of twenty-two patients. J Am Acad Dermatol. 1996;34(5 Pt 1):765–71. https://doi.org/10.1016/s0190-9622(96)90010-9.
14. van de Kerkhof PC, Pasch MC, Scher RK, Kerscher M, Gieler U, Haneke E, Fleckman P. Brittle nail syndrome: a pathogenesis-based approach with a proposed grading system. J Am Acad Dermatol. 2005;53(4):644–51. https://doi.org/10.1016/j.jaad.2004.09.002.

Chronic Paronychia

32

Yuna Oh and Shari R. Lipner

32.1 Description of Disease

Chronic paronychia is defined as nail fold inflammation lasting more than 6 weeks in duration [1]. Unlike acute paronychia, which typically arises from a bacterial or fungal infection, chronic paronychia stems primarily from repeated exposure to irritants and allergens, leading to a complex cycle of inflammation characterized by erythema, edema, fibrosis, and subsequent retraction of nail folds [1, 2]. The persistent inflammation compromises the protective barrier of the nail fold, often leading to secondary infections or fungal colonization. *Candida* spp. and *Pseudomonas aeruginosa* are the most commonly cultured organisms [2, 3]. Several medications have been implicated in drug-induced paronychia, either acute or chronic. The reported drug culprits include antiretroviral protease inhibitors (indinavir and lamivudine), epidermal growth factor receptor (EGFR) inhibitors (cetuximab, gefitinib, and lapatinib), EGFR tyrosine kinase inhibitors (gefitinib, erlotinib, and osimertinib), and retinoids (isotretinoin, etretinate, and acitretin) [1, 4–9].

32.2 Epidemiology

Although epidemiologic studies on chronic paronychia are limited, some report that it is more prevalent in females, with a reported female-to-male ratio of 3:1 [10, 11]. While chronic paronychia may affect individuals of any age, adults between 20 and 50 years old are most commonly affected [1, 12].

32.3 Risk Factors

Establishing definitive risk factors for chronic paronychia remains challenging given its multifactorial nature. Nonetheless, frequent exposure to water, detergents, chemicals (acids, alkalis), and mechanical friction associated with occupations,

S. R. Lipner, *Atlas of Nail Disorders Across All Skin Colors*,
https://doi.org/10.1007/978-3-031-74272-9_32

including dishwashing, cleaning, hairdressing, and gardening significantly increases risk [2, 7, 8, 10]. Patients with hand eczema and psoriasis, who have a compromised skin barrier, may be more susceptible to chronic paronychia [7, 13]. Although *Candida* spp. and other organisms are often cultured, they are thought to be colonizers from a compromised protective barrier [14, 15]. In an open randomized double-blind study including 45 adults with chronic paronychia, 2 of the 18 patients who were positive for *Candida* spp. at baseline were treated with topical steroids rather than an antifungal and had clinical cure and negative follow-up culture [14], suggesting that *Candida* spp. in this study were colonizers rather than pathogens. Immunosuppressive conditions, including diabetes, HIV, or malignancy, increase the risk of secondary colonization and/or complications [7].

32.4 Clinical Features

Chronic paronychia may involve one finger but typically affects multiple fingers, often on the dominant hand, likely due to frequent use in day-to-day activities [2, 3, 16]. In the largest cross-sectional analysis of paronychia to date including 2,512 paronychia cases (acute and chronic), 228 cases (15.5%) affected the thumb, followed by the third finger (181 cases, 12.3%). These findings align with smaller studies that included only isolated chronic paronychia patients [3, 16, 17]. The condition generally follows a protracted course marked by recurring, self-limited episodes of acute exacerbation. The proximal and/or lateral nail fold appear red, swollen, and irritated, often with disruption or absence of cuticles. This can progress to thickening and fibrosis of the nail fold with repeated flares [10]. Fluctuance is rare in chronic paronychia in contrast to acute paronychia [11]. Beau's lines may appear as a result of temporary interruptions in nail growth. Onycholysis, ridging, yellow discoloration, and rounding of the nail plate may be observed [18].

32.5 Clinical Features in Skin of Color

In darker skin tones, the erythema and swelling may be less pronounced, and less obvious changes, including nail fold thickening and subtle discoloration, may be more important diagnostic clues in the skin of color patients.

32.6 Requirements for Diagnosis

Diagnosis is primarily clinical, based on characteristic appearance and symptoms lasting over 6 weeks in duration. The differential diagnosis of chronic paronychia includes acute paronychia, candidiasis, and herpetic whitlow, as well as inflammatory conditions, including psoriasis or dyshidrotic eczema. Wound culture may be appropriate if there is a strong suspicion of nail fold infection (either primary or secondary) or in refractory cases [18]. If only a single digit is involved, the possibility of malignancy, including squamous cell carcinoma should be considered [1, 7, 13]. Additionally, other conditions including foreign body, subungual fibroma, and glomus tumor can be considered for the differential diagnosis of chronic paronychia in appropriate clinical settings. While imaging modalities, including X-ray, ultrasound, or MRI are not required for diagnosis, they may help rule out osteomyelitis, abscess, or glomus tumor [18–22]. In rare cases, a biopsy of the affected tissue may be performed to rule out malignancy or other conditions mimicking chronic paronychia [23–25].

32.7 Cases

Figures 32.1, 32.2, 32.3, 32.4, 32.5, 32.6, 32.7, 32.8 and 32.9 demonstrate the presentation of chronic paronychia in a clinical setting.

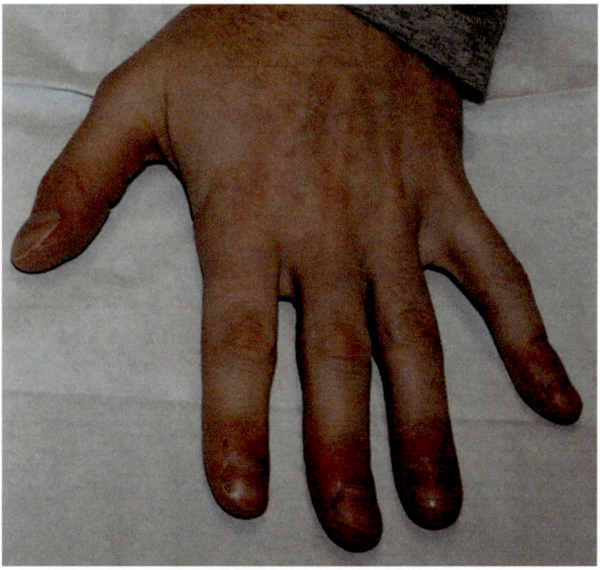

Fig. 32.1 32-Year-old male, Fitzpatrick type I, chronic paronychia, with eroded and erythematous proximal nail folds secondary to onychotillomania

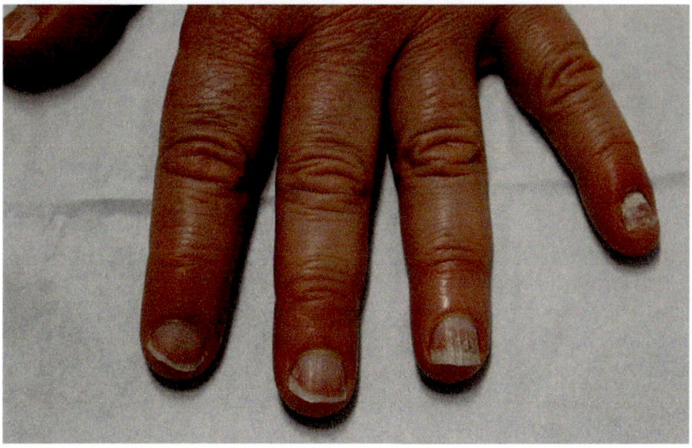

Fig. 32.2 66-Year-old female, Fitzpatrick type II, chronic paronychia, with erythema involving the nail folds. There is also onychorrhexis involving the left fourth fingernail and leukonychia involving the left fifth fingernail

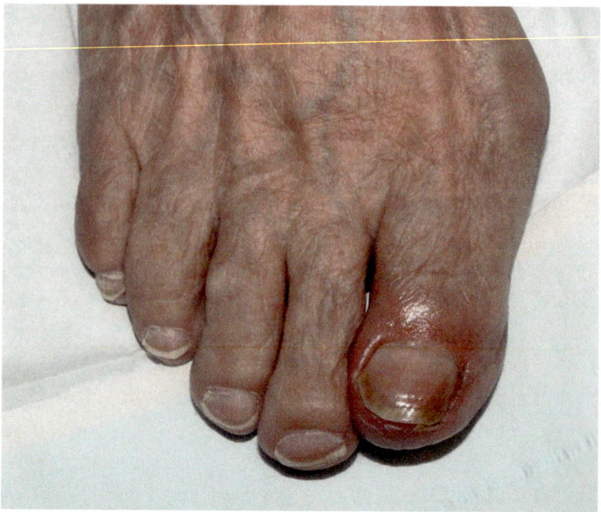

Fig. 32.3 80-Year-old female, Fitzpatrick type II, with erythema and swelling of the proximal and lateral nail folds of the right great toenail. There is also a bunion and toe overlap

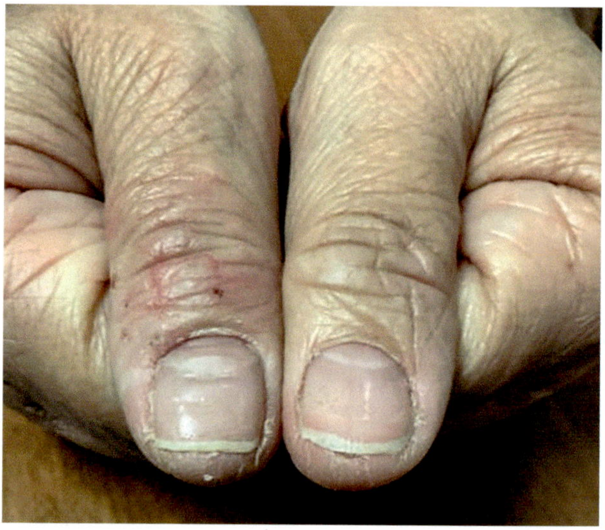

Fig. 32.4 61-Year-old female, Fitzpatrick type III, chronic paronychia, with erythema and erosions of the proximal nail fold of the right thumbnail. There is also cuticle retraction, enlarged lunula, and Beau's lines involving the right thumbnail. There is a background of xerotic skin on the thumbs

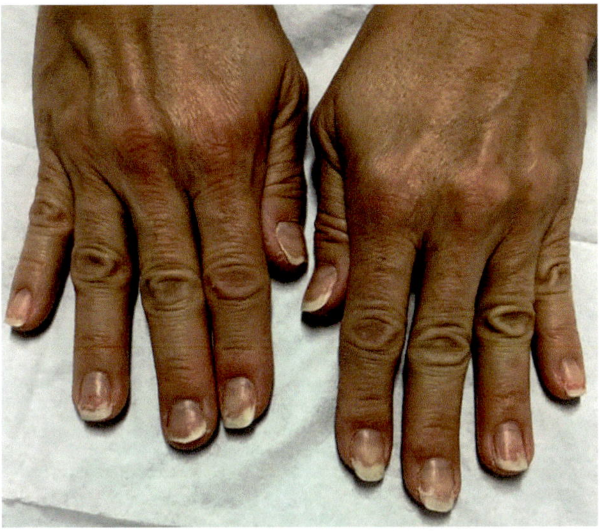

Fig. 32.5 56-Year-old female, Fitzpatrick type III, chronic paronychia, with subtle erythema of the proximal nail folds. There is also onycholysis and splitting of the fingernails

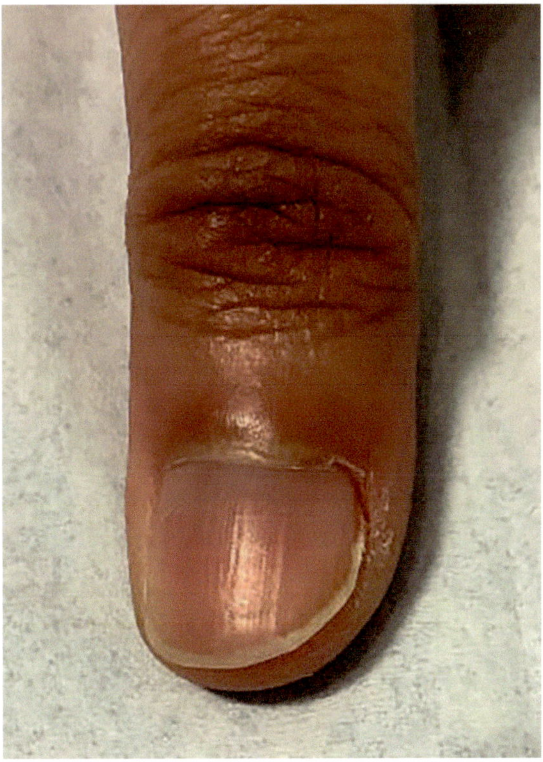

Fig. 32.6 39-year-old female, Fitzpatrick type IV, chronic paronychia, with minimal erythema of the proximal nail fold of the right thumbnail

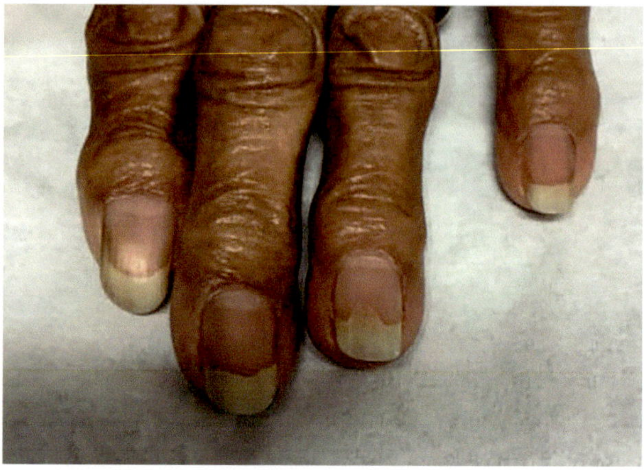

Fig. 32.7 76-Year-old female, Fitzpatrick type IV, chronic paronychia, with slight edema of the proximal nail folds and onycholysis of the fingernails

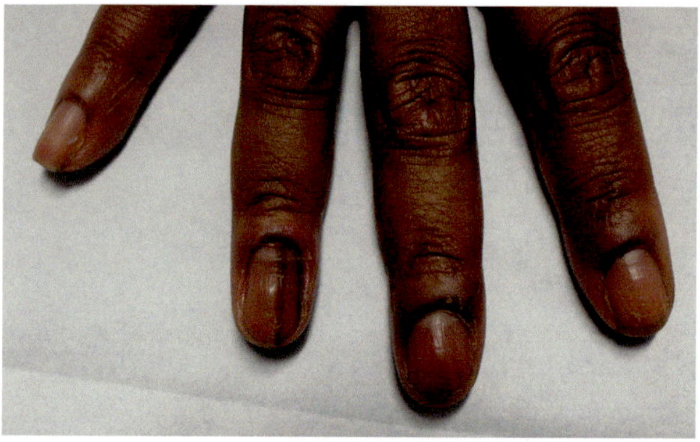

Fig. 32.8 58-Year-old female, Fitzpatrick type V, with edema and erythema of the proximal nail folds of the right third and fourth fingers. There are also gray to brown longitudinal bands involving the right third and fourth fingernails

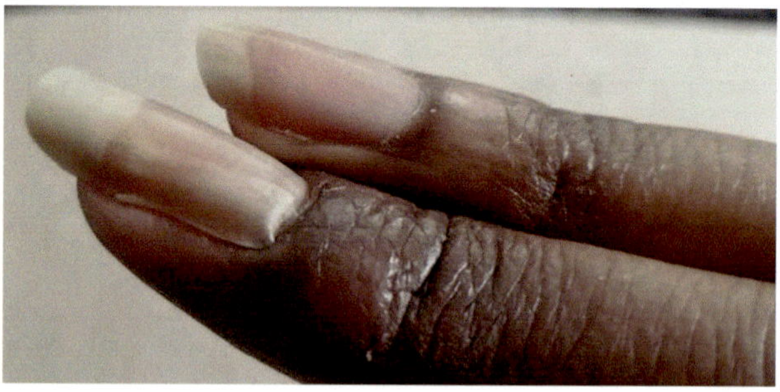

Fig. 32.9 43-Year-old female, Fitzpatrick type VI, with lateral onycholysis, minimal erythema, and swelling of the proximal nail folds of the right third fingernail

References

1. Leggit JC. Acute and chronic paronychia. Am Fam Physician. 2017;96(1):44–51.
2. Shemer A, Daniel CR. Common nail disorders. Clin Dermatol. 2013;31(5):578–86. https://doi.org/10.1016/j.clindermatol.2013.06.015.
3. Bahunuthula RK, Thappa DM, Kumari R, Singh R, Munisamy M, Parija SC. Evaluation of role of Candida in patients with chronic paronychia. Indian J Dermatol Venereol Leprol. 2015;81(5):485–90. https://doi.org/10.4103/0378-6323.158635.

4. Habif TP. Clinical dermatology: a color guide to diagnosis and therapy. 6th ed. Elsevier; 2016.
5. Capriotti K, Capriotti JA, Lessin S, et al. The risk of nail changes with taxane chemotherapy: a systematic review of the literature and meta-analysis. Br J Dermatol. 2015;173(3):842–5. https://doi.org/10.1111/bjd.13743.
6. Lacouture ME, Anadkat MJ, Bensadoun RJ, et al. Clinical practice guidelines for the prevention and treatment of EGFR inhibitor-associated dermatologic toxicities. Support Care Cancer. 2011;19(8):1079–95. https://doi.org/10.1007/s00520-011-1197-6.
7. Relhan V, Bansal A. Acute and chronic paronychia revisited: a narrative review. J Cutan Aesthet Surg. 2022;15(1):1. https://doi.org/10.4103/JCAS.JCAS_30_21.
8. Baran RL, editor. Advances in nail disease and management. Springer International Publishing; 2021. https://doi.org/10.1007/978-3-030-59997-3.
9. Gupta MK, Lipner SR. Review of chemotherapy-associated paronychia. Int J Dermatol. 2022;61(4):410–5. https://doi.org/10.1111/ijd.15740.
10. Scher and Daniel's nails: diagnosis, surgery, therapy. Springer Nature; 2019.
11. Dulski A, Edwards CW. Paronychia. In: StatPearls. StatPearls Publishing; 2024. Accessed January 30, 2024, http://www.ncbi.nlm.nih.gov/books/NBK544307/.
12. James WD, Elston DM, Treat J, Rosenbach M, Neuhaus IM. Andrews' Diseases of the skin: clinical dermatology. 13th ed. Elsevier; 2020.
13. Shafritz AB, Coppage JM. Acute and chronic paronychia of the hand. J Am Acad Orthop Surg. 2014;22(3):165–74. https://doi.org/10.5435/JAAOS-22-03-165.
14. Tosti A, Piraccini BM, Ghetti E, Colombo MD. Topical steroids versus systemic antifungals in the treatment of chronic paronychia: an open, randomized double-blind and double dummy study. J Am Acad Dermatol. 2002;47(1):73–6. https://doi.org/10.1067/mjd.2002.122191.
15. Daniel CR, Daniel MP, Daniel CM, Sullivan S, Ellis G. Chronic paronychia and onycholysis: a thirteen-year experience. Cutis. 1996;58(6):397–401.
16. Sharquie KE, Noaimi AA, Galib SA. Treatment of chronic paronychia: a double blind comparative clinical trial using singly vaseline, nystatin and fucidic acid ointment. JCDSA. 2013;03(04):250–5. https://doi.org/10.4236/jcdsa.2013.34038.
17. Dorko E, Jautová J, Pilipčinec E, Tkáčiková L. Occurrence of Candida strains in cases of paronychia. Folia Microbiol. 2004;49(5):591–5. https://doi.org/10.1007/BF02931539.
18. Lee DK, Lipner SR. Optimal diagnosis and management of common nail disorders. Ann Med. 2022;54(1):694–712. https://doi.org/10.1080/07853890.2022.2044511.
19. Pang HN, Yi-Liang Lee J, Beng-Hoi TA. Pincer nails complicated by distal phalangeal osteomyelitis. J Plast Reconstruct Aesth Surg. 2009;62(2):254–7. https://doi.org/10.1016/j.bjps.2007.10.009.
20. Grover C, Bansal S, Varma A, Jakhar D. Radiological imaging in nail unit disorders (Part I)—Modalities used. Indian Dermatol Online J. 2022;13(4):449. https://doi.org/10.4103/idoj.idoj_3_22.
21. Lipner SR, Scher RK. Subungual glomus tumors: Underrecognized clinical findings in neurofibromatosis 1. J Am Acad Dermatol. 2021;84(6):e269. https://doi.org/10.1016/j.jaad.2020.08.129.
22. Lee DK, Hill RC, Desai AD, Lipner SR. Utility of imaging in diagnosing subungual glomus tumors: a single-center retrospective study. J Am Acad Dermatol. 2024.:S0190962224005826; https://doi.org/10.1016/j.jaad.2024.03.044.
23. Jack C, El Helou T. Non-healing ulcerative paronychia. Lancet. 2017;389(10080):1740. https://doi.org/10.1016/S0140-6736(16)32400-X.
24. Lee CC, Wu YH. Paronychia-like digital metastases of osteosarcoma. Int J Dermatol. 2017;56(1):104–5. https://doi.org/10.1111/ijd.13394.
25. Ko J-H, Young A, Wang K-H. Paronychia-like digital cutaneous metastasis. Br J Dermatol. 2014;171(3):663–5. https://doi.org/10.1111/bjd.13025.

Traumatic Onycholysis

33

Rachel E. Reingold, Rachel C. Hill, and Shari R. Lipner

33.1 Description of Disease

Traumatic onycholysis refers to the lifting of the distal nail plate from the nail bed due to various environmental factors that introduce overt or subtle mechanical force. It is speculated that the nail plate maintains connection to the nail bed via the distal onychocorneal band. Interruption of this band or from other supportive structures (lateral nail folds, hyponychium) via traumatic shearing, blunt force (slamming finger in door), or microtrauma (rubbing against shoe material) initiates the development of onycholysis [1, 2]. Traumatic onycholysis is exacerbated via continued exposure to trauma from microtraumas, including ill-fitting shoes, frequent typing, manual labor, or child care, and is made worse with long nails, frequent under-nail cleaning by patients, harsh manicure techniques, or exposure to water work or caustic irritants [3–5]. With prolonged exposure to these environmental factors over 6 weeks, the nail bed may undergo keratinization making nail plate reattachment unlikely [2, 3]. Further, superimposed infection (fungal, bacterial, or viral) may impede proper nail attachment/re-growth [3, 4]. Traumatic toenail onycholysis from ill-fitting/narrow toe-box shoes is sometimes categorized into a group of clinical findings referred to as asymmetric gait nail unit signs [6]. Onycholysis can be staged from I to V based on the range of separation with stages I–III representing various measures of onycholysis measured via the distal nail plate from hyponychium, to stage IV with total onycholysis and, stage V with full destruction and subsequent cornification of the nail bed [3].

33.2 Epidemiology

33.2.1 Sex

The overall prevalence and sex distribution of traumatic onycholysis specifically has not been reported. Some studies have speculated that onycholysis may be more common in women due to the proximity of the fingers to the vaginal and

S. R. Lipner, *Atlas of Nail Disorders Across All Skin Colors*,
https://doi.org/10.1007/978-3-031-74272-9_33

gastrointestinal tract [6]. Women are also more likely to have exposure to traumatic nail injury via manicures and are more frequently offered or exposed to "at home" remedies via cosmetologists or friends which could exacerbate the condition (i.e., nail soaks and traumatic filing/nail injury) [6].

33.2.2 Age

There are no reports highlighting a predilection for age as trauma can occur at any age. However, those with prolonged/frequent microtraumas are likely to be adults based on the types of activities that introduce these risks. In a retrospective study of 60 patients at a tertiary hospital in India, the mean age of patients was 37 years (range: 6–68 years), suggesting that patients of all ages, including the extremes of age, are susceptible to traumatic onycholysis [7].

33.2.3 Risk Factors

While few risk factors for traumatic onycholysis have been formally studied, it tends to be more common in women and those with long nails [2]. Additionally, those with hallux valgus (bunions) have high rates of traumatic onycholysis given frequent, painless friction from shoes and elevation of the first toe [8]. Onycholysis may also be a clinical clue to systemic conditions, including thyroid disease, iron deficiency, anemia, or syphilis [4].

33.3 Clinical Features

Clinically, the nail plate is lifted off the nail bed and will classically appear as an opaque to mildly translucent cream-to-white color with a linear, horizontal proximal line of detachment. This white nail discoloration appears to extend proximally, often standing out in comparison to the non-avulsed, translucent, healthy nail that often has a pink hue indicative of proper vascularization [1]. Whether fingernails or toenails are more frequently affected by traumatic onycholysis is unknown. Hand dominance in relation to traumatic onycholysis has not been formally studied, but likely the first three digits of the dominant hand are affected most frequently. Clinical clues on history and physical examination may include the chronic, painless onset of onycholysis with symmetry or bilaterality, with unaffected nails generally appearing healthy in the absence of other nail conditions. If chronic, evidence of fungal or bacterial colonization may be present with associated color changes (cream, yellow, green, black) and may indicate the presence of dermatophytes, *Pseudomonas aeruginosa*, or candida. However, with onycholysis, bacterial, fungal, or viral colonization is secondary to the conducive, moist, warm environment rather than the primary cause of traumatic onycholysis in otherwise healthy individuals [1]. Onychoscopy can support a diagnosis of traumatic onycholysis when visualization of the nail bed reveals an opaque white coloration with a clear horizontal demarcation between the white lifted and healthy nail [1].

33.4 Clinical Features in Skin of Color

There are no reports addressing the variations in clinical features of traumatic onycholysis in patients with skin of color. However, in one case series, five skin of color patients with traumatic onycholysis had splinter hemorrhages and non-erythematous nail edges on dermoscopy [7]. Of note, trauma (usually repetitive, chronic trauma) often induces longitudinal melanonychia secondary to melanocyte activation [9].

33.5 Requirements for Diagnosis

Traumatic onycholysis is largely a clinical diagnosis requiring thorough history taking, with a focus on known acute/historical traumas, as well as occupational or activity of daily living exposures to repetitive or significant mechanical trauma. Differential diagnoses include inflammatory dermatoses (nail psoriasis or nail lichen planus) or infection (onychomycosis or *P. aeruginosa* colonization) [5]. Traumatic onycholysis requires exclusion of other conditions via history, review of systems, clinical/dermoscopy examination findings (assessing for splinter hemorrhages, pitting, oil spots, or other lesions on skin seen in psoriasis vs. subungual hyperkeratosis seen in onychomycosis), and possible nail clipping for fungal/bacterial elements and histopathology. Systemic causes of onycholysis, including thyroid disease, iron deficiency, anemia, and/or syphilis, should also be ruled out via laboratory testing.

33.6 Cases

Figures 33.1, 33.2, 33.3, 33.4, 33.5, and 33.6 demonstrate the presentation of traumatic onycholysis in a clinical setting.

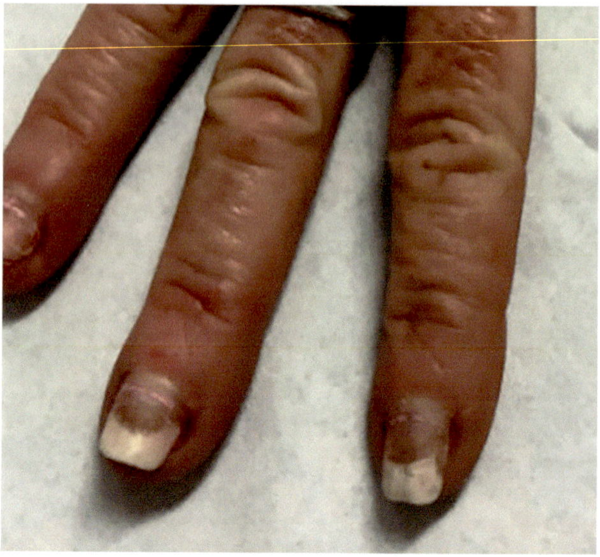

Fig. 33.1 57-Year-old female, Fitzpatrick type II, traumatic onycholysis, with separation of the nail plate from the nail bed and linear, transverse demarcation between the white nail plate and healthy, pink nail plate involving the right first and second fingernails

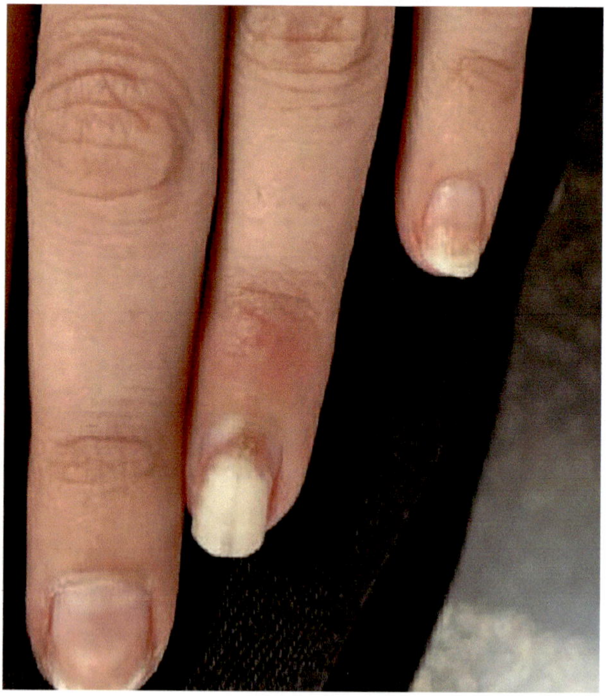

Fig. 33.2 32-Year-old female, Fitzpatrick type II, traumatic onycholysis, with separation of the nail plate from the nail bed and loss of healthy, pink nail plate involving the left fourth fingernail and more subtle similar findings involving the left fifth fingernail

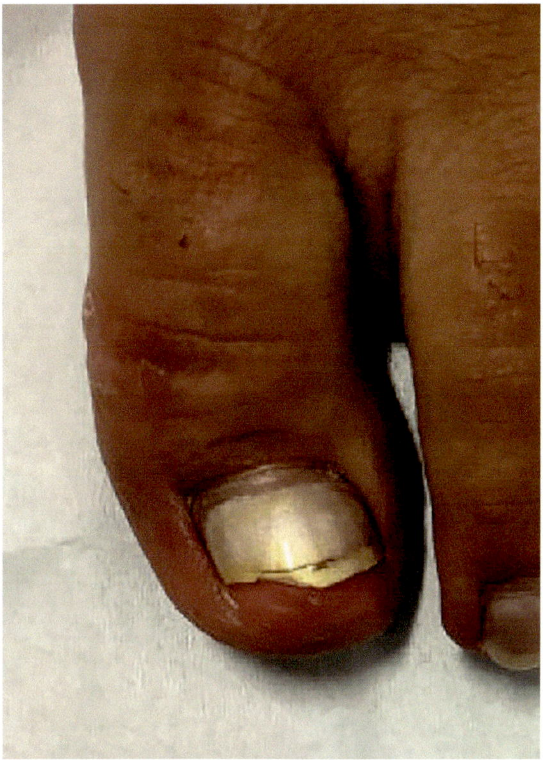

Fig. 33.3 32-Year-old female, Fitzpatrick type III, traumatic onycholysis, with loss of a portion of the distal, lifted, white nail plate affecting left great toenail

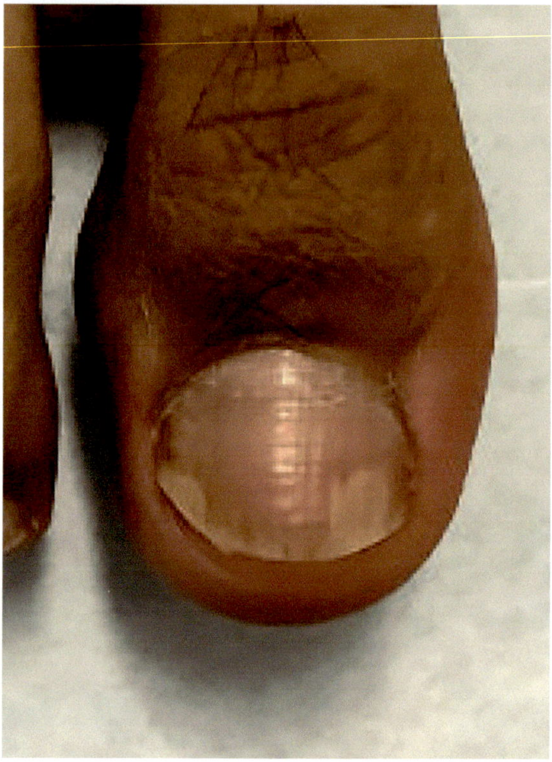

Fig. 33.4 29-Year-old male, Fitzpatrick type IV, traumatic onycholysis, with symmetric detached nail plate with white discoloration of the right great toenail

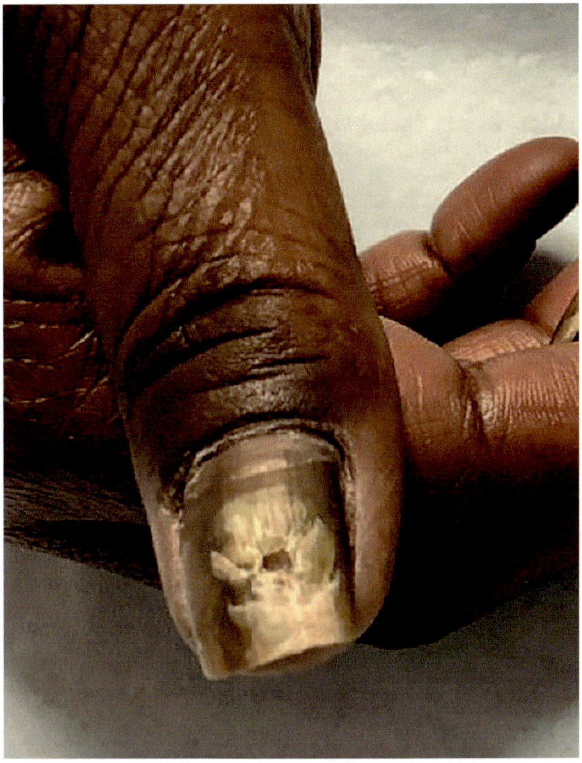

Fig. 33.5 64-Year-old female, Fitzpatrick type V, traumatic onycholysis, with xanthonychia and loss of portion of the nail plate affecting the right thumbnail

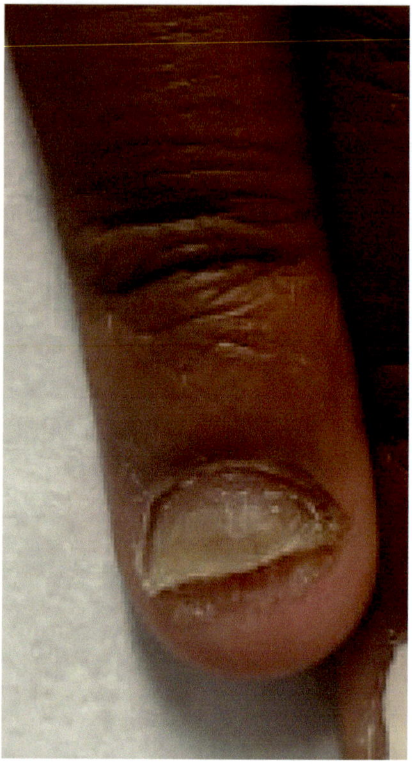

Fig. 33.6 32-Year-old female, Fitzpatrick type V, traumatic onycholysis, with partially detached nail plate, and linear, horizontal proximal line of detachment involving the right fourth fingernail

References

1. Piraccini BM, Alessandrini A, Starace M. Onychoscopy: Dermoscopy of the Nails. Dermatol Clin. 2018;36(4):431–8. https://doi.org/10.1016/j.det.2018.05.010.
2. Tucker JR. Nail Deformities and Injuries. Prim Care. 2015;42(4):677–91. https://doi.org/10.1016/j.pop.2015.08.005.
3. Shemer A, Daniel CR 3rd. Common nail disorders. Clin Dermatol. 2013;31(5):578–86. https://doi.org/10.1016/j.clindermatol.2013.06.015.
4. Kechijian P. Onycholysis of the fingernails: evaluation and management. J Am Acad Dermatol. 1985;12(3):552–60. https://doi.org/10.1016/s0190-9622(85)70077-1.
5. Vélez NF, Jellinek NJ. Simple onycholysis: a diagnosis of exclusion. J Am Acad Dermatol. 2014;70(4):793–4. https://doi.org/10.1016/j.jaad.2013.09.061.
6. Zaias N, Escovar SX, Zaiac MN. Finger and toenail onycholysis. J Eur Acad Dermatol Venereol. 2015;29(5):848–53. https://doi.org/10.1111/jdv.12862.
7. Ankad BS, Gupta A, Alekhya R, Saipriya M. Dermoscopy of onycholysis due to nail psoriasis, onychomycosis and trauma: a cross sectional study in skin of color. Indian Dermatol Online J. 2020;11(5):777–83. https://doi.org/10.4103/idoj.IDOJ_475_19.
8. Giménez-López R, Barrios-Pitarque C. Cross-sectional study of the prevalence of hyperextension of the first metatarsophalangeal joint and its relationship to onycholysis in women with hallux valgus. BMC Musculoskel Disord. 2024;25(1):111. https://doi.org/10.1186/s12891-024-07219-1.
9. Leung AKC, Lam JM, Leong KF, Sergi CM. Melanonychia striata: clarifying behind the Black Curtain. A review on clinical evaluation and management of the 21st century. Int J Dermatol. 2019;58(11):1239–45. https://doi.org/10.1111/ijd.14464.

34 Onychocryptosis

Noelle Desir and Shari R. Lipner

34.1 Description of Disease

Onychocryptosis, or ingrown nail, is a common nail pathology that occurs when the nail plate grows into the periungual dermis causing inflammation and potentially causing infection. Prevalence in the general population ranges from 2.5% to 5% [1]. Onychocryptosis may cause significant pain, discomfort, and disability if left untreated [2]. The hallux nails, or great toenails, are the most frequently affected [3]. Onychocryptosis may present at any age, but most often presents in adolescents and in older adults [1, 4]. Mild disease can frequently be treated with conservative management and surgical approaches are often reserved for moderate to severe disease [1]. Patients who underwent treatment have reported high levels of overall satisfaction [5].

34.2 Epidemiology

There is sparse data on the epidemiology of onychocryptosis. Underreporting is expected because patients experiencing mild symptoms are not likely to seek care [6].

34.2.1 Sex

It is unclear if sex plays a role in the development of onychocryptosis. A representative sample of the South Korean National Health Information Database of one million participants, 2004–2013, reported that 53.8% of female vs. 46.2% of male patients presented with onychocryptosis ($P < 0.001$) [4]. In contrast, other studies assert a male predominance ranging from a nearly 2:1 ratio in a prospective study of 133 patients evaluated for operative management, to as high as 3:1 ratio in a separate prospective study of 249 patients with onychocryptosis evaluated for surgery [7, 8].

S. R. Lipner, *Atlas of Nail Disorders Across All Skin Colors*,
https://doi.org/10.1007/978-3-031-74272-9_34

34.2.2 Age

While onychocryptosis affects patients of all ages, there is a bimodal age distribution, presenting in the first and third decade and then after the fifth decade of life [1, 4, 9, 10]. A prospective cohort study of 66 female and 74 male adolescents reported that nearly 40% of all 21-year-olds presenting with a nail disorder had onychocryptosis [11]. In contrast, a single-center cross-sectional study of 170 podiatric patients with onychocryptosis in Spain reported mean age of 54 years [12].

34.2.3 Other Factors

The prevalence of onychocryptosis in the general population ranges from 2.5% to 5% and it is more common in diabetic patients (13–32%) [1, 13]. Diabetic patients and patients with impaired arterial circulation and decreased sensation may present with severe cases (i.e., secondary infection) [14]. Some studies have suggested that bone deformity, especially acquired valgus or varus deformity and flat foot, are associated with onychocryptosis, but this relationship has been debated [2, 4]. A retrospective case-control study of the radiographic findings of 81 patients and 100 healthy controls showed no difference in hallux valgus angle, intermetatarsal angle, and interphalangeal angle between groups ($P = 0.123$, $P = 0.198$, and $P = 0.925$, respectively). The distribution of foot anatomy between groups was also similar ($P = 0.97$), suggesting no relationship between anatomic variants and onychocryptosis [15]. Isotretinoin therapy for acne vulgaris may be associated with the development of onychocryptosis. A 2019 case report of an 18-year-old male treated for acne vulgaris with isotretinoin describes the development of bilateral onychocryptosis of the great toenails during month four out of six of isotretinoin therapy. His onychocryptosis eventually required surgical intervention which resolved his symptoms [16]. These findings are consistent with a separate 2016 case report of a 19-year-old male who developed onychocryptosis of the first and second toenails bilaterally while on isotretinoin therapy for acne vulgaris [17]. While the mechanism behind the association between isotretinoin and onychocryptosis is poorly understood, it is thought to be a consequence of exuberant periungual granulation tissue formation in some patients while on isotretinoin therapy [17].

34.3 Risk Factors

Improper nail trimming is a well-established risk factor for the development of onychocryptosis. Nail trimming that results in "rounded" corners may lead to the formation of a nail barb or spicule that traumatizes the adjacent periungual dermis [1, 3, 18]. As the nail plate grows, a spicule of the lateral/distal nail may anchor itself into the periungual tissue [1, 19]. Trimming of the spicule often causes soft tissue trauma resulting in further pain. Therefore, it is recommended that toenails are trimmed straight across [1]. A similar mechanism of ingrown toenail formation is seen in patients with onychomycosis with accompanying hyperkeratosis resulting in an unstable nail plate with nail spicules that may anchor into the surrounding skin [10].

Tight-fitting footwear is another risk factor for ingrown toenail formation. Trauma from toe compression may cause shrinkage of the distal nail bed which may impede nail growth. This association is strengthened by evidence of decreased incidence of onychocryptosis in barefoot populations [20]. Obesity may facilitate the formation of onychocryptosis by a similar pathophysiological mechanism as compression, as increased soft tissue habitus increases constriction of the foot by footwear. Similarly, disorders that increase lower extremity edema (diabetes, thyroid, cardiac, and renal disease) may mimic the effect of obesity on the nail unit [1]. Hyperhidrosis may result in periungual skin maceration which increases nail plate malleability and facilitates skin perforation [19]. Another risk factor for the development of ingrown toenails is nail thickness, though some studies suggest that the increased malleability of thin and flattened nails increases the risk of onychocryptosis [11, 21].

34.4 Clinical Features

The diagnosis of onychocryptosis is often a straightforward one. Pain is a universal finding with some patients also presenting with edema or erythema [1]. The classification of onychocryptosis is traditionally divided into three stages: mild (stage I) is characterized by nail fold swelling, edema, erythema, and pain exacerbated by pressure, moderate (stage II) is characterized by the features of stage I and active or acute infection, and severe (stage III) is characterized by the features of stage 2 and chronic inflammation and formation of epithelialized granulation tissue with marked nail fold hypertrophy [22]. Since assessing the exact stage can be subjective, staging is more often used for research purposes, rather than in clinical practice [1].

34.5 Clinical Features in Skin of Color

Clinical features of onychocryptosis in skin of color have not been previously described. The 1990 United States National Health Survey reported a decreased prevalence of onychocryptosis in African American populations compared to Caucasians in nearly all age groups; however, other studies show no association between race and onychocryptosis [3, 23]. In addition to classical clinical findings, darker-skinned patients may have gray-brown longitudinal bands due to melanocytic activation.

34.6 Requirements for Diagnosis

Onychocryptosis is a clinical diagnosis. There are no standardized diagnostic criteria for diagnosis of onychocryptosis. Key clinical findings include periungual pain worsened by pressure and nail fold swelling and/or erythema caused by impingement of the nail fold by the nail plate. Worsening pain with pressure is a sign that can be elicited on physical examination, and nail fold impingement can often be visualized.

34.7 Cases

Figures 34.1, 34.2, 34.3, 34.4, 34.5, and 34.6 demonstrate the presentation of glomus tumors in a clinical setting.

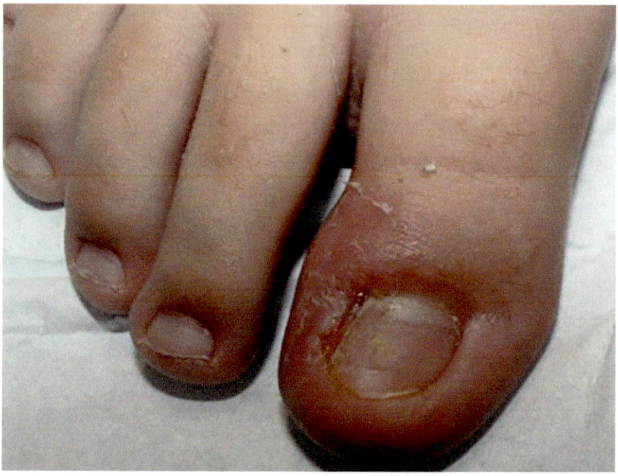

Fig. 34.1 13-Year-old female, Fitzpatrick type II, onychocryptosis, with erythema of the lateral nail fold of the left great toenail, s/p phenol matricectomy, with recurrence of symptoms

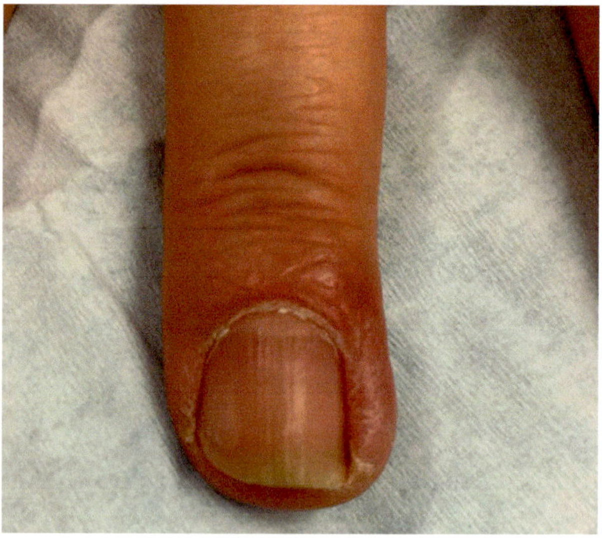

Fig. 34.2 57-Year-old female, Fitzpatrick type II, onychocryptosis, with overcurvature of the left third fingernail with erythema and hypertrophy of the lateral nail fold

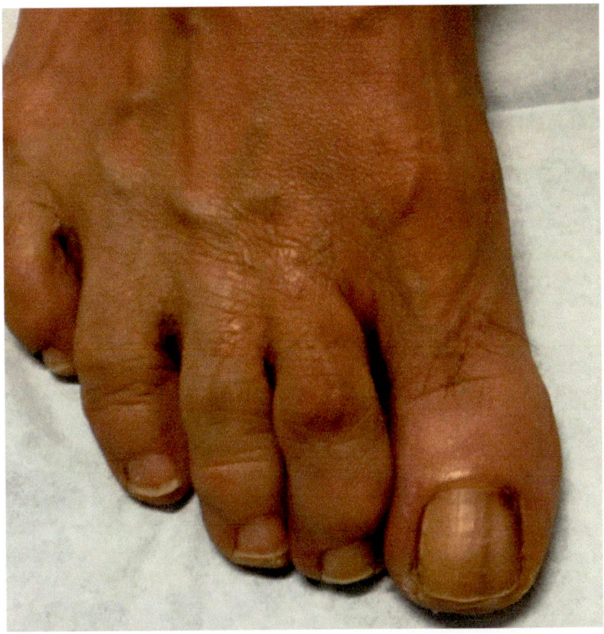

Fig. 34.3 63-Year-old female, Fitzpatrick type III, onychocryptosis, with impingement of the right great toenail into the lateral nail fold. There is also a 1 mm light brown longitudinal band

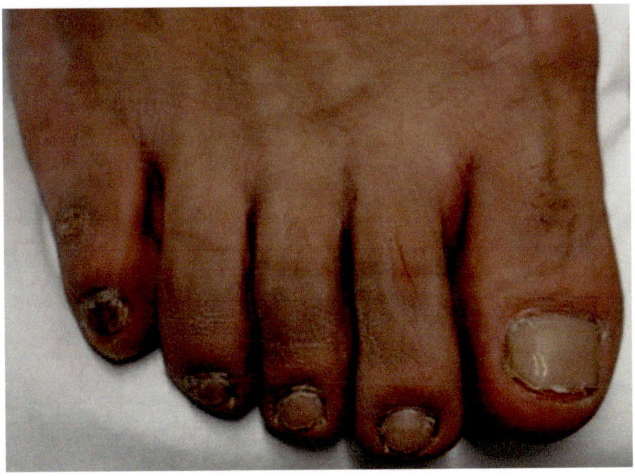

Fig. 34.4 55-Year-old, Fitzpatrick type IV, onychocryptosis, with impingement of the right great toenail into the medial nail fold. The patient reported loss of sensation in the right great toe

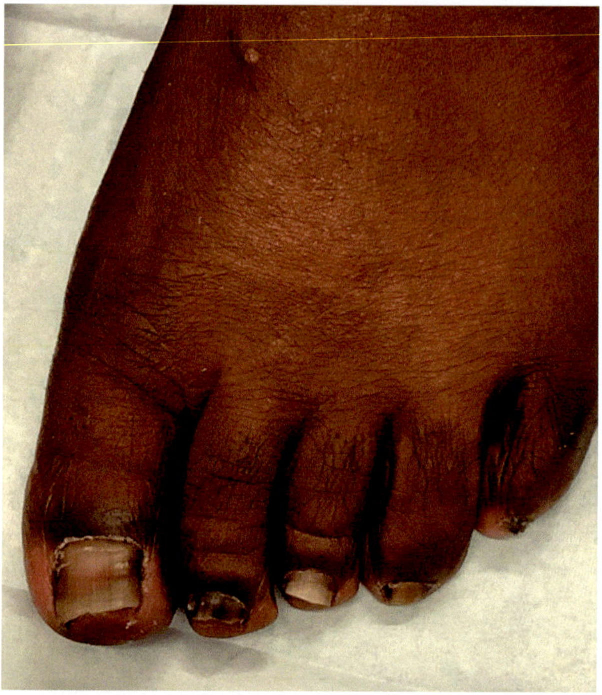

Fig. 34.5 73-Year-old, Fitzpatrick type V, onychocryptosis, with impingement of the left great toenail into the medial and lateral nail folds. There are gray-brown longitudinal bands involving the left great toenail, as well as other toenails

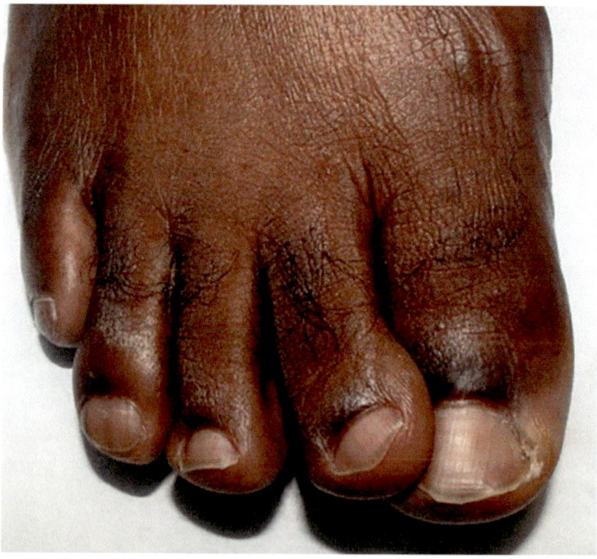

Fig. 34.6 44-Year-old male, Fitzpatrick type VI, onychocryptosis, with very tender right great toenail and nail plate impingement into the medial nail fold. There is significant toe overlap between the first and second toes

References

1. Geizhals S, Lipner SR. Review of onychocryptosis: epidemiology, pathogenesis, risk factors, diagnosis and treatment. Dermatol Online J. 2019;25(9):13030/qt9985w2n0.
2. Bryant A, Knox A. Ingrown toenails: the role of the GP. Aust Fam Physician. 2015;44(3):102–5.
3. DeLauro NM, DeLauro TM. Onychocryptosis. Clin Podiatr Med Surg. 2004;21(4):617–30, vii. https://doi.org/10.1016/j.cpm.2004.05.009.
4. Cho SY, Kim YC, Choi JW. Epidemiology and bone-related comorbidities of ingrown nail: a nationwide population-based study. J Dermatol. 2018;45(12):1418–24. https://doi.org/10.1111/1346-8138.14659.
5. Stewart CR, Algu L, Kamran R, et al. Patient satisfaction with treatment for onychocryptosis: a systematic review. Skin Appendage Disord. 2020;6(5):272–9. https://doi.org/10.1159/000508927.
6. Borges APP, Pelafsky VPC, Miot LDB, Miot HA. Quality of life with ingrown toenails: a cross-sectional study. Dermatol Surg. 2017;43(5):751–3. https://doi.org/10.1097/DSS.0000000000000954.
7. van der Ham AC, Hackeng CA, Yo TI. The treatment of ingrowing toenails. A randomised comparison of wedge excision and phenol cauterisation. J Bone Joint Surg Br. 1990;72(3):507–9. https://doi.org/10.1302/0301-620X.72B3.2341458.
8. Barreiros H, Matos D, Goulão J, Serrano P, João A, Brandão FM. Using 80% trichloroacetic acid in the treatment of ingrown toenails. An Bras Dermatol. 2013;88(6):889–93. https://doi.org/10.1590/abd1806-4841.20132296.
9. Eekhof JA, Van Wijk B, Knuistingh Neven A, van der Wouden JC. Interventions for ingrowing toenails. Cochrane Database Syst Rev. 2012;2012(4):CD001541. https://doi.org/10.1002/14651858.CD001541.pub3.
10. Khunger N, Kandhari R. Ingrown toenails. Indian J Dermatol Venereol Leprol. 2012;78(3):279–89. https://doi.org/10.4103/0378-6323.95442.
11. Pico AM, Verjano E, Mayordomo R. Relation between nail consistency and incidence of ingrown toenails in young male runners. J Am Podiatr Med Assoc. 2017;107(2):137–43. https://doi.org/10.7547/15-121.
12. Mosquera-Fernández A, Díaz-Rodríguez M, González-Martín C, Platero-Arboiro M, Souto-Rey V, Balboa-Barreiro V. Hábitos podológicos en personas con alteraciones ungueales. Gaceta medica de Mexico. 2017;153(7):810–7. https://doi.org/10.24875/GMM.17003023.
13. Vural S, Bostanci S, Koçyigit P, Çaliskan D, Baskal N, Aydin N. Risk factors and frequency of ingrown nails in adult diabetic patients. J Foot Ankle Surg. 2018;57(2):289–95. https://doi.org/10.1053/j.jfas.2017.10.006.
14. Perper M, Tosti A. Chapter 6. Nail diseases in the elderly. In: Tosti A, Piraccini BM, editors. Nail disorders. 1st ed. Elsevier; 2018. p. 52–3.
15. Kose O, Celiktas M, Kisin B, Ozyurek S, Yigit S. Is there a relationship between forefoot alignment and ingrown toenail? A case-control study. Foot Ankle Spec. 2011;4(1):14–7. https://doi.org/10.1177/1938640010382293.
16. Sivaraj K, Friedman J, Morrell D. Onychocryptosis and asymptomatic external urethritis as complications of oral isotretinoin therapy. BMJ Case Rep. 2019;12(8):e231387. https://doi.org/10.1136/bcr-2019-231387.
17. Figueiras Dde A, Ramos TB, Marinho AK, Bezerra MS, Cauas RC. Paronychia and granulation tissue formation during treatment with isotretinoin. An Bras Dermatol. 2016;91(2):223–5. https://doi.org/10.1590/abd1806-4841.20163817.
18. Park DH, Singh D. The management of ingrowing toenails. BMJ. 2012;344:e2089. https://doi.org/10.1136/bmj.e2089.
19. Heidelbaugh JJ, Lee H. Management of the ingrown toenail. Am Fam Physician. 2009;79(4):303–8.

20. Günal I, Koşay C, Veziroğlu A, Balkan Y, Ilhan F. Relationship between onychocryptosis and foot type and treatment with toe spacer. A preliminary investigation. J Am Podiatr Med Assoc. 2003;93(1):33–6. https://doi.org/10.7547/87507315-93-1-33.
21. Langford DT, Burke C, Robertson K. Risk factors in onychocryptosis. Br J Surg. 1989;76(1):45–8. https://doi.org/10.1002/bjs.1800760114.
22. Heifetz CJ. Operative management of ingrown toenail. Mo Med. 1945;42:213–6.
23. Dunn JE, Link CL, Felson DT, Crincoli MG, Keysor JJ, McKinlay JB. Prevalence of foot and ankle conditions in a multiethnic community sample of older adults. Am J Epidemiol. 2004;159(5):491–8. https://doi.org/10.1093/aje/kwh071.

Pincer Nails

35

Jose W. Ricardo and Shari R. Lipner

35.1 Description of Disease

Pincer nail (PN) refers to an excessive transverse curvature of the nail plate [1, 2]. The overcurvature progresses from proximal to distal, following the nail plate longitudinal axis, resulting in impingement of the distal nail bed [1–3]. The condition most commonly affects the hallux toenails [4]. In 2001, Baran et al. [1] noted that PNs occur from an osteophyte at the base of the distal phalanx elevating the nail plate and causing the lateral nail margins to roll inward. More recently, it has been suggested that osteophyte formation at the distal phalanx is not the cause of PN, but rather a consequence of the nail plate overcurvature [5, 6]. This theory is supported by the differing physical properties of the "hard" dorsal nail plate and the "plastic" ventral nail plate [7]. An unknown factor is thought to cause shrinkage or constriction of the nail bed, affecting the ventral nail plate, but not the dorsal nail plate. The difference between the affected ventral site and unaffected dorsal site causes an inward twisting of the lateral nail margins that exerts traction over the distal tuft of the distal phalanx, resulting in osteophyte formation [3, 6, 7]. PN is distinct from onychocryptosis, a symptomatic condition in which the nail plate shape remains unchanged [6, 8].

35.2 Epidemiology

35.2.1 Sex

In Jemec et al.'s survey-based study including 567 patients admitted to general medical and surgical wards, the incidence of PNs in fingernails was 0.9% [9]. The overall incidence of PNs in toenails remains unknown, although it is presumed to be significantly higher since the condition is infrequently observed in fingernails [3]. The condition most commonly affects women, with a clinical study by Lee et al. including 35 PN cases, reporting an estimated female-to-male ratio of 2:1 (23 women and 12 men) [10].

S. R. Lipner, *Atlas of Nail Disorders Across All Skin Colors*,
https://doi.org/10.1007/978-3-031-74272-9_35

35.2.2 Age

Mechanical force disturbance, namely lack of upward forces, plays a role in PN formation [11]. In a case-control study including 12 bilateral PN cases and 12 age- and sex-controlled healthy controls, the pressure on the hallux of the PN group was lower than that of the control group (bare feet: 1010.0 ± 309.0 vs. 1318 ± 226.2 g/ cm^2, $P < 0.01$) [12]. PNs are thought to occur more frequently in older adults, possibly due to their engaging in less regular walking [13]. In Lee et al.'s clinical study, the mean age was 52.09 ± 17.26 years (range: 10–77) [10].

35.2.3 Other Factors

There are inherited and acquired forms of PNs [1]. Hereditary PNs are typically symmetric, with disease onset often occurring during childhood [1]. Cases of autosomal-dominant [14] and autosomal-recessive [15] inheritance patterns have been reported. Acquired PN is often asymmetric. It is associated with underlying systemic conditions, including gastrointestinal disease [9], Kawasaki disease [16, 17], amyotrophic lateral sclerosis [18], and systemic lupus erythematosus [19]; when these conditions are treated, spontaneous resolution often occurs. PNs affecting both fingernails and toenails symmetrically should raise suspicion of a systemic etiology [20]. Iatrogenic PNs may occur due to beta-blockers use [20, 21] or placement of arteriovenous fistula for hemodialysis [22]. The latter may lead to unilateral PN deformity which is thought to arise due to increased venous pressures and microcirculatory ischemia [22]. Other causes of PN include onychomycosis [10], psoriasis, and nail tumors, including onychomatricoma [23] and myxoid cyst [1].

35.3 Risk Factors

Several mechanical factors can contribute to PN formation. Wearing ill-fitting shoes and being bedridden are associated with PN development in toenails [1, 12]. Osteoarthritis and inappropriate trimming of nails can lead to PN deformity in both fingernails and toenails [1, 12]. Female sex and advanced age are also risk factors. All other causes of PNs covered in Sect. 35.2.3 are also considered risk factors for this condition.

35.4 Clinical Features

Based on morphology, there are three clinical types of PNs: the "common" PN, the tile-shaped nail, and the plicated nail [1]. The most common type is the "common" PN, in which nail plate overcurvature progresses from proximal to distal in the longitudinal axis [1]. This overcurvature results in the lateral margins rolling inward, causing impingement of the distal nail bed and resulting in a trumpet-like shape of the nail plate [1]. The tile-shaped nail type presents with a parallel transverse overcurvature along the nail's longitudinal axis and is usually a less severe form than the "common" variant [1]. The plicated type is characterized by a sharp bending of one or both lateral nail margins that may impinge into the lateral nail folds causing granulation tissue formation [1]. Among the 35 PN cases described in Lee et al.'s study, 83% had the "common" type, 14% had the plicated type, and 3% had the tile-shaped type [10]. Pain may occur with PNs but it is not a consistent symptom, as opposed to ingrown nails which are invariably painful [1].

35.5 Clinical Features in Skin of Color

The specific clinical characteristics of PNs in individuals with darker skin tones have not been previously documented. PN deformity can predispose the nail unit to repeated trauma, potentially leading to frictional melanonychia, a type of melanocytic activation prevalent in individuals with skin of color [24].

35.6 Requirements for Diagnosis

The diagnosis of PNs relies primarily on clinical assessment of nail morphology. Symptoms, including pain and functional limitations, may or may not be present [1]. A comprehensive medical history can aid in identifying a potential hereditary pattern, as well as in identifying occupational risk factors, including wearing poorly fitted shoes, participating in sports, or engaging in repetitive manual work. When the diagnosis is unclear, a histopathologic examination of nail clippings can help rule out onychomycosis and nail psoriasis. Radiographs of the hands and feet are useful for excluding osteoarthritis and identifying the presence of osteophytes. Transillumination helps in ruling out a digital myxoid pseudocyst [25]. Histopathologic evaluation of the avulsed nail plate or excised tumor can help rule out an onychomatricoma.

35.7 Cases

Figures 35.1, 35.2, 35.3, 35.4, 35.5, 35.6, and 35.7 depict the clinical presentation of pincer nails.

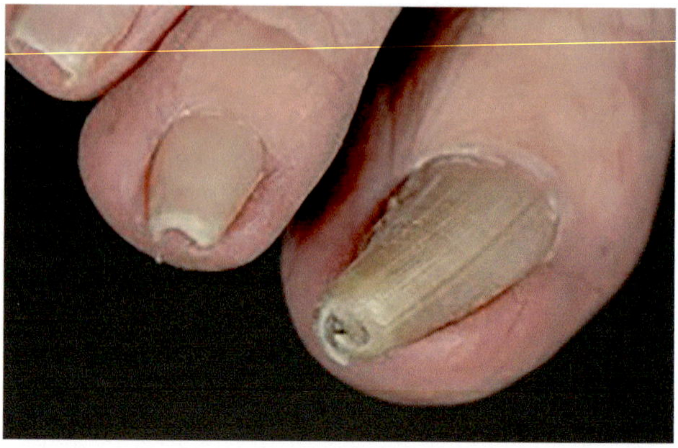

Fig. 35.1 Fitzpatrick type I, pincer nail, with "common" pincer nail of the right first and second toenails. The right first toenail has severe transverse overcurvature of the nail plate resulting in a trumpet-like appearance. The right second toenail has moderate transverse overcurvature (*from* Schneiderman and Grossman [26]; *with permission*)

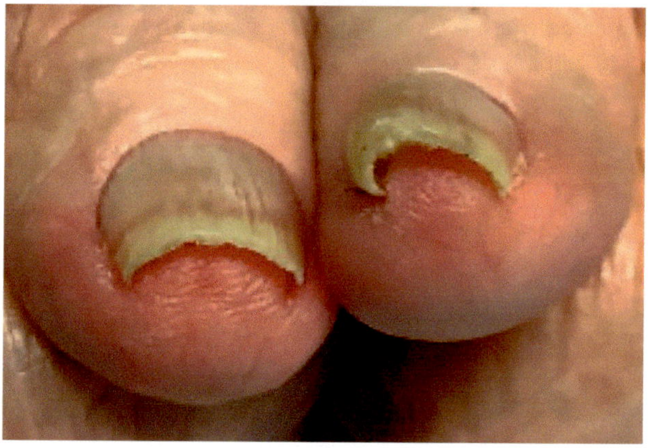

Fig. 35.2 73-Year-old female, Fitzpatrick type II, pincer nails, with transverse overcurvature and distal onycholysis of the bilateral thumbnails. The left thumbnail exhibits a plicated nail with a sharp bend on the medial nail margin. The right thumbnail shows a "common" pincer nail morphology

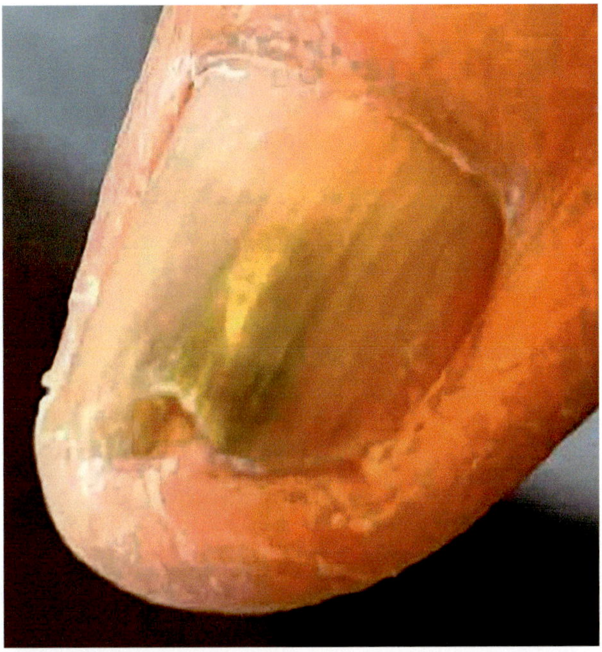

Fig. 35.3 65-Year-old female, Fitzpatrick type II, pincer nail, with right thumbnail showing "common" pincer nail with symmetric transverse overcurvature of the nail plate and a greenish-yellow discoloration indicative of superimposed green nail syndrome

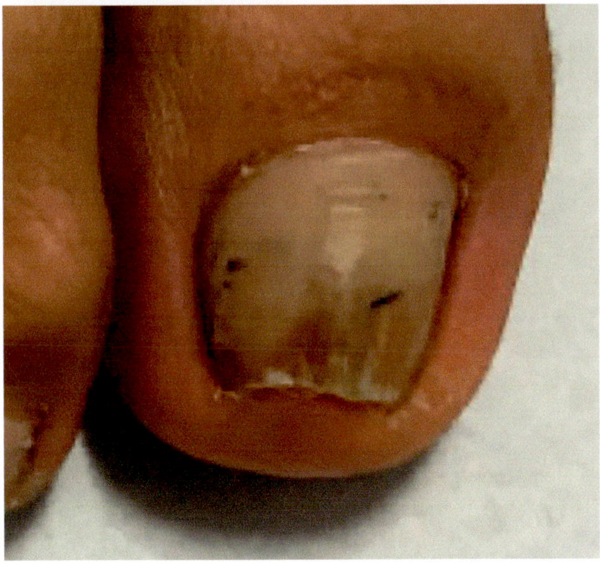

Fig. 35.4 49-Year-old male, Fitzpatrick type III, pincer nail, with symmetric transverse overcurvature and progressive distal narrowing of the nail plate width of the left great toenail, characteristic of a "common" pincer nail. The distal nail plate has diffuse faint brown-red discoloration, indicative of a subungual hematoma

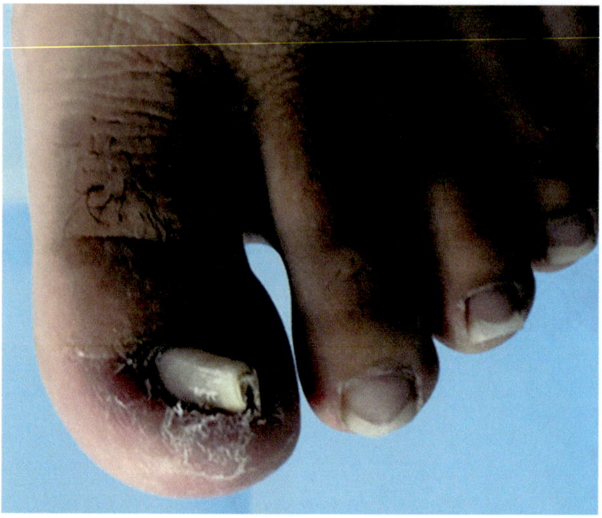

Fig. 35.5 45-Year-old male, Fitzpatrick type IV, pincer nail. Left first toenail shows "common" PN deformity with severe transverse curvature of the nail plate, forming a trumpet-like appearance with a lateral deviation (*from* Huang et al. [27]; *with permission*)

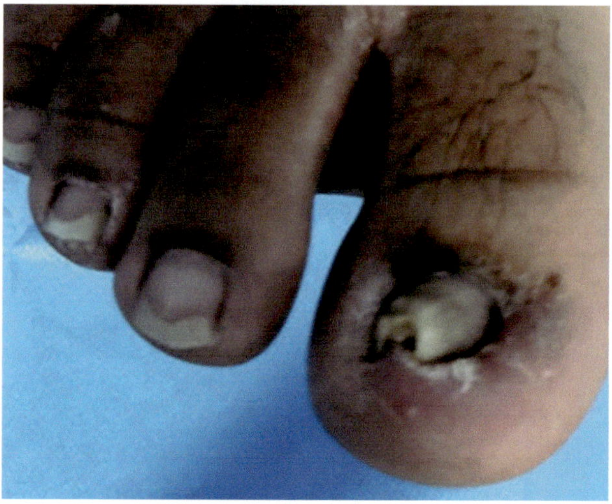

Fig. 35.6 45-Year-old male, Fitzpatrick type IV, pincer nail. Right first toenail displays excessive transverse curvature and distal narrowing of the nail plate, resulting in impingement on the distal nail bed (*from* Huang et al. [27]; *with permission*)

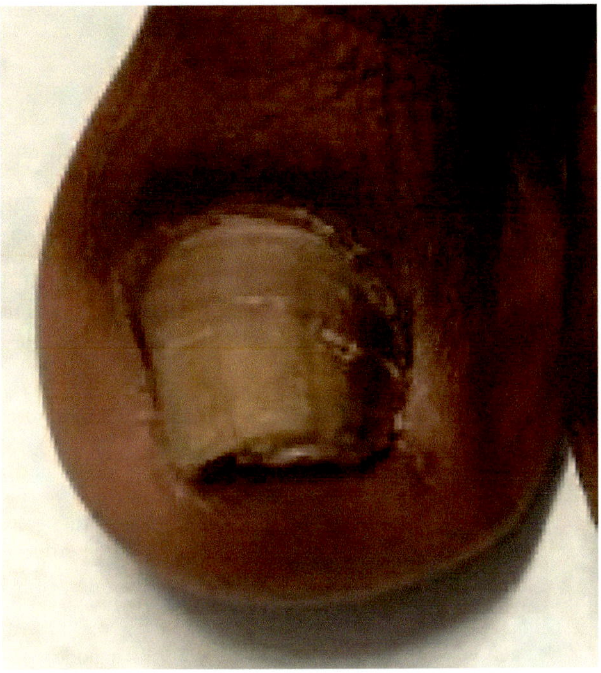

Fig. 35.7 54-Year-old female, Fitzpatrick type V, pincer nail, with the left great toenail showing "common" pincer nail with mild transverse overcurvature and distal narrowing of the nail plate, along with gray longitudinal bands due to melanocytic activation

References

1. Baran R, Haneke E, Richert B. Pincer nails: definition and surgical treatment. Dermatologic Surg. 2001;27(3):261–6.
2. Grover C, Yadav S, Gupta R. An uncommon cause of pincer nail. J Cutan Aesthet Surg. 2023;16(2):159–62.
3. Plusje LG. Pincer nails: a new surgical treatment. Dermatologic Surg. 2001;27(1):41–3.
4. Huang C, Huang R, Yu M, et al. Pincer nail deformity: clinical characteristics, causes, and managements. Biomed Res Int. 2020;2020:2939850.
5. Kim JY, Park SY, Jin SP, Yoon HS, Cho S, Park HS. Quick and easy correction of a symptomatic pincer nail using a shape memory alloy device. Dermatologic Surg. 2013;39(10):1520–6.
6. Kosaka M, Kusuhara H, Mochizuki Y, Mori H, Isogai N. Morphologic study of normal, ingrown, and pincer nails. Dermatologic Surg. 2010;36(1):31–8.
7. Forslind B, Thyresson N. On the structure of the normal nail. A scanning electron microscope study. Arch Dermatol Forsch. 1975;251(3):199–204.
8. Pearson HJ, Bury RN, Wapples J, Watkin DF. Ingrowing toenails: is there a nail abnormality? A prospective study. J Bone Joint Surg Br. 1987;69(5):840–2.
9. Jemec GB, Kollerup G, Jensen LB, Mogensen S. Nail abnormalities in nondermatologic patients: prevalence and possible role as diagnostic aids. J Am Acad Dermatol. 1995;32(6):977–81.
10. Lee JI, Lee YB, Oh ST, Park HJ, Cho BK. A clinical study of 35 cases of pincer nails. Ann Dermatol. 2011;23(4):417–23.
11. Sano H, Shionoya K, Ogawa R. Finger nail configuration is influenced by mechanical forces on finger pads. J Dermatol. 2013;40(12):1056–7.
12. Sano H, Shionoya K, Ogawa R. Foot loading is different in people with and without pincer nails: a case control study. J Foot Ankle Res. 2015;8:43.
13. Kasuya A, Tokura Y. Preservative and surgical interventions to treat ingrown nail and pincer nail. J Cutan Immunol Allergy. 2018;1(5):165–9.

14. Chapman RS. Letter: overcurvature of the nails--an inherited disorder. Br J Dermatol. 1973;89(3):317–8.
15. Mimouni D, Ben-Amitai D. Hereditary pincer nail. Cutis. 2002;69(1):51–3.
16. Matsumura O, Nakagishi Y. Pincer nails upon convalescence from Kawasaki disease. J Pediatr. 2022;246:279.
17. Vanderhooft SL, Vanderhooft JE. Pincer nail deformity after Kawasaki's disease. J Am Acad Dermatol. 1999;41(2 Pt 2):341–2.
18. Fujita Y, Fujita T. Pincer nail deformity in a patient with amyotrophic lateral sclerosis. Neurol Int. 2014;6(4):5716.
19. Majeski C, Ritchie B, Giuffre M, Lauzon G. Pincer nail deformity associated with systemic lupus erythematosus. J Cutan Med Surg. 2005;9(1):2–5.
20. Bostanci S, Ekmekci P, Akyol A, Peksari Y, Gurgey E. Pincer nail deformity: inherited and caused by a beta-blocker. Int J Dermatol. 2004;43(4):316–8.
21. Greiner D, Schofer H, Milbradt R. Reversible transverse overcurvature of the nails (pincer nails) after treatment with a beta-blocker. J Am Acad Dermatol. 1998;39(3):486–7.
22. Clark EG, Burns KD. Pincer nails following arteriovenous fistula creation. Kidney Int. 2015;88(4):918.
23. Singal A, Arora R. Nail as a window of systemic diseases. Indian Dermatol Online J. 2015;6(2):67–74.
24. Lee DK, Chang MJ, Desai AD, Lipner SR. Clinical and dermoscopic findings of benign longitudinal melanonychia due to melanocytic activation differ by skin type and predict likelihood of nail matrix biopsy. J Am Acad Dermatol. 2022;87(4):792–9.
25. Gupta MK, Lipner SR. Transillumination for improved diagnosis of digital myxoid cysts. Cutis. 2020;105(2):82.
26. Schneiderman PI, Grossman ME. The clinician's guide to dermatologic differential diagnosis. Cham: Springer; 2022. https://doi.org/10.1007/978-3-030-63527-5.
27. Huang C, Zhao Y, Guo W, Yu M, Li R, Zhu Z. An L-shaped flap for the correction of pincer nail deformity: a case report. Australas J Dermatol. 2020;61:253–6. https://doi.org/10.1111/ajd.13275.

Onychauxis

36

Eden Axler and Shari R. Lipner

36.1 Description of Disease

Onychauxis, localized hypertrophy of the nail plate, is characterized by thickened, hyperkeratotic, and discolored nails, often accompanied by subungual hyperkeratosis and loss of translucency [1]. Onychauxis is often caused by traumatic onychodystrophy, involving chronic nail malformations resulting from repetitive external injuries [2]. Clinically, onychauxis presents similarly to onychomycosis, leading to frequent misdiagnosis and inappropriate treatment with antifungal therapy [2]. Common complications of onychauxis include distal onycholysis, increased susceptibility to onychomycosis, and pain due to constant pressure on surrounding tissues [3].

36.2 Epidemiology

36.2.1 Age

Onychauxis is more prevalent in the geriatric population as it is associated with the natural aging process [1]. Conditions that are more prevalent in older adults, such as arteriosclerosis, can contribute to the development of onychauxis even in the absence of obvious vascular compromise, leading to slower nail growth and greater susceptibility to lower extremity trauma [1]. Additionally, histological changes in the nail plate, such as the presence of increased "pertinax bodies," which represent remnants of keratinocyte nuclei, are more pronounced in older individuals and contribute to nail plate hardening [1]. These alterations can lead to thicker and harder toenails, often accompanied by calluses and corns in the toenail region.

S. R. Lipner, *Atlas of Nail Disorders Across All Skin Colors*,
https://doi.org/10.1007/978-3-031-74272-9_36

36.3 Risk Factors

36.3.1 Trauma

Trauma, particularly from ill-fitting footwear, can lead to the development of onychauxis. Increased toenail trauma may also be due to structural abnormalities, including hallux valgus, hammer and mallet toes, Morton's toe, adductovarus fifth toe, hallux extensus, hallux limitus/rigidus, digiti flexi, foot-to-shoe incompatibility, hallux rigidus, hallux valgus, and overlapping and underlapping toes [1, 4]. Continuous pressure and friction on the nails, especially from shoes that do not fit properly, can cause onycholysis and trigger the formation of hyperkeratotic tissue in the periungual folds or lateral nail grooves [5]. In a prospective study by Pinheiro et al. [3] including 82 cases of onychodystrophy, 47.6% had a history of nail injury, and 91.5% had a podiatric deformity (any of hallux valgus/erectus; hammer or mallet toes) [3].

36.3.2 Neurologic Factors

Nerve-related conditions can contribute to the development of onychauxis. Complex regional pain syndrome, peripheral neuropathy, hemiplegia, and dysfunction of the median nerve can influence the onset of onychauxis [4]. Therefore, there may be an interplay of immobilization, unequal mechanical forces, and neural factors in the pathogenesis of onychauxis [4].

36.4 Clinical Features

Onychauxis is characterized by hyperkeratotic and discolored nails. The affected nails often exhibit a thickened appearance, accompanied by a loss of translucency of the nail plate. Additionally, subungual hyperkeratosis is a common finding in individuals with onychauxis [1].

36.4.1 Dermoscopic Features

Dermoscopy can aid in the diagnosis of onychauxis. In the prospective study by Pinheiro et al. [3] including 82 cases of onychodystrophy, dermoscopic findings of total hazy homogeneous background (20%) and partial hazy homogeneous background (11.5%) were associated with increased odds of onychauxis by approximately 15- and 14-fold, respectively. Regular macular or onycholysis pattern (12%) and distal fine line pattern (7.8%) were also features associated with traumatic onychodystrophy ($P < 0.001$) [3].

36.5 Clinical Features in Skin of Color

In individuals with darker skin tones, longitudinal melanonychia often accompanies other characteristic nail findings.

36.6 Requirements for Diagnosis

Onychauxis diagnosis is made clinically. Historical assessment includes inquiring about history of trauma to the nails, footwear, occupational risk factors, or pertinent medical conditions, including hemiplegia or neurologic conditions. Physical examination includes inspecting the foot for structural abnormalities including overlapping toes, Morton's toe, and hallux varus. Infectious or inflammatory causes, including onychomycosis and psoriasis, can be excluded using a nail plate clipping with histopathological examination.

36.7 Cases

Figures 36.1, 36.2, 36.3, 36.4, 36.5, and 36.6 demonstrate the presentation of Onychauxis in a clinical setting.

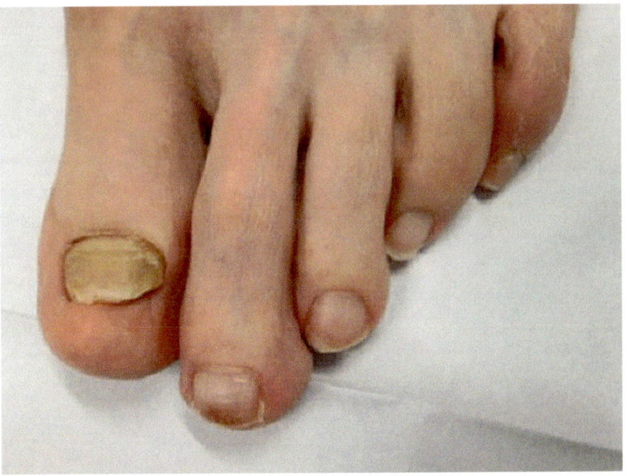

Fig. 36.1 60-Year-old male, Fitzpatrick type II, onychauxis, with xanthonychia and nail plate thickening of the left great toenail. Clipping with histopathology and PAS staining was negative for fungal elements. Morton's toe deformity is also present

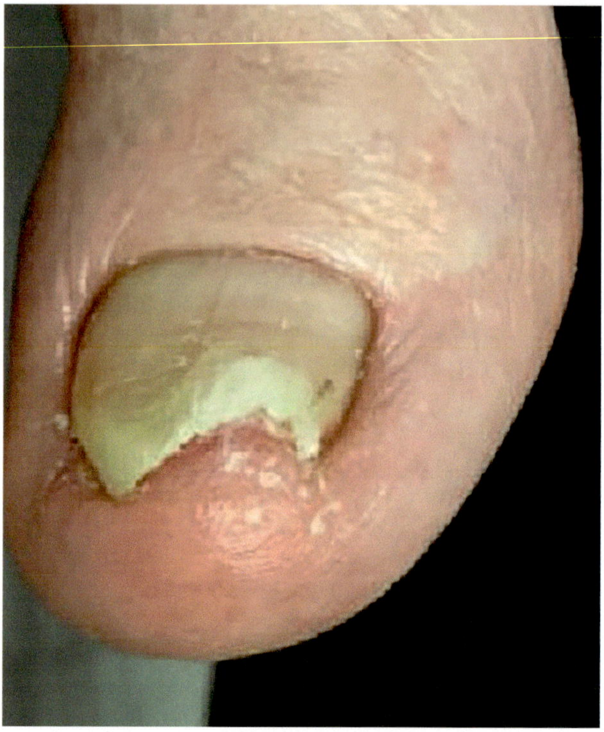

Fig. 36.2 79-Year-old female, Fitzpatrick type II, onychauxis, with thickening and increased transverse curvature of the right great toenail

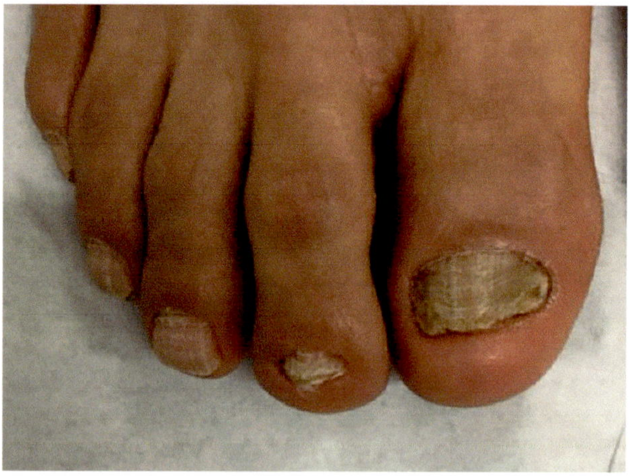

Fig. 36.3 78-Year-old male, Fitzpatrick type III, onychauxis, with xanthonychia and loss of transparency of the right great toenail. A clipping with histopathology and PAS staining was negative for fungal elements

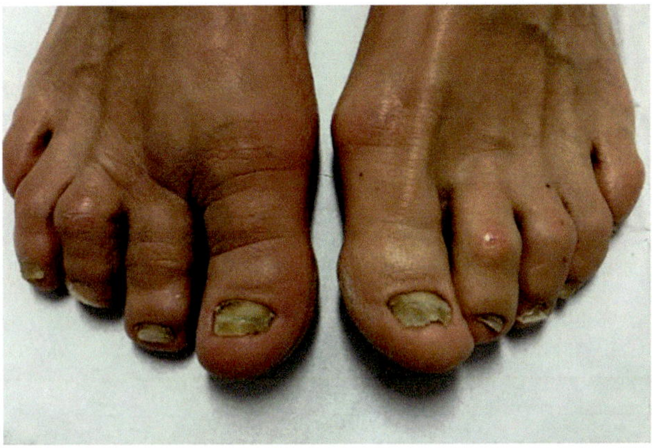

Fig. 36.4 75-Year-old female, Fitzpatrick type III, onychauxis, with hyperkeratosis and xanthonychia of all ten toenails. A clipping with histopathology and PAS staining was negative for fungal elements

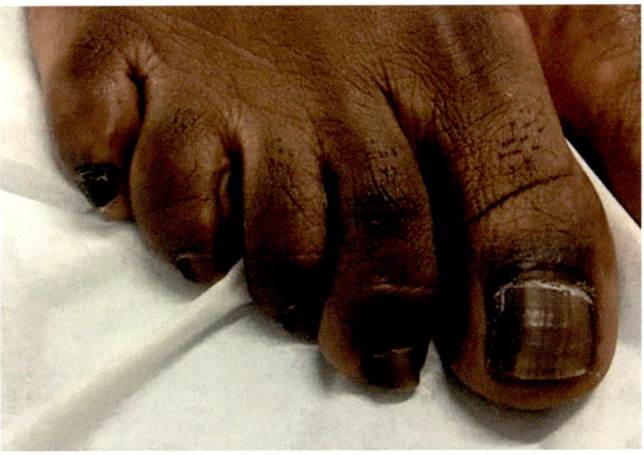

Fig. 36.5 67-Year-old female, Fitzpatrick type VI, onychauxis, with thickening and longitudinal melanonychia of the right toenails. Morton's toe and hammer toe deformity are present

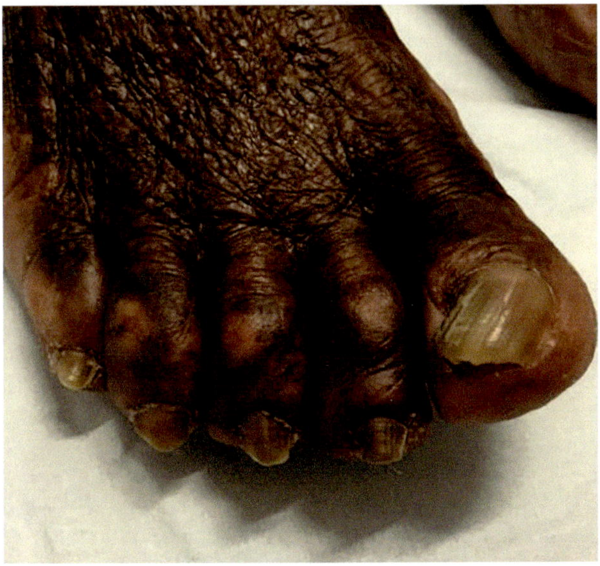

Fig. 36.6 101-Year-old female, Fitzpatrick type VI, onychauxis, with thickening and loss of transparency of the right toenails. There is additionally onychogryphosis of the right great toenail, hallux valgus deformity, and hammer toes. A clipping with histopathology and PAS staining was negative for hyphae

References

1. Cohen PR, Scher RK. Geriatric nail disorders: diagnosis and treatment. J Am Acad Dermatol. 1992;26(4):521–31. https://doi.org/10.1016/0190-9622(92)70075-q.
2. Ho D, Mamalis A, Jagdeo J. Successful treatment of traumatic onychodystrophy and associated pterygium unguis with fractionated carbon dioxide laser: case report and review of the literature. J Drugs Dermatol. 2016;15(11):1461–4.
3. Ramos Pinheiro R, Dias Domingues T, Sousa V, Galhardas C, Apetato M, Lencastre A. A comparative study of onychomycosis and traumatic toenail onychodystrophy dermoscopic patterns. J Eur Acad Dermatol Venereol. 2019;33(4):786–92. https://doi.org/10.1111/jdv.15358.
4. Rana J, Vlahovic TC. Nails as dynamic, not static, entities-rethinking the approach to nail disorders. JAMA Dermatol. 2024;160(6):595–6. https://doi.org/10.1001/jamadermatol.2024.0400.
5. Baran R. The nail in the elderly. Clin Dermatol. 2011;29(1):54–60. https://doi.org/10.1016/j.clindermatol.2010.07.008.

Part VIII

Benign Melanonychia

Subungual Hematoma

37

Eden Axler and Shari R. Lipner

37.1 Description of Disease

Subungual hematoma refers to the accumulation of blood under the nail plate due to acute or chronic trauma to a fingernail or toenail. The injury results in the rupture of blood vessels in the nail bed, leading to the accumulation of blood between the nail bed and the nail plate [1]. Patients may experience pain or pressure in the affected area. Subungual hematomas grow out with nail plate growth (toenails 12–18 months, fingernails 6–9 months).

37.2 Epidemiology

Subungual hematoma may occur in any individual who experiences direct trauma to a nail. In a prospective study by Metin et al. [2]. including 47 subungual hematoma cases, mean age was 45 years (age range: 9–67), and 72.5% were men. The most common location was the big toenail [2]. Overall, 64% of patients reported a history of trauma [2].

37.2.1 Patients with Fractures

Subungual hematoma may coincide with distal phalanx fractures, nail avulsion, or fingertip avulsions. In a prospective study including 47 patients presenting to the emergency room with a subungual hematoma, 44% of those with a hematoma involving more than 50% of the nail plate surface area also had a concurrent fracture, necessitating repair of the nail bed in all cases [3].

S. R. Lipner, *Atlas of Nail Disorders Across All Skin Colors*,
https://doi.org/10.1007/978-3-031-74272-9_37

37.2.2 Children

Children are susceptible to nail unit injuries due to their typically high activity levels. Fingernail injuries contribute to over two-thirds of pediatric hand injuries, often resulting from crushing incidents involving doors or windows (77%). Additionally, fractures of the distal phalanx occur in over half of the cases, with the middle finger most frequently affected [4]. In a retrospective study including 457 children aged 0–18 who sustained nail bed injuries, 62.6% were male. Door crush injuries accounted for the highest proportion (59.5%) of overall causes. These injuries predominantly occurred at home (46.4%), followed by the playground (28.4%), public areas (17.5%), and school (7.7%) [5].

37.2.3 Military Personnel

Injuries to the fingers and nails significantly affect military personnel. During 2014, there were 68,553 ambulatory visits related to hand injuries in nondeployed soldiers alone. On average, approximately 13.7 non-combat-related hand injuries occurred per month, making up 4.4% of total emergency department visits. Most cases resulted from finger trauma due to vehicle doors, hatches, or direct contact with weapons [6].

37.3 Risk Factors

While no studies have specifically identified risk factors for subungual hematoma, factors that may increase the likelihood of experiencing trauma to a digit include substantial physical activity (occupational or recreational), poorly fitted footwear, structural foot abnormalities, and peripheral neuropathy. Athletes, especially those participating in contact sports such as soccer, basketball, and football may have risk due to repetitive trauma to the toes. Additionally, subungual hematomas are more prevalent in warmer climates, where individuals tend to go barefoot or wear open-toed shoes more frequently [7]. Coagulation disorders, anticoagulant medication usage, blood thinners, and other conditions that prevent blood clotting, may also increase likelihood of subungual hematoma development [7].

37.4 Clinical Features

Subungual hematoma typically presents as a distinct color change or irregular patch beneath the nail plate, ranging from red to black depending on the age of the injury [2, 8]. In a prospective study including 90 subungual hematomas by Mun et al. [9], color varied based on duration of disease: pink (1.1 weeks), purple (4.4 weeks), pink–purple (3.0 weeks), red–purple (5.0 weeks), red–brown (6.7 weeks), purple–brown (3.2 weeks), red–black (8.9 weeks), purple–black (9.0 weeks), brown–black (17.6 weeks), and black (16.0 weeks) [9]. In a prospective study including 59 cases of subungual hematoma, 73% exhibited an area of clear proximal plate, with no patients displaying a longitudinal pigmented band extending from the cuticle to the distal nail plate as seen in longitudinal melanonychia [10]. Subungual hematoma was accompanied by nail dystrophy, including loss of nail translucency, discoloration, or deformity (thickened or cracked nail), in 54% of cases [10]. In the study by Mun et al. [9] including 90 cases of subungual hemorrhage, nail plate destruction or dystrophy was noted in 16% of cases [9]. Overall, 39% of cases localized to the great toenail, with one digit involved in 41 patients and multiple digits in 23 patients. Nail involvement was distributed across the proximal third, distal two-thirds, or entire nail in varying proportions depending on the extent of injury. Pain or tenderness was present in 22% of cases, with only 21% recalling overt trauma at the site of hemorrhage [9].

37.4.1 Dermoscopic Features

Onychoscopy is a useful tool for the diagnosis of subungual hematoma. On dermoscopy, subungual hematoma typically presents as a red–purple–brown patch with a homogeneous color, with globules at the proximal edge and a linear distribution at the distal edge, along with peripheral fading [11]. In Mun et al.'s study including 90 subungual hematoma cases, dermoscopy showed a homogeneous pattern in 92% of cases, followed by a globular pattern (42%) and streaks (39%) [9]. Peripheral fading and periungual hemorrhage were observed in 54% and 22% of cases, respectively [9]. Similarly, in a prospective study by Metin et al. [2] analyzing dermoscopic features of 47 subungual hematoma cases, the most frequently observed color was purple–black (53%), followed by blue–white (26%) and granular leukonychia (19%) [2]. All hematomas exhibited homogeneous patterns, with globular pattern in 53% and streaks in 30%. A majority of nails (89%) exhibited multiple colors, including purple–black (53%), red–black (32%), brown (28%), black (28%), blue–white (26%), red (21.2%), gray-black (17%), and purple (6%) [2]. Acute hematomas can be differentiated from chronic traumatic hematomas by the presence of well-circumscribed reddish dots, globules, or streaks at the distal edge, along with a red–purple to black coloration, while chronic hematomas may display red–brown coloration with linear patterns and splinter hemorrhages [11]. In a prospective study comparing 71 cases of subungual hematomas with 11 cases of subungual melanocytic lesions using optical coherence tomography (OCT), subungual hematomas exhibited sharply defined black sickle-shaped areas ($P < 0.001$) or globular regions with a hyperreflective margin ($P = 0.002$), along with a gray center ($P = 0.013$), hyperreflective lines in the periphery ($P = 0.031$), peripheral fading ($P = 0.029$), and red dots within the area ($P = 0.001$) [12]. However, use of OCT to differentiate between subungual hematomas and melanomas requires further study.

37.5 Clinical Features in Skin of Color

In individuals with darker skin tones, the color of the hematoma may not be as apparent initially due to the melanin present in the skin. Instead of the typical dark red or purple appearance seen in lighter skin, it might appear more brown or black.

37.6 Requirements for Diagnosis

Diagnosis of subungual hematoma relies on thorough clinical evaluation, including a detailed history to identify recent acute or chronic, trauma, vigorous physical activity, or medications that increase bleeding risk. As 50% of nail bed injuries may be associated with an accompanying fracture, in cases of severe injury (>50% of nail bed affected), radiographs are necessary to evaluate the injured digit for potential fractures or dislocations [13]. Dermoscopy serves as a valuable tool for confirming the diagnosis, while nail matrix biopsy is generally unnecessary. In some cases, it may be difficult to differentiate subungual hematoma from subungual melanoma. Most cases of subungual hematoma exhibit a clear proximal area of nail plate and grow out with nail plate growth, distinguishing it from melanonychia due to melanin [10]. Serial photography can be used to monitor the resolution of the hematoma [14]. However, approximately 15% of cases of subungual hematoma do not migrate with nail growth, and nail malignancies may also bleed. Therefore, nail unit biopsy may be necessary to rule out malignancy in equivocal cases [9, 15]. If the nail plate detaches, patients can be reassured that a new one will typically grow back normally. If more than 25–50% of the nail bed is affected by the hematoma, trephination, or creation of a small hole in the nail plate, may be required to relieve pressure and drain fluid from beneath the nail [13]. Trephination using electrocautery or nail boring can safely be employed if the hematoma is <24 h old and covers <25–50% of the nail plate's surface [16]. A sterile disposable curette (2 or 3 mm) or a sterile disposable biopsy punch (1.5–3 mm) can be applied tangentially to puncture the nail without the need for squeezing to minimize pain [17].

37.7 Cases

Figures 37.1, 37.2, 37.3, 37.4, 37.5, and 37.6 depict the clinical presentation of subungual hematoma.

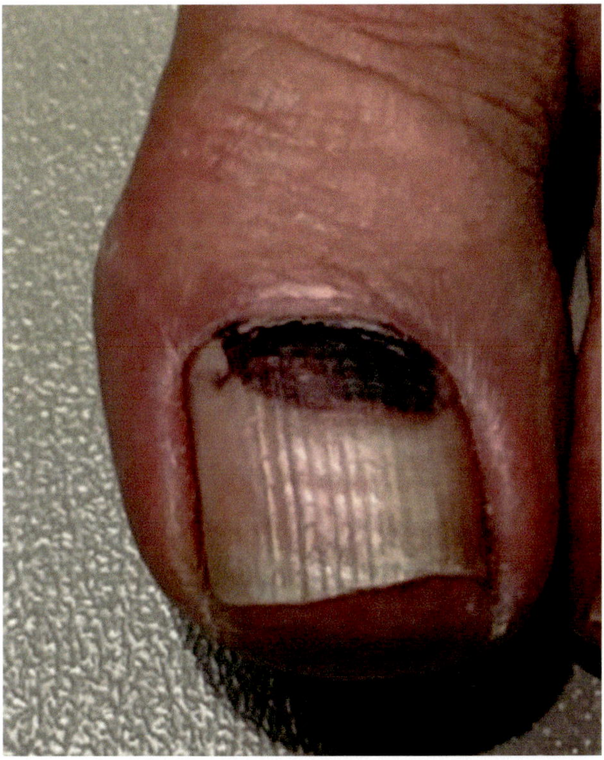

Fig. 37.1 68-Year-old male, Fitzpatrick type II, subungual hematoma, with black-purple discoloration of the right great toenail

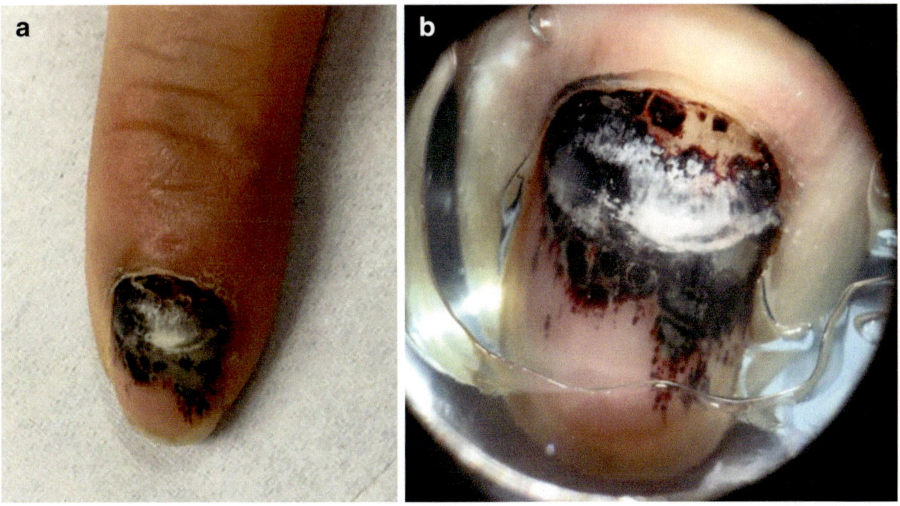

Fig. 37.2 (**a** and **b**) 59-Year-old female, Fitzpatrick type II, subungual hematoma, with black/violaceous discoloration of the nail plate, proximal onycholysis, and transverse leukonychia. On dermoscopy, transverse leukonychia, homogenous areas, globules, and streaks are appreciated

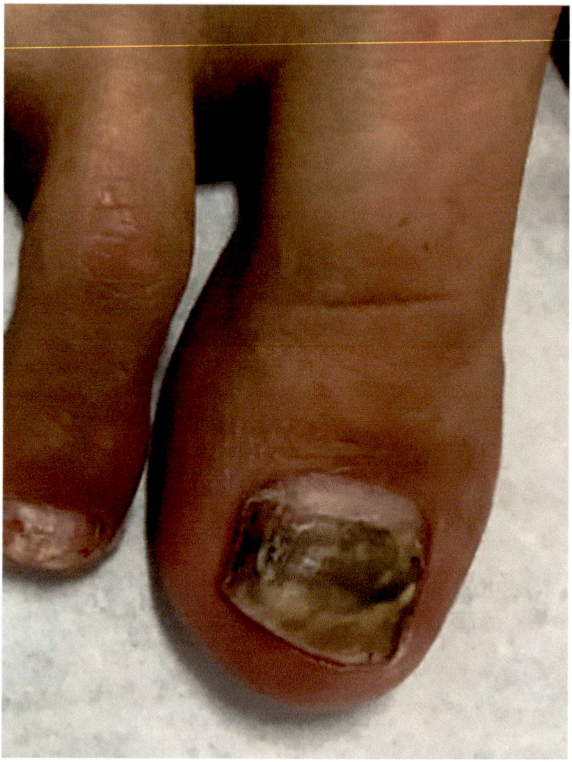

Fig. 37.3 33-Year-old female, Fitzpatrick type III, subungual hematoma, right great toenail with onycholysis and brown-yellow discoloration of the distal nail plate

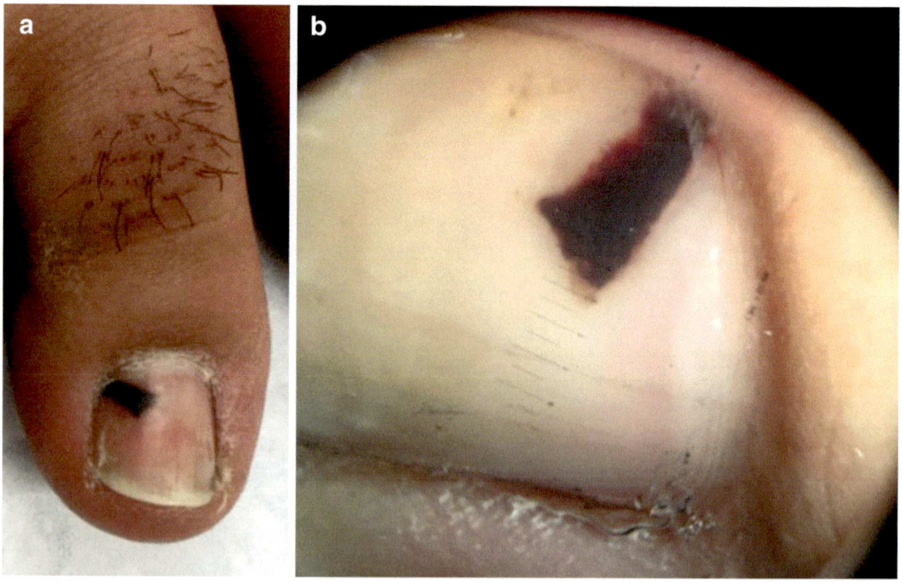

Fig. 37.4 (**a** and **b**) 25-Year-old female, Fitzpatrick type IV, subungual hematoma, with black-violaceous pigment seen through nail plate. On dermoscopy, purple-red color, homogenous areas, and peripheral fading are appreciated

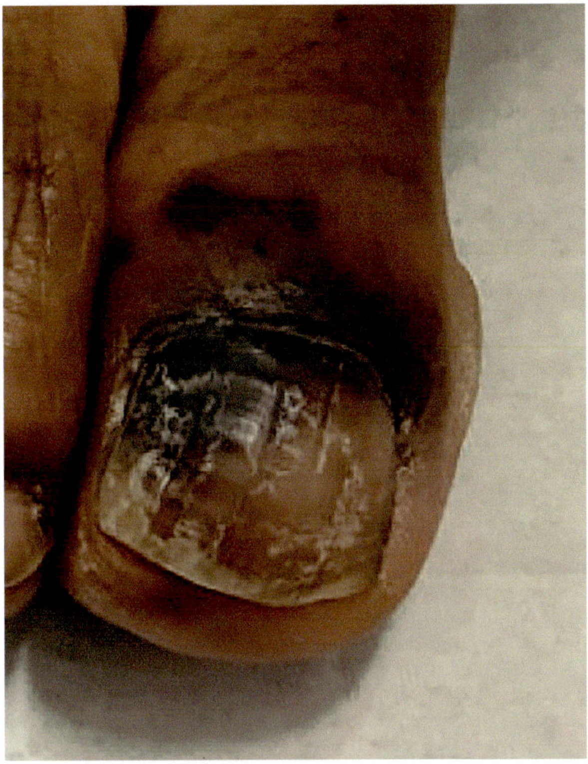

Fig. 37.5 61-Year-old female, Fitzpatrick type V, subungual hematoma, with brown-black discoloration of the left great toenail

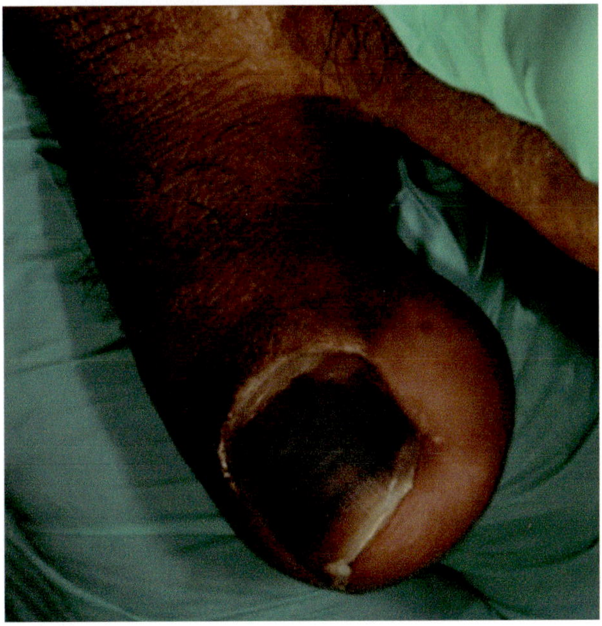

Fig. 37.6 64-Year-old male, Fitzpatrick type VI, subungual hematoma, with purple-black discoloration of the left great toenail (*from* Akella et al. [7]; CC-BY 4.0, https://creativecommons.org/licenses/by/4.0)

References

1. Pingel C, McDowell C. Subungual hematoma drainage. In: StatPearls. StatPearls Publishing LLC; 2023.
2. Metin MS, Elmas ÖF. Dermoscopic diagnosis of subungual hematoma: new observations. Postepy Dermatol Alergol. 2020;37(4):490–4. https://doi.org/10.5114/ada.2020.98235.
3. Simon RR, Wolgin M. Subungual hematoma: association with occult laceration requiring repair. Am J Emerg Med. 1987;5(4):302–4. https://doi.org/10.1016/0735-6757(87)90356-1.
4. Braga SJ. Fingernail injury in children. Hand Surg Rehabil. 2024;43S:101512. https://doi.org/10.1016/j.hansur.2023.01.001.
5. James V, Heng TYJ, Yap QV, Ganapathy S. Epidemiology and outcome of nailbed injuries managed in children's emergency department: a 10-year single-center experience. Pediatr Emerg Care. 2022;38(2):e776–83. https://doi.org/10.1097/pec.0000000000002400.
6. Wells ME, Scanaliato JP, Kusnezov NA, Nesti LJ, Dunn JC. The burden of fingertip trauma on the US military. Hand Clin. 2021;37(1):155–65. https://doi.org/10.1016/j.hcl.2020.09.010.
7. Akella A, Daniel AR, Gould MB, Mangal R, Ganti L. Subungual Hematoma. Cureus. 2023;15(11):e48952. https://doi.org/10.7759/cureus.48952.
8. Braun RP, Baran R, Le Gal FA, et al. Diagnosis and management of nail pigmentations. J Am Acad Dermatol. 2007;56(5):835–47. https://doi.org/10.1016/j.jaad.2006.12.021.
9. Mun JH, Kim GW, Jwa SW, et al. Dermoscopy of subungual haemorrhage: its usefulness in differential diagnosis from nail-unit melanoma. Br J Dermatol. 2013;168(6):1224–9. https://doi.org/10.1111/bjd.12209.
10. Phillips M, Oakley A. Macroscopic and dermoscopic evaluation used to differentiate subungual haemorrhage from melanocytic lesions. J Prim Health Care. 2020;12(4):368–72. https://doi.org/10.1071/hc20092.
11. Piraccini BM, Alessandrini A, Starace M. Onychoscopy: dermoscopy of the nails. Dermatol Clin. 2018;36(4):431–8. https://doi.org/10.1016/j.det.2018.05.010.
12. Hobelsberger S, Laske J, Aschoff R, Beissert S. Examination of subungual hematomas and subungual melanocytic lesions by using optical coherence tomography and dermoscopy. Dermatology. 2022;238(6):1130–8. https://doi.org/10.1159/000524347.
13. Hawken JB, Giladi AM. Primary management of nail bed and fingertip injuries in the emergency department. Hand Clin. 2021;37(1):1–10. https://doi.org/10.1016/j.hcl.2020.09.001.
14. Chelidze K, Ko D, Lipner SR. The nail hematoma selfie. J Am Acad Dermatol. 2018;78(6):e137–8. https://doi.org/10.1016/j.jaad.2017.12.047.
15. Mannava KA, Mannava S, Koman LA, Robinson-Bostom L, Jellinek N. Longitudinal melanonychia: detection and management of nail melanoma. Hand Surg. 2013;18(1):133–9. https://doi.org/10.1142/s0218810413300015.
16. Perper M, Tosti A. Chapter 6. Nail diseases in the elderly. In: Tosti A, editor. Nail disorders. Elsevier; 2019. p. 49–54.
17. De Villeneuve Bargemon JB, Niddam S, Morand A, Mattei JC, Jaloux C. A simple painless technique to drain subungual hematoma. J Am Acad Dermatol. 2021;85(5):e283–5. https://doi.org/10.1016/j.jaad.2020.03.062.

Benign Melanocytic Activation 38

Eden Axler and Shari R. Lipner

38.1 Description of Disease

Melanocytic activation is a type of longitudinal melanonychia (LM) that results from increased pigmentation in the nail matrix epithelium and nail plate without a corresponding increase in melanocyte count [1, 2]. Melanocytic activation typically presents as a gray longitudinal band, involving a single nail or multiple nails. In adults, melanocytic activation is by far the most common cause of melanonychia [2]. Physiologically, trauma, infection, or inflammation can activate nail matrix melanocytes, leading to increased pigment production [3, 4]. Melanocyte activation initiates melanin synthesis, and melanin-rich melanosomes are then transferred to differentiating matrix cells via dendrites. These cells migrate distally and eventually transform into nail plate onychocytes, resulting in visible pigmentation within the nail plate [4].

38.2 Epidemiology

In a prospective study of 100 patients with LM who underwent nail matrix biopsy, 49% of patients were diagnosed with melanocytic activation [5]. In a retrospective study of 248 cases of clinically diagnosed LM due to melanocytic activation by Lee et al., 76% were female with a mean age of 49.81 years (range: 18–86 years) [6].

38.2.1 Fitzpatrick Skin Type

Melanocytic activation is more prevalent in individuals with skin of color, particularly among darker-pigmented ethnicities such as Blacks, Asians, Middle Easterners, and Hispanics. Prevalence rates vary across different racial groups, with 1% of Caucasians affected, 10%–20% of Japanese and Asians affected, and up to

S. R. Lipner, *Atlas of Nail Disorders Across All Skin Colors*,
https://doi.org/10.1007/978-3-031-74272-9_38

77%–100% among African Americans affected [4, 7]. In the retrospective study by Lee et al. [6], 65% of individuals were identified as Fitzpatrick skin type III–IV [6]. Individuals with lighter skin types (Fitzpatrick I–II) had a higher likelihood of a family history of melanoma compared to those with darker skin types [6].

38.2.2 Children

Melanocytic activation is also reported in children, but less commonly than in adults. In a retrospective analysis of 40 pediatric patients ages 16 and younger with LM who underwent nail biopsy, 23% of cases were due to melanocytic activation [8].

38.3 Risk Factors

38.3.1 Systemic Risk Factors

Melanocytic activation may occur due to hormonal changes during pregnancy or due to Laugier–Hunziker–Baran syndrome, Nelson syndrome, human immunodeficiency virus (HIV), or graft versus host disease (GVHD). Systemic conditions, including systemic lupus erythematosus, Addison's disease, Cushing's disease, hyperthyroidism, acromegaly, alkaptonuria, hemosiderosis, hyperbilirubinemia, or porphyria may also induce melanocyte activation [3, 4, 9, 10].

38.3.2 Neoplasms

Melanocytic activation can be triggered by non-melanocytic neoplasms, including squamous cell carcinoma, onychomatricoma, onycholemmal cyst, basal cell carcinoma, subungual fibrous histiocytoma, verruca vulgaris, and subungual keratosis [4].

38.3.3 Inflammatory Disorders

Inflammatory skin conditions, including nail psoriasis, nail lichen planus, amyloidosis, and chronic paronychia, can induce melanocytic activation [4].

38.3.4 Local and Regional Risk Factors

Melanocytic activation can be triggered by trauma to the nail, including nail picking, nail biting, or carpal tunnel syndrome [11]. A case series documented six patients with history of onychotillomania who presented with LM due to melanocytic activation [12]. Additionally, friction from shoes can lead to melanocytic activation, typically in the lateral fourth and fifth toenails [4, 11].

38.3.5 Iatrogenic Risk Factors

Phototherapy, electron beam therapy, X-rays, and radiodermatitis are potential causes of melanocytic activation. The melanonychia pattern may be diffuse, transverse, or longitudinal [4].

38.4 Clinical Features

Clinically, LM due to melanocytic activation presents as a longitudinal gray or brown band extending the length of the nail plate and typically affects multiple nails [4]. The first three digits, particularly of the dominant hand, are most frequently involved, likely because they are most often used during daily activities. Frictional melanonychia typically localizes to the lateral sides of the fourth and/or fifth toenails. LM due to melanocytic activation may be a consequence of onychotillomania, which also presents with concurrent transverse grooves, generalized or patchy rough areas, macrolunula, washboard nails, or pterygium. When due to onychophagia, LM will present with shortened nails with ragged distal borders [13, 14].

38.4.1 Clinical Features of Dermoscopy

On dermoscopy, melanocytic activation presents as a gray background with regular gray lines in terms of color, thickness, and spacing [13].

38.5 Clinical Features in Skin of Color

In the retrospective analysis by Lee et al. [6], patients with Fitzpatrick skin types III/VI had lower band brightness ($P < 0.0001$) and wider bands ($P = 0.0125$) compared to those with skin types I/II [6]. On dermoscopic examination, individuals with Fitzpatrick skin types III/VI vs. skin types I/II ($P = 0.0232$) were more likely to have brown lines and a brown background rather than gray lines on a gray backdrop [6].

38.6 Requirements for Diagnosis

Melanocytic activation may be hard to differentiate from nail unit melanoma [6]. If the LM appears narrow, with regular lines under dermoscopy, and remains stable over time, patients can be reassured, and the LM monitored. Presence of bands on multiple nails is reassuring of a benign etiology. If the band is evolving or symptomatic, a nail unit biopsy is necessary [2]. In the retrospective study of LM by Lee et al. [6], biopsied vs. non-biopsied patients less often had involvement of multiple digits ($P = 0.0008$), a higher mean bandwidth percentage ($P = 0.0213$), reduced band brightness ($P = 0.0003$), and more often exhibited evolution of nail changes, such as darkening and widening of bands ($P < 0.0001$) [6]. On histopathology, melanocytes appear normal. The presence of dendritic extensions of melanocytes may be visible alongside dermal melanophages [3]. Fontana staining may be required to confirm the presence of melanin [2].

38.7 Cases

Figures 38.1, 38.2, 38.3, 38.4, 38.5, 38.6, and 38.7 demonstrate the presentation of benign melanocytic activation in clinical practice.

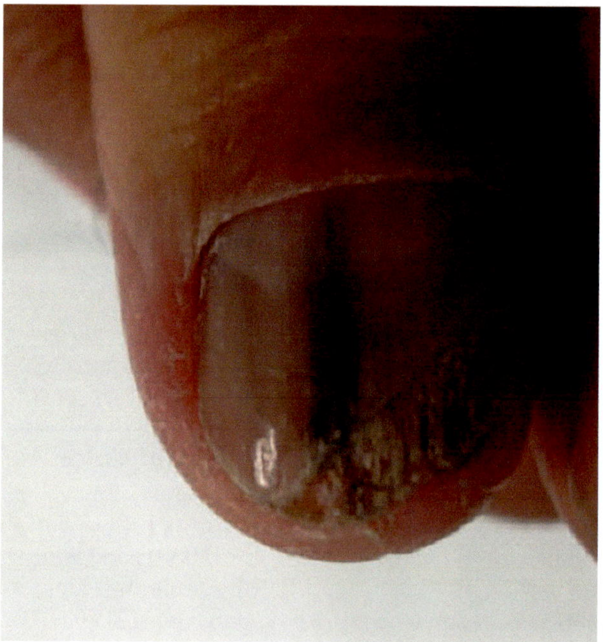

Fig. 38.1 88-Year-old male, Fitzpatrick type II, melanocytic activation, with 2 mm dark brown band involving the right thumbnail. There are also ridges on the distal part of the nail plate

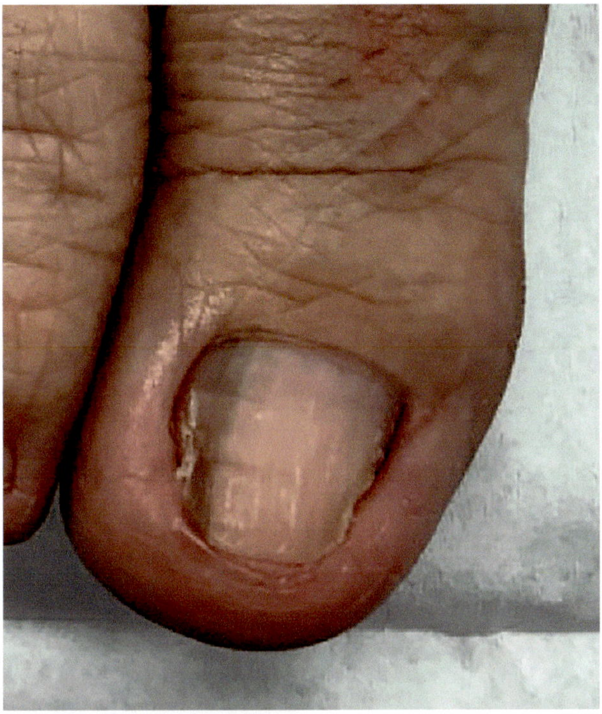

Fig. 38.2 68-Year-old female, Fitzpatrick type II, melanocytic activation, with 2 mm gray/brown longitudinal band involving the right great toenail

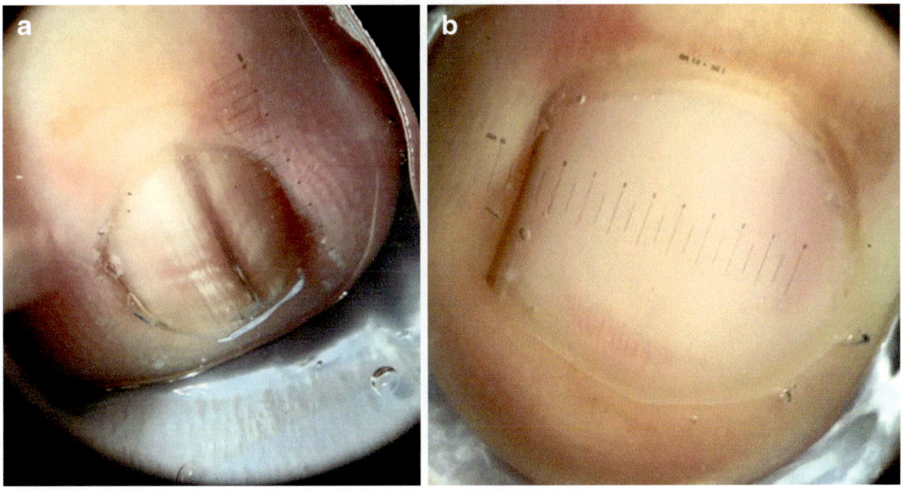

Fig. 38.3 (**a** and **b**) Dermoscopy of a 58-year-old female, Fitzpatrick type II, melanocytic activation. A brown background with regular brown bands is appreciated

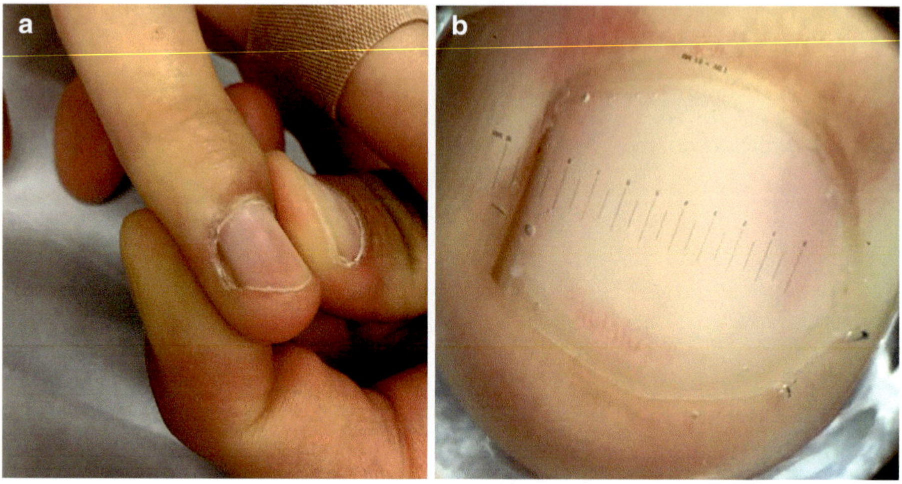

Fig. 38.4 (**a**) 36-Year-old female, Fitzpatrick type III, melanocytic activation, with 1 mm brown band involving the right fourth fingernail. (**b**) On dermoscopy, parallel brown lines on a light brown background are appreciated

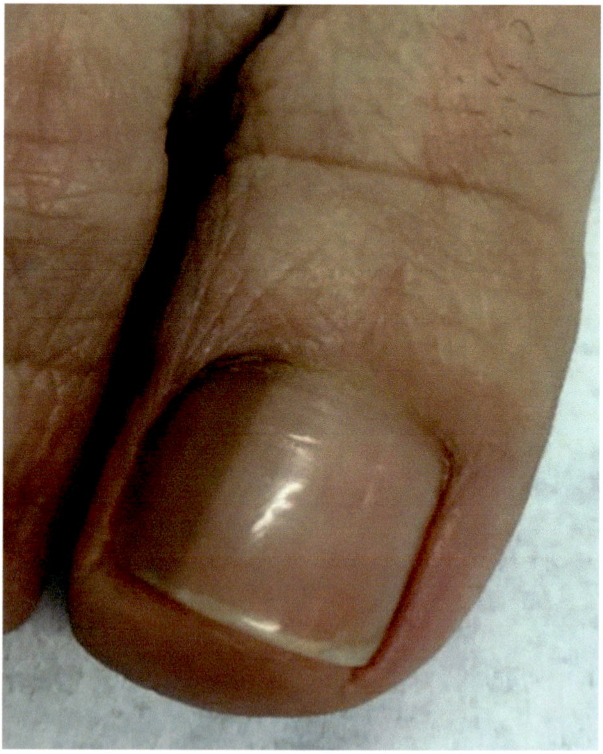

Fig. 38.5 63-Year-old female, Fitzpatrick type III, melanocytic activation, with 5 mm longitudinal light brown band involving the right great toenail

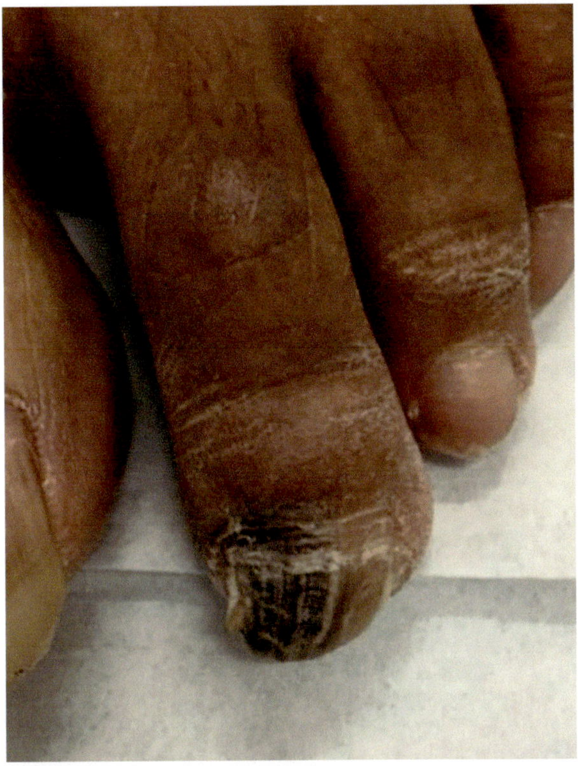

Fig. 38.6 77-Year-old female, Fitzpatrick type V, melanocytic activation, with brown longitudinal band and nail plate thickening involving the left second toenail

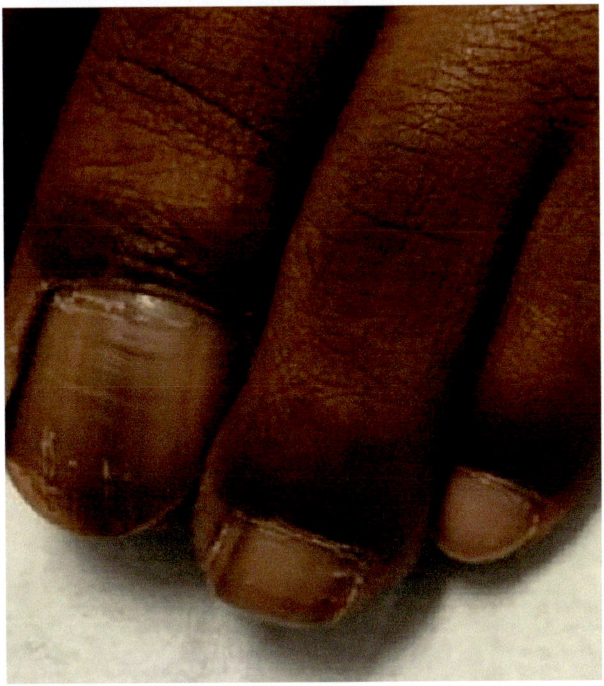

Fig. 38.7 60-Year-old female, Fitzpatrick type V, melanocytic activation, with homogenous gray to brown bands involving the left first and second toenails

References

1. Jefferson J, Rich P. Melanonychia. Dermatol Res Pract. 2012;2012:952186. https://doi.org/10.1155/2012/952186.
2. Di Chiacchio N, Ruben BS, Loureiro WR. Longitudinal melanonychias. Clin Dermatol. 2013;31(5):594–601. https://doi.org/10.1016/j.clindermatol.2013.06.007.
3. Güneş P, Göktay F. Melanocytic lesions of the nail unit. Dermatopathology (Basel). 2018;5(3):98–107. https://doi.org/10.1159/000490557.
4. Singal A, Bisherwal K. Melanonychia: etiology, diagnosis, and treatment. Indian Dermatol Online J. 2020;11(1):1–11. https://doi.org/10.4103/idoj.IDOJ_167_19.
5. Hirata SH, Yamada S, Enokihara MY, et al. Patterns of nail matrix and bed of longitudinal melanonychia by intraoperative dermatoscopy. J Am Acad Dermatol. 2011;65(2):297–303. https://doi.org/10.1016/j.jaad.2010.06.009.
6. Lee DK, Chang MJ, Desai AD, Lipner SR. Clinical and dermoscopic findings of benign longitudinal melanonychia due to melanocytic activation differ by skin type and predict likelihood of nail matrix biopsy. J Am Acad Dermatol. 2022;87(4):792–9. https://doi.org/10.1016/j.jaad.2022.06.1165.
7. André J, Lateur N. Pigmented nail disorders. Dermatol Clin. 2006;24(3):329–39. https://doi.org/10.1016/j.det.2006.03.012.
8. Goettmann-Bonvallot S, André J, Belaich S. Longitudinal melanonychia in children: a clinical and histopathologic study of 40 cases. J Am Acad Dermatol. 1999;41(1):17–22. https://doi.org/10.1016/s0190-9622(99)70399-3.
9. Gupta AK, De Doncker P, Scher RK, et al. Itraconazole for the treatment of onychomycosis. Int J Dermatol. 1998;37(4):303–8. https://doi.org/10.1046/j.1365-4362.1998.00360.x.
10. Zhang S, Liu X, Cai L, Zhang J, Zhou C. Longitudinal melanonychia and subungual hemorrhage in a patient with systemic lupus erythematosus treated with hydroxychloroquine. Lupus. 2019;28(1):129–32. https://doi.org/10.1177/0961203318812685.
11. Anolik RB, Shah K, Rubin AI. Onychophagia-induced longitudinal melanonychia. Pediatr Dermatol. 2012;29(4):488–9. https://doi.org/10.1111/j.1525-1470.2011.01496.x.
12. Baran R. Nail biting and picking as a possible cause of longitudinal melanonychia: a study of 6 cases. Dermatologica. 2009;181(2):126–8. https://doi.org/10.1159/000247900.
13. Starace M, Alessandrini A, Brandi N, Piraccini BM. Use of nail dermoscopy in the management of melanonychia: review. Dermatol Pract Concept. 2019;9(1):38–43. https://doi.org/10.5826/dpc.0901a10.
14. Shin JO, Roh D, Son JH, et al. Onychophagia: detailed clinical characteristics. Int J Dermatol. 2022;61(3):331–6. https://doi.org/10.1111/ijd.15861.

Nail Matrix Nevus

39

Eden Axler and Shari R. Lipner

39.1 Description of Disease

Nail matrix nevus is a type of benign melanocytic proliferation that presents as longitudinal melanonychia (LM) [1]. Nail matrix nevus may be congenital or acquired and is localized to a fingernail or toenail [2, 3]. Histopathologically, there is a melanocytic proliferation organized into nests. Nail matrix nevus variants include junctional, compound, or intradermal.

39.2 Epidemiology

Since nail matrix nevi are most often clinically monitored, with nail matrix biopsies only performed when there is concern for malignancy, their prevalence is unknown [3]. In a prospective study of 100 biopsy-confirmed LM cases, 21% were nail matrix nevi [4].

39.2.1 Age

Nail matrix nevi most commonly occur in children. In a meta-analysis of pediatric LM by Tsai et al. [5] including 731 LM cases, the most common diagnosis was nail matrix nevus (86.3%, $P = 0.005$) [5]. In a prospective study by Tosti et al. [3] of 100 patients with single-band LM, 22 patients had nail matrix nevi, with 50% aged 1–13 years (mean age 6.6 years) [3]. In a prospective study of 40 pediatric patients with LM who underwent nail biopsy, 19 cases were nail matrix nevi (junctional in 17 cases and compound in 2) [6]. In a retrospective study of 174 cases of biopsy-confirmed LM, 56.1% of LM in children were nail matrix nevus, vs. 34.3% in adults ($P = 0.005$) [7]. In a retrospective, single-center review of 28 Asian patients with biopsy-confirmed nail matrix nevi diagnosed 2012–2015, 71% were in children and 29% were in adults [8].

S. R. Lipner, *Atlas of Nail Disorders Across All Skin Colors*,
https://doi.org/10.1007/978-3-031-74272-9_39

39.3 Risk Factors

There are no known risk factors for development of nail matrix nevus.

39.4 Clinical Features

In children, nail matrix nevus presents clinically as LM and may exhibit signs that would be concerning for nail unit melanoma in adults, including dark brown or black color, width >3 mm, and pigment involving the nail folds. In the prospective study by Tosti et al., 17 cases were localized to the fingernails and 5 to the toenails, with 45% of cases localized to the thumbnail [3]. On clinical examination, 14 patients exhibited a dark-brown band with linear streaks of darker pigmentation, which frequently extended to the proximal nail fold and cuticle. Eight patients presented with light brown, uniform bands. Four patients showed mild nail surface irregularities, with no reported pain or sensory disturbances [3]. In a retrospective analysis of 29 biopsy-confirmed pediatric nail matrix nevus by Lee et al. [9], pigment involving the periungual skin was present in 45%, nail dystrophy was present in 41%, 48% of bands were dark brown, 7% were light brown, and 45% were black. LM of children diagnosed with nail matrix nevus were darker in color compared to LM due to functional melanonychia or lentigo ($P < 0.0001$) [9]. In a retrospective study of 28 biopsy-confirmed cases of nail matrix nevus, average bandwidth was 37.6% of the nail plate width (range 2.6–100%), nine bands were dark brown, 19 were light brown, with Hutchinson sign present in 25% [8]. In a retrospective study including 19 cases of biopsy-confirmed LM, 6 were >4 mm wide, with three cases of total melanonychia, and seven with periungual pigmentation [6].

Dermoscopy plays an important role in diagnosing nail matrix nevus. A distinctive dermoscopic feature observed in nail matrix nevus is longitudinal brush pigmentation (LBP), characterized by linear and parallel pigmentation along the hyponychium [10]. Additional dermoscopic features frequently observed are irregular line patterns characterized by variations in color, width, and globules. In a prospective study of 69 congenital and 161 congenital-type nail matrix nevus cases, dermoscopy showed irregular longitudinal microlines in 64% of cases, resembling subungual melanoma in adults. LBP was more common in congenital nail matrix nevus (39.1%) compared to congenital-type nail matrix nevus (23%) ($P = 0.012$). Additionally, congenital nail matrix nevus cases more often had periungual pigmentation ($P = 0.029$) and pigment involving the surrounding skin ($P = 0.027$) than congenital-type nail matrix nevus [11]. In a prospective study of 16 children with nail matrix nevi aged 4–12 years examined with dermoscopy, 31% showed an irregular pattern of lines with variations in color and width, with line disruption in 25% and globules in 19% [12]. In a prospective study of 15 biopsy-confirmed pediatric cases of nail matrix nevus, 100% exhibited LBP. Additionally, irregular patterns with color variations and irregular lines were present with dermoscopy in all cases. Globular pigmentation was present in 40% of cases [10]. In a retrospective study of 20 children and eight adults with biopsy-confirmed nail matrix nevus, all hyponychial pigmentations demonstrated an LBP pattern under dermoscopy [8]. In the retrospective analysis by Lee et al. [9] including 29 cases of pediatric nail matrix nevus, dermoscopy showed an irregular pattern in 72.41%, globules in 27.59%, and pigment involving the surrounding skin in 44.83% [9].

39.5 Clinical Features in Skin of Color

Nail matrix nevus may be difficult to diagnose in patients with skin of color since LM due to melanocytic activation can present similarly and concurrently.

39.6 Requirements for Diagnosis

Pediatric LM can generally be managed with a watch-and-wait approach. Certain indicators of nail unit melanoma in adults include sudden appearance of LM, brown to black bands that are irregular, nail dystrophy, and pigment involving the surrounding skin, which may be common in pediatric patients [13]. For example, in the prospective study by Lee et al. [8] including 28 cases of biopsied nail matrix nevus, the width of LM averaged 47% of the nail width in pediatric cases vs. 14% in adults. Pigment involving the surrounding skin was present in 30% of pediatric cases, with five presenting with hyponychial pigmentation [8]. Most nail experts agree that conservative management, including follow-up with serial clinical examination, dermoscopy, and photography at-three to six month intervals, is appropriate for pediatric LM, with biopsy reserved for cases of development of concerning signs or symptoms (changing color, increase in pigmentation >50% of the nail width, bleeding, or pain) [13, 14].

If biopsy is performed, histology of junctional nevi show polygonal or rounded melanocytes that are organized in nests along the dermoepidermal junction. Many melanocytes in these nevi contain melanin granules, with small nuclei and sometimes a small nucleolus [3]. There are few melanophages present in the papillary dermis. In compound nevi, melanocytes are arranged in nests at the dermoepidermal junction and in clusters at the papillary dermis, often surrounding blood vessels and nerves. Melanocytes in compound nevi are round to oval, with moderate to abundant cytoplasm and few melanin granules [3]. In the retrospective analysis by Lee et al. [9] including 29 cases of pediatric nail matrix nevus, retraction artifacts around nests were present in 69.23%, abundant pale or eosinophilic cytoplasm in 69.23%, and hyperchromatic nuclei were present in 69.23% upon biopsy [9].

39.7 Cases

Figures 39.1, 39.2, 39.3, 39.4, 39.5, and 39.6 depict the clinical presentation of nail matrix nevus.

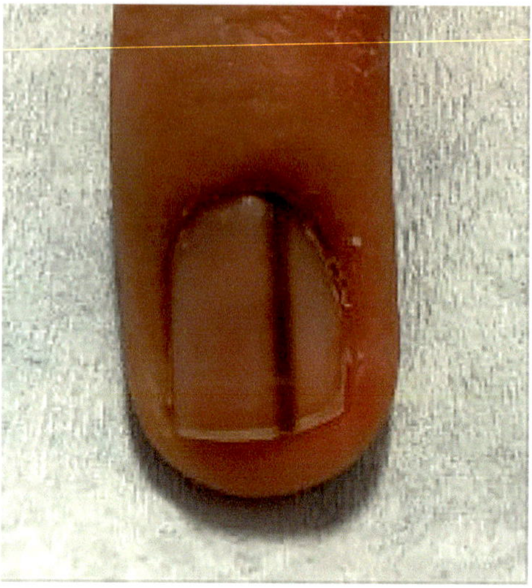

Fig. 39.1 27-Year-old female, Fitzpatrick type II, histopathologically confirmed nail matrix nevus, with 1 mm brown longitudinal band involving the right fourth fingernail

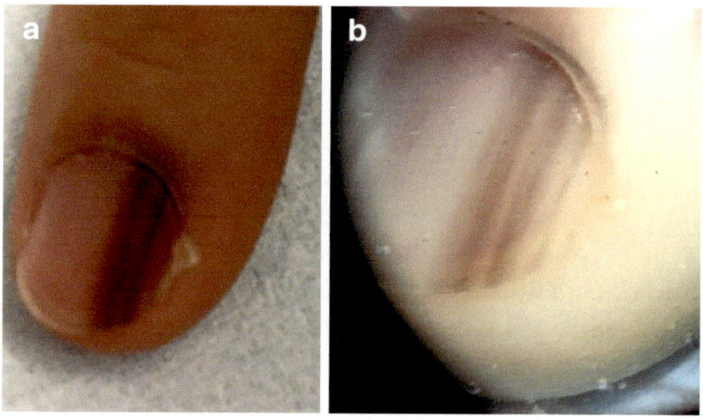

Fig. 39.2 (**a**) 47-Year-old male, Fitzpatrick type II, histopathologically confirmed nail matrix nevus, with 3.5 mm dark-brown longitudinal band involving the right fifth fingernail. (**b**) On dermoscopy, brown background with brown bands with regular color, but irregular spacing and thickness

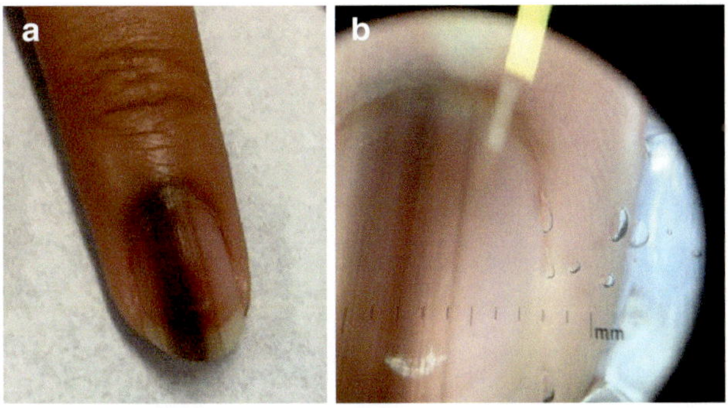

Fig. 39.3 (**a**) 22-Year-old female, Fitzpatrick type III, histopathologically confirmed junctional nail matrix nevus, with 5 mm dark-brown longitudinal band involving the left second fingernail. (**b**) Dermoscopy shows a brown background and irregular lines in terms of color, spacing, and thickness

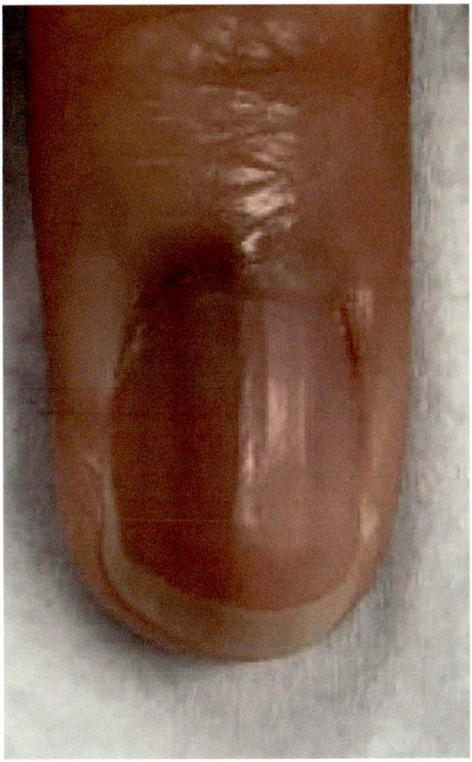

Fig. 39.4 34-Year-old female, Fitzpatrick type III, histopathologically confirmed nail matrix nevus, with a 2.4 mm gray-brown longitudinal band involving the left third fingernail

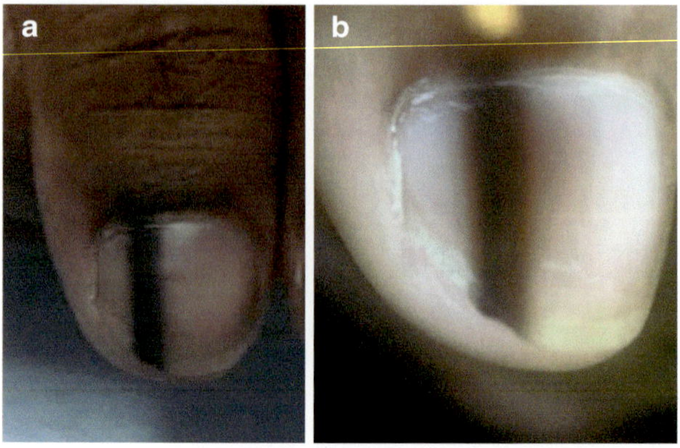

Fig. 39.5 (**a**) 38-Year-old female, Fitzpatrick type V, histopathologically confirmed nail unit junctional nevus, with a 4.5 mm dark brown longitudinal band involving the right thumbnail. (**b**) Dermoscopy shows a brown background with irregular lines in terms of color and thickness

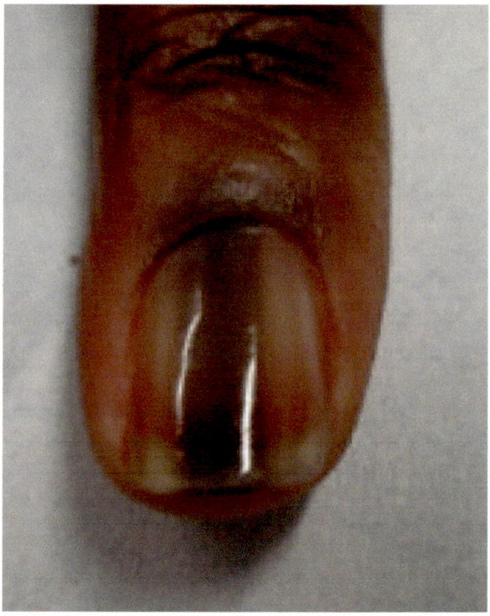

Fig. 39.6 48-Year-old female, Fitzpatrick type VI, histopathologically confirmed nail matrix nevus, with a 4 mm gray-brown homogenous band involving the right second fingernail

References

1. Husain S, Scher RK, Silvers DN, Ackerman AB. Melanotic macule of nail unit and its clinicopathologic spectrum. J Am Acad Dermatol. 2006;54(4):664–7. https://doi.org/10.1016/j.jaad.2005.11.1098.
2. Nevares-Pomales OW, Sarriera-Lazaro CJ, Barrera-Llaurador J, et al. Pigmented lesions of the nail unit. Am J Dermatopathol. 2018;40(11):793–804. https://doi.org/10.1097/dad.0000000000001106.
3. Tosti A, Baran R, Piraccini BM, Cameli N, Fanti PA. Nail matrix nevi: a clinical and histopathologic study of twenty-two patients. J Am Acad Dermatol. 1996;34(5 Pt 1):765–71. https://doi.org/10.1016/s0190-9622(96)90010-9.
4. Hirata SH, Yamada S, Enokihara MY, et al. Patterns of nail matrix and bed of longitudinal melanonychia by intraoperative dermatoscopy. J Am Acad Dermatol. 2011;65(2):297–303. https://doi.org/10.1016/j.jaad.2010.06.009.
5. Tsai SY, Hamilton CE, Mologousis MA, Hawryluk EB. Melanoma-like features in pediatric longitudinal melanonychia: a systematic review and meta-analysis. Pediatr Dermatol. 2024;41(4):613–20. https://doi.org/10.1111/pde.15597.
6. Goettmann-Bonvallot S, André J, Belaich S. Longitudinal melanonychia in children: a clinical and histopathologic study of 40 cases. J Am Acad Dermatol. 1999;41(1):17–22. https://doi.org/10.1016/s0190-9622(99)70399-3.
7. Lyu A, Hou Y, Wang Q. Retrospective analysis of longitudinal melanonychia: a Chinese experience. Front Pediatr. 2022;10:1065758. https://doi.org/10.3389/fped.2022.1065758.
8. Lee JH, Lim Y, Park JH, et al. Clinicopathologic features of 28 cases of nail matrix nevi (NMNs) in Asians: comparison between children and adults. J Am Acad Dermatol. 2018;78(3):479–89. https://doi.org/10.1016/j.jaad.2017.08.052.
9. Lee J, Bae JH, Oh SJ, et al. Clinical and histopathologic features of pediatric longitudinal melanonychia: a multicenter retrospective study. J Am Acad Dermatol. 2023;88(6):1393–6. https://doi.org/10.1016/j.jaad.2023.02.019.
10. Lee J, Park S, Lee D, Jang KT, Kwon EJ. Longitudinal brush pigmentation on the hyponychium, a dermoscopic feature observed in pediatric nail matrix nevi. J Am Acad Dermatol. 2021;84(6):1758–60. https://doi.org/10.1016/j.jaad.2020.11.012.
11. Pham F, Boespflug A, Duru G, et al. Dermatoscopic and clinical features of congenital or congenital-type nail matrix nevi: a multicenter prospective cohort study by the International Dermoscopy Society. J Am Acad Dermatol. 2022;87(3):551–8. https://doi.org/10.1016/j.jaad.2022.01.028.
12. Stefanaki C, Soura E, Sgouros D, et al. Nail matrix naevi in children: a prospective study. J Eur Acad Dermatol Venereol. 2020;34(4):e203–e5. https://doi.org/10.1111/jdv.16154.
13. Smith RJ, Rubin AI. Pediatric nail disorders: a review. Curr Opin Pediatr. 2020;32(4):506–15. https://doi.org/10.1097/mop.0000000000000921.
14. Scher RK, Lipner SR. Pediatric melanomas often mimic benign skin lesions. J Am Acad Dermatol. 2017;76(4):e131. https://doi.org/10.1016/j.jaad.2016.10.046.

Lentigo

40

Eden Axler and Shari R. Lipner

40.1 Description of Disease

Subungual lentigo presents as a dark brown to black longitudinal band on a single fingernail or toenail [1]. It is a benign melanonychia subtype. On histopathology, there is melanocyte proliferation in the basal layer of the epidermis without nest formation [1, 2].

40.2 Epidemiology

Subungual lentigo is relatively common. In a prospective study of 275 patients with longitudinal melanonychia (LM) who underwent nail biopsy, subungual lentigo was diagnosed in 11.6% of cases [1].

40.2.1 Children

Subungual lentigo may be relatively more common in children than in adults [2]. In a retrospective study that assessed 172 biopsy-confirmed cases of adult ($n = 66$) and pediatric ($n = 106$) LM, lentigo was diagnosed in 5.6% of pediatric patients and 3.0% of adults [3]. In a prospective study of 40 children under 16 years old presenting with LM who underwent nail biopsy, the diagnosis was nevus in 47.4% of cases, lentigo in 30.0%, and functional melanonychia in 22.5% [4]. In a retrospective study of 30 children ages 18 years or younger who presented with LM and underwent nail biopsy, 66.6% of cases were subungual lentigines [5].

S. R. Lipner, *Atlas of Nail Disorders Across All Skin Colors*,
https://doi.org/10.1007/978-3-031-74272-9_40

40.3 Risk Factors

There are no known risk factors for the development of subungual lentigo.

40.4 Clinical Features

Subungual lentigo presents as an asymptomatic brown to black longitudinal band involving a single digit, with a width rarely >5 mm, and may affect fingernails or toenails [6].

40.4.1 Clinical Features of Dermoscopy

Dermoscopy of subungual lentigo is characterized by a gray background with gray lines and a regular overall distribution of width, lines, and spacing. Rarely, dermoscopy of subungual lentigo may demonstrate irregular lines and may be difficult to distinguish from melanoma in situ [7].

40.5 Clinical Features in Skin of Color

Subungual lentigo may be difficult to diagnose in patients with skin of color since longitudinal melanonychia due to melanocytic activation can present similarly.

40.6 Requirements for Diagnosis

If the width of the LM is relatively narrow, with regular lines on dermoscopy and stable over time, the patient can be reassured and the LM monitored. The definitive diagnosis of subungual lentigo requires a biopsy and is needed to rule out a nail unit melanoma, which can present similarly. Histological examination may show normal melanocytes that may exhibit mild cytological atypia [8]. There is an observable increase in the number of melanocytes, often reaching 10–31 melanocytes/mm located predominantly in the basal layer, without evidence of confluence or nests [9, 10]. Subungual lentigo histopathology contrasts with that of the normal nail, in which nail matrix melanocytes are located above the basal layer.

40.7 Cases

Figures 40.1, 40.2, 40.3, 40.4, 40.5, 40.6, and 40.7 demonstrate the presentation of subungual lentigo in clinical practice.

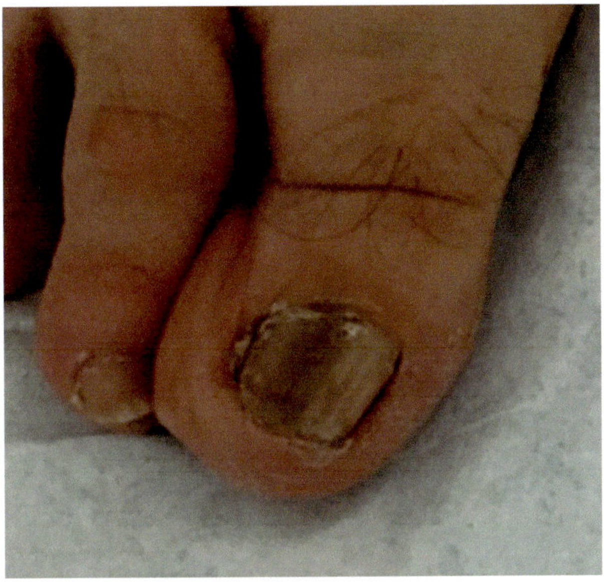

Fig. 40.1 69-Year-old female, Fitzpatrick type II, biopsy-proven subungual lentigo, presenting with a 4 mm gray-brown longitudinal band involving the right great toenail

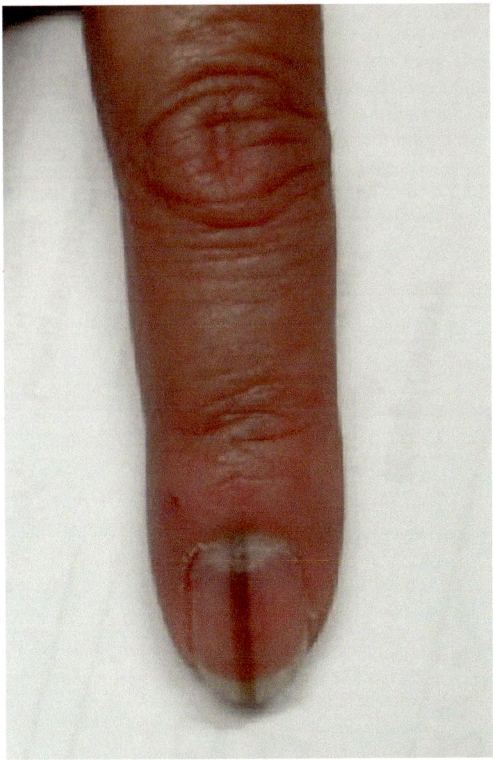

Fig. 40.2 71-Year-old female, Fitzpatrick type II, biopsy-proven subungual lentigo, presenting with a 3 mm longitudinal brown band involving the left second fingernail

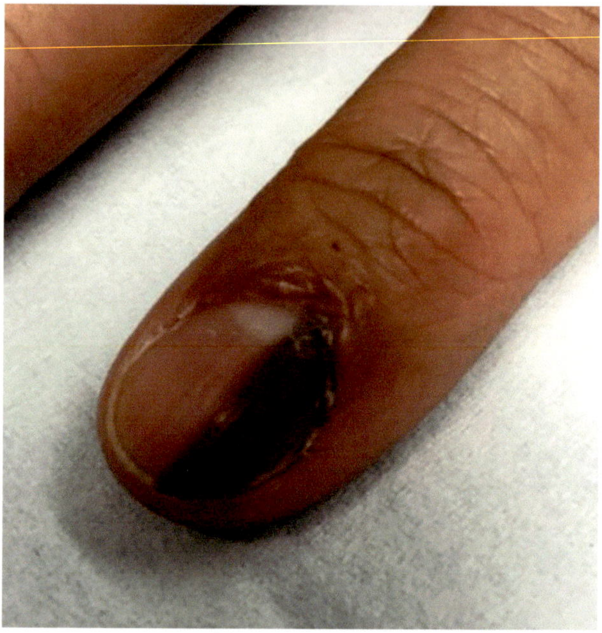

Fig. 40.3 45-Year-old male, Fitzpatrick type III, biopsy-proven subungual lentigo, presenting with a 5.7 mm longitudinal brown band involving the right second fingernail

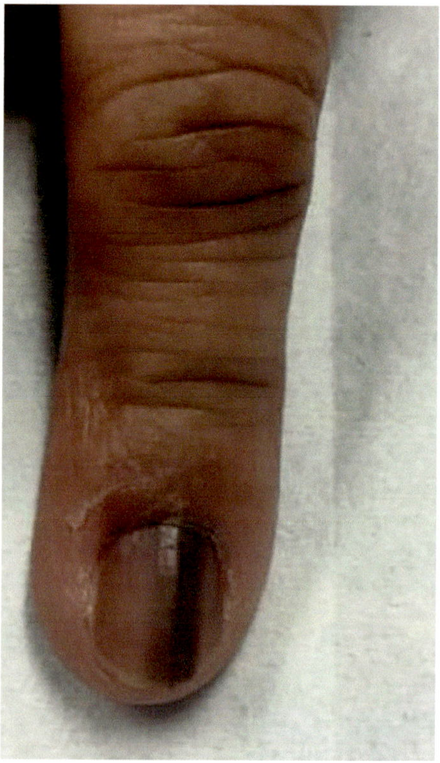

Fig. 40.4 64-Year-old female, Fitzpatrick type III, biopsy-proven subungual lentigo, presenting with a 3 mm dark brown longitudinal band involving the left fifth fingernail

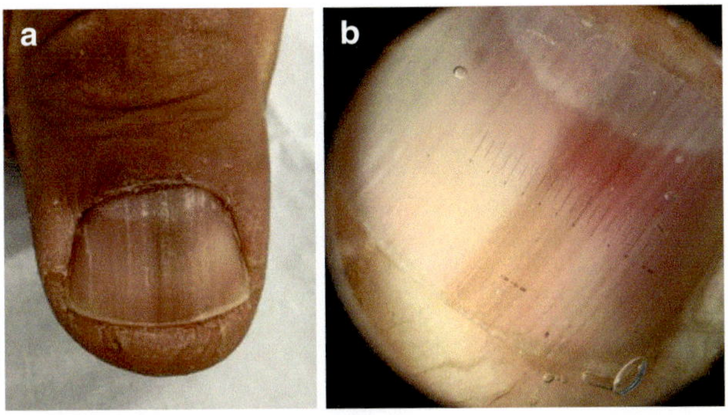

Fig. 40.5 (**a**) 63-Year-old male, Fitzpatrick type IV, biopsy-proven subungual lentigo, presenting with 3 mm gray–brown longitudinal band involving the right thumbnail. (**b**) 63-year-old male, Fitzpatrick skin type IV, biopsy-proven subungual lentigo. Dermoscopy showing a brown background and regular lines in terms of color, width, and spacing

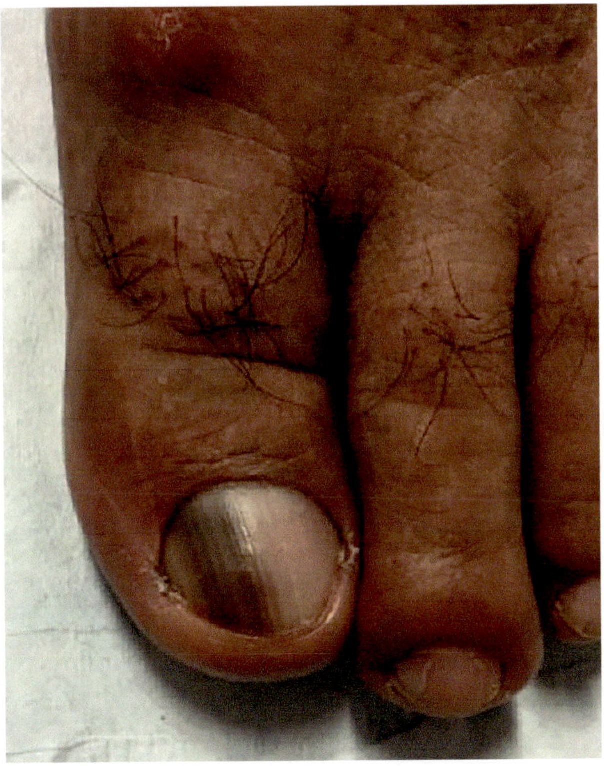

Fig. 40.6 62-Year-old male, Fitzpatrick type V, biopsy-proven subungual lentigo, presenting with a 7 mm brown longitudinal band involving the left great toenail

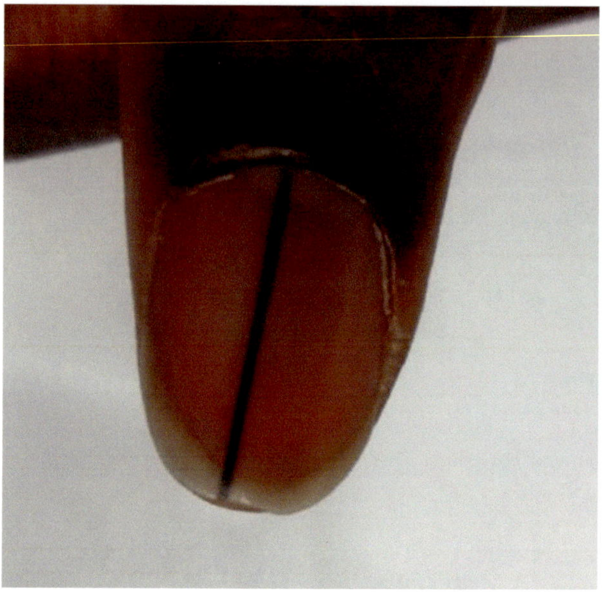

Fig. 40.7 75-Year-old female, Fitzpatrick type VI, biopsy-proven subungual lentigo, presenting with a longitudinal brown to black band involving the right second fingernail

References

1. Jin H, Kim JM, Kim GW, et al. Diagnostic criteria for and clinical review of melanonychia in Korean patients. J Am Acad Dermatol. 2016;74(6):1121–7.
2. Ruben BS. Pigmented lesions of the nail unit: clinical and histopathologic features. Semin Cutan Med Surg. 2010;29(3):148–58.
3. Lyu A, Hou Y, Wang Q. Retrospective analysis of longitudinal melanonychia: a Chinese experience. Front Pediatr. 2022;10:1065758.
4. Goettmann-Bonvallot S, André J, Belaich S. Longitudinal melanonychia in children: a clinical and histopathologic study of 40 cases. J Am Acad Dermatol. 1999;41(1):17–22.
5. Cooper C, Arva NC, Lee C, et al. A clinical, histopathologic, and outcome study of melanonychia striata in childhood. J Am Acad Dermatol. 2015;72(5):773–9.
6. Alessandrini A, Dika E, Starace M, Chessa MA, Piraccini BM. Diagnosis of melanonychia. Dermatol Clin. 2021;39(2):255–67.
7. Rich P. Longitudinal melanonychia. UpToDate; 2022 [updated 2024 Jan] [cited 2024 Feb 04]. https://www.uptodate.com/contents/longitudinal-melanonychia#:~:text=The%20most%20common%20type%20of,multiple%20bands%20affecting%20multiple%20nails.
8. Güneş P, Göktay F. Melanocytic lesions of the nail unit. Dermatopathology (Basel). 2018;5(3):98–107.
9. Gradinaru TC, Mihai M, Beiu C, Tebeica T, Giurcaneanu C. Melanonychia - clues for a correct diagnosis. Cureus. 2020;12(1):e6621.
10. Singal A, Bisherwal K. Melanonychia: etiology, diagnosis, and treatment. Indian Dermatol Online J. 2020;11(1):1–11.

Part IX

Leukonychia

Punctate Leukonychia

41

Kaya L. Curtis and Shari R. Lipner

41.1 Description of Disease

Leukonychia is defined as white discoloration of the nail(s). Leukonychia is classified into five morphologic presentations, including punctate leukonychia, transverse leukonychia, longitudinal leukonychia, partial leukonychia, and total leukonychia [1]. Leukonychia is further classified by the involved anatomical structure [2]. Apparent leukonychia occurs due to changes in the nail bed, true leukonychia occurs due to pathology in the nail matrix or nail plate, and pseudoleukonychia involves only the surface of the nail plate [1]. As a general diagnostic principle, the white discoloration in apparent leukonychia disappears with pressure and does not move distally with nail growth. On the other hand, the white discoloration in true leukonychia and pseudoleukonychia does not disappear with pressure and moves distally with nail growth. It is helpful to keep these principles in mind when evaluating a patient with leukonychia, in order to identify the anatomic region that is pathologic. Punctate leukonychia is characterized by white spots on the nail(s). The most common subtype of punctate leukonychia is punctate true leukonychia, followed by punctate pseudoleukonychia [1].

41.2 Epidemiology

Patients of all ages may be affected by punctate leukonychia. Punctate true leukonychia frequently presents in pediatric patients secondary to trauma [1], whereas punctate pseudoleukonychia frequently presents in female patients secondary to nail cosmetics. Punctate pseudoleukonychia may also occur in patients with risk factors for onychomycosis, including older and immunosuppressed patients.

S. R. Lipner, *Atlas of Nail Disorders Across All Skin Colors*,
https://doi.org/10.1007/978-3-031-74272-9_41

41.3 Risk Factors

Punctate true leukonychia is most frequently caused by trauma (e.g., onychophagia and cryotherapy for periungual verruca treatment) [1, 3]. Inflammatory disorders including alopecia areata, psoriasis, and lichen planus are also associated with punctate true leukonychia [4–7]. Punctate pseudoleukonychia is frequently caused by superficial white onychomycosis and trauma from nail cosmetics [1, 8, 9]. Frequent use of artificial nails (including gel nails or acrylic nails) or nail polish remover may lead to nail keratin degranulation resulting in punctate pseudoleukonychia [10]. Punctate pseudoleukonychia may occur secondary to exposure to exogenous compounds, such as 2-ethyl-cyanoacrylate glue [11].

41.4 Clinical Features

Punctate leukonychia is characterized by 1–3 mm white spots on the nail plate. These white spots move distally with nail growth [12]. The pattern of punctate leukonychia may change with nail growth [1]. Punctate leukonychia is most frequently caused by trauma and therefore typically affects a few nails. Punctate leukonychia secondary to nail cosmetic-induced trauma may involve all of the fingernails or toenails. White spots seen in punctate pseudoleukonychia secondary to onychomycosis may eventually coalesce into transverse white bands (transverse leukonychia) [13, 14]. Punctate leukonychia is asymptomatic [1].

41.5 Clinical Features in Skin of Color

Distinct clinical presentations of punctate leukonychia in skin of color have not been characterized. White discoloration may be more difficult to visualize in patients with higher Fitzpatrick skin types. Longitudinal melanonychia may be present particularly in adult skin of color patients, as trauma responsible for punctate leukonychia may also result in melanocytic activation.

41.6 Requirements for Diagnosis

Punctate leukonychia is a clinical diagnosis dependent on the observation of small white spots on the nail plate(s). Dermoscopy may aid in visualization. White discoloration does not fade with pressure for punctate true leukonychia and punctate pseudoleukonychia [12]. A history of trauma, especially frequent nail manicures, is a supportive feature. Other etiologies are considered in patients without a history of trauma. For patients with punctate leukonychia of the toenails, a history of tinea pedis or household contacts with onychomycosis should raise suspicion for punctate pseudoleukonychia secondary to superficial onychomycosis. Concurrent specific skin findings should raise suspicion for punctate leukonychia secondary to inflammatory diseases, including psoriasis or lichen planus.

41.7 Cases

Figures 41.1, 41.2, 41.3, 41.4, 41.5, 41.6, 41.7, 41.8, and 41.9 demonstrate the presentation of punctate leukonychia in a clinical setting.

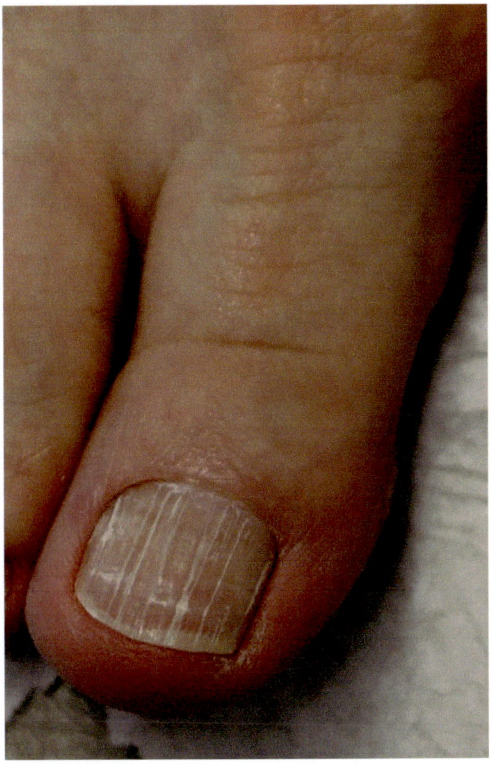

Fig. 41.1 52-Year-old female, Fitzpatrick type I, punctate leukonychia, with onychorrhexis and white spots on the nail plate of the right great toenail

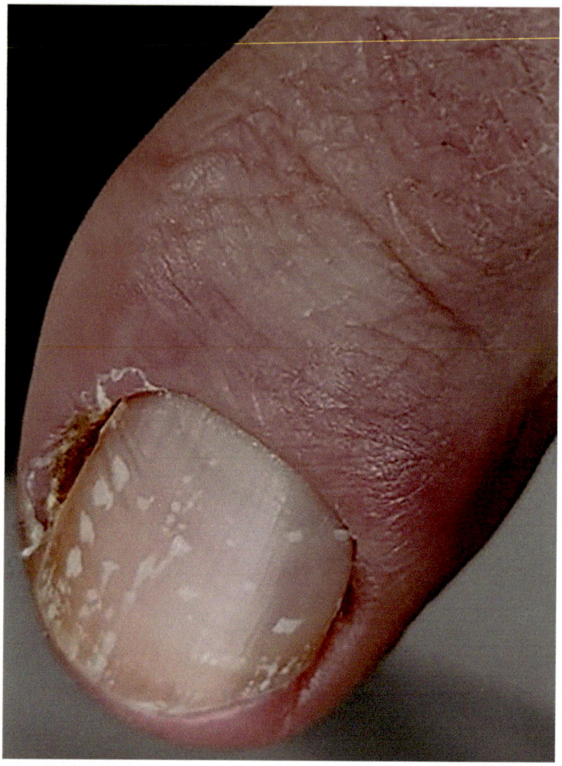

Fig. 41.2 48-Year-old female, Fitzpatrick type II, punctate leukonychia, with white spots on the nail plate of the left great toenail

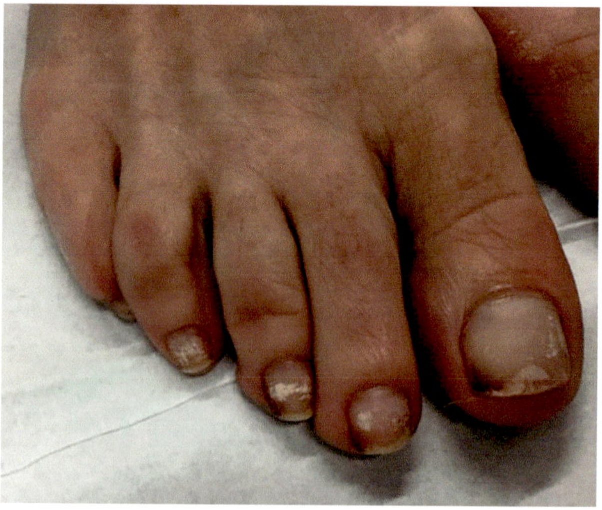

Fig. 41.3 69-Year-old female, Fitzpatrick type II, punctate leukonychia, with white spots on the nail plates of the right toenails

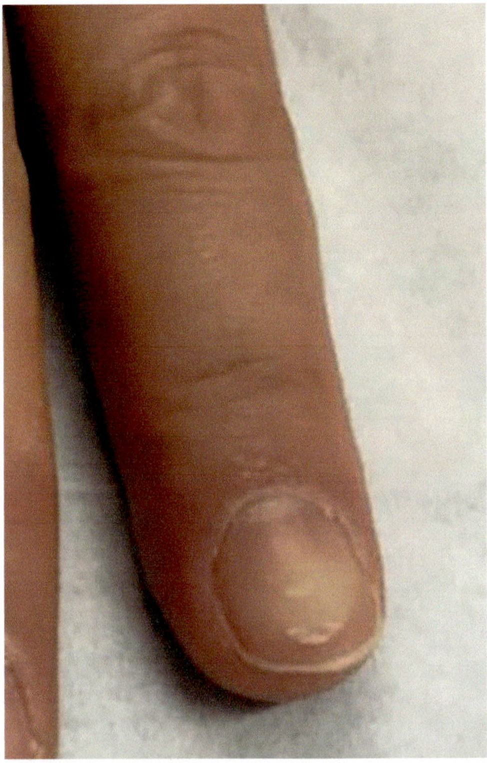

Fig. 41.4 26-Year-old female, Fitzpatrick type III, punctate leukonychia, with white spots on the nail plate of the left fifth fingernail

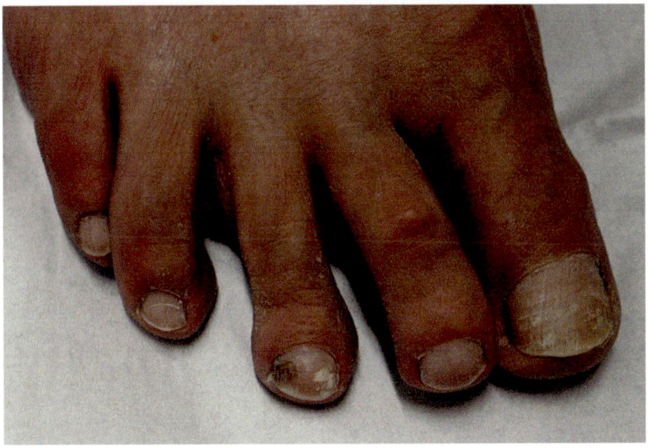

Fig. 41.5 76-Year-old male, Fitzpatrick type III, punctate leukonychia, with white spots on the distal nail plates of the right great toenail and right third toenail

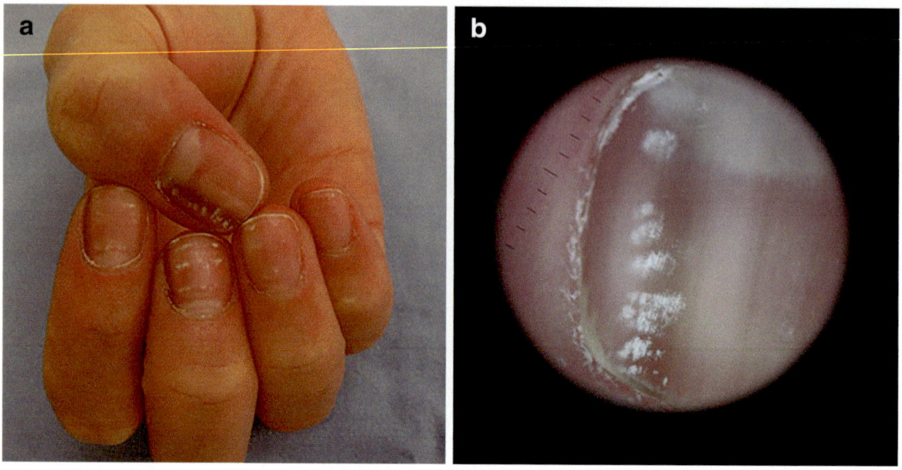

Fig. 41.6 (**a**) Adult patient, Fitzpatrick type III, punctate leukonychia, with white spots on the nail plates of the right fingernails and gray–brown longitudinal band (longitudinal melanonychia) of the right thumbnail. (**b**) Adult patient, Fitzpatrick type III, punctate leukonychia, with white spots and gray–brown longitudinal band (longitudinal melanonychia) of the right thumbnail. Dermoscopy of (**a**). (*courtesy of* Dr. Nilton Gioia Di Chiacchio, MD, PhD)

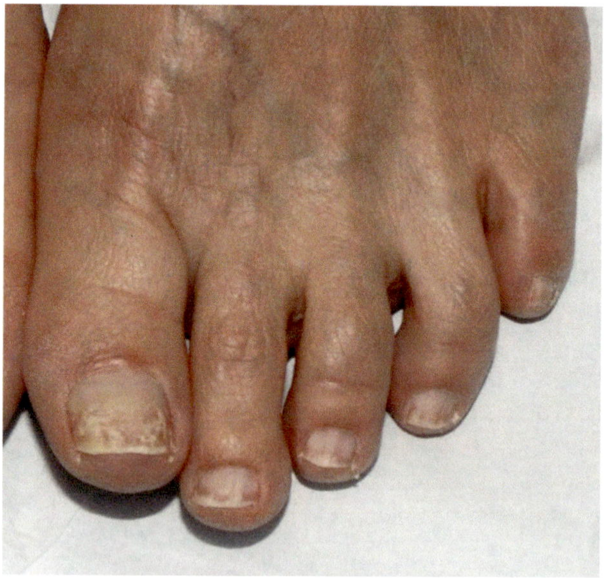

Fig. 41.7 64-Year-old female, Fitzpatrick type IV, punctate leukonychia, with white spots on the left toenails

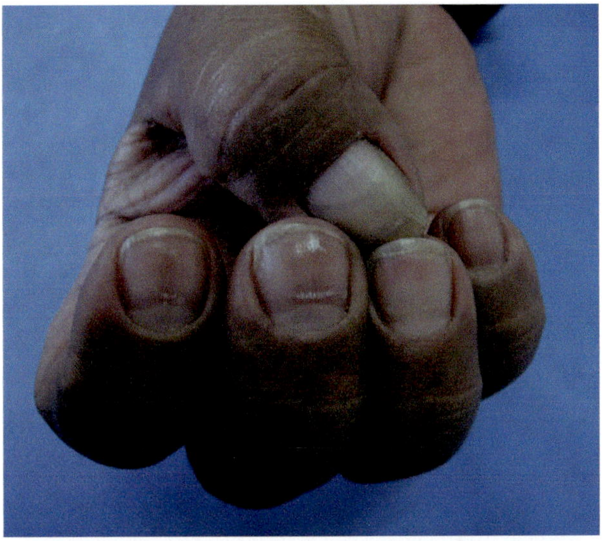

Fig. 41.8 Adult patient, Fitzpatrick type IV, punctate leukonychia, with white spots on the right fingernails (*courtesy of* Dr. Nilton Gioia Di Chiacchio, MD, PhD)

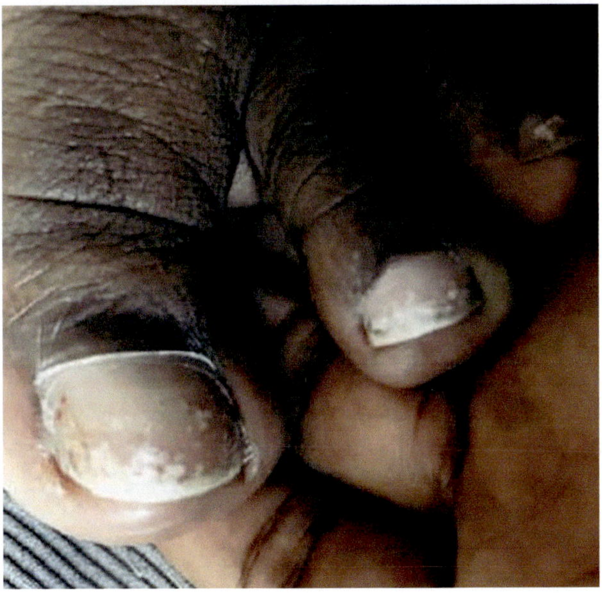

Fig. 41.9 44-Year-old female, Fitzpatrick type VI, punctate leukonychia, with onycholysis and white spots on the left great toenail, left second toenail, and left third toenail

References

1. Iorizzo M, Starace M, Pasch MC. Leukonychia: what can white nails tell us? Am J Clin Dermatol. 2022;23(2):177–93.
2. Grossman M, Scher RK. Leukonychia: review and classification. Int J Dermatol. 1990;29(8):535–41.
3. Fıçıcıoğlu S, Korkmaz S. Onychophagia induced melanonychia, splinter hemorrhages, leukonychia, and pterygium inversum unguis concurrently. Case Rep Dermatol Med. 2018;2018:3230582.
4. Elmas OF. Uncovering subtle nail involvement in lichen planus with dermoscopy: a prospective, controlled study. Postepy Dermatol Alergol. 2020;37(3):396–400.
5. Bae SH, Lee MY, Lee JB. Distinct patterns and aetiology of chromonychia. Acta Derm Venereol. 2018;98(1):108–13.
6. Dotz WI, Lieber CD, Vogt PJ. Leukonychia punctata and pitted nails in alopecia areata. Arch Dermatol. 1985;121(11):1452–4.
7. Chelidze K, Lipner SR. Nail changes in alopecia areata: an update and review. Int J Dermatol. 2018;57(7):776–83.
8. van Gelderen de Komaid A, Borges de Kestelman M, Duran EL. Etiology and clinical characteristics of mycotic leukonychia. Mycopathologia. 1996;136(1):9–15.
9. Gupta AK, Baran R, Summerbell RC. Fusarium infections of the skin. Curr Opin Infect Dis. 2000;13(2):121–8.
10. Chessa MA, Iorizzo M, Richert B, et al. Pathogenesis, clinical signs and treatment recommendations in brittle nails: a review. Dermatol Ther (Heidelb). 2020;10(1):15–27.
11. Ena P, Mazzarello V, Fenu G, Rubino C. Leukonychia from 2-ethyl-cyanoacrylate glue. Contact Derm. 2000;42(2):105–6.
12. Lipner SR, Scher RK. Evaluation of nail lines: color and shape hold clues. Cleve Clin J Med. 2016;83(5):385–91.
13. Moreno-Coutino G, Toussaint-Caire S, Arenas R. Clinical, mycological and histological aspects of white onychomycosis. Mycoses. 2010;53(2):144–7.
14. Rathore T, Millington GW. Mycotic pseudoleukonychia affecting the fingernails. Clin Exp Dermatol. 2010;35(5):558–9.

Transverse Leukonychia

42

Kaya L. Curtis and Shari R. Lipner

42.1 Description of Disease

Transverse leukonychia (also known as leukonychia striata) is characterized by white horizontal bands on the nail plate. There are three anatomic subtypes, including transverse true leukonychia, transverse apparent leukonychia, and transverse pseudoleukonychia. Transverse leukonychia is sometimes used interchangeably with Mees' lines, though some authors reserve the term Mees' lines for transverse true leukonychia secondary to arsenic poisoning [1]. Muehrcke's lines are a type of transverse apparent leukonychia associated with systemic disease. The pathogenesis in transverse true leukonychia is abnormal nail matrix keratinization, whereas transverse apparent leukonychia (Muehrcke's lines) is caused by vascular abnormalities in the nail bed [2].

42.2 Epidemiology

Epidemiologic studies on transverse leukonychia have not been conducted. However, since transverse leukonychia is associated with systemic diseases and chemotherapeutic drugs, transverse leukonychia is likely more prevalent among adult patients.

42.3 Risk Factors

There are many etiologies of transverse leukonychia. Transverse true leukonychia may be caused by trauma (e.g., from manicures, picking away chipped nail polish, or pressure from shoes) [3–5]. There are a multitude of systemic diseases that may cause transverse true leukonychia, including systemic lupus erythematosus, infectious diseases (e.g., COVID-19 infection, herpes zoster, and pleural empyema),

S. R. Lipner, *Atlas of Nail Disorders Across All Skin Colors*,
https://doi.org/10.1007/978-3-031-74272-9_42

hematologic disorders (e.g., acute myeloid leukemia and sickle cell anemia), heart failure, and catabolic stress due to high altitude (Everest nails) [6]. Chemotherapeutic drugs may cause transverse leukonychia of multiple nails [7]. The most commonly implicated chemotherapeutics include cyclophosphamide, doxorubicin, and vincristine [8]. Toxic causes of transverse true leukonychia include arsenic (Mees' lines), strontium, and thallium [9–12]. Local chemical exposures, such as herbicides may also cause transverse true leukonychia [13, 14]. Risk factors for transverse apparent leukonychia (Muehrcke's lines) include hypoalbuminemia, kidney disease, rheumatoid arthritis, and systemic retinoids [6]. Muehrcke's lines resolve when the associated systemic disease is treated [15]. Transverse pseudoleukonychia may be observed in cases of superficial onychomycosis and proximal subungual onychomycosis [16].

42.4 Clinical Features

Transverse leukonychia is characterized by 1–2 mm bands on the nail plate running parallel to the distal lunula. Mees' lines secondary to arsenic poisoning typically present 2 months after exposure [2]. Muehrcke's lines are multiple pale transverse white bands running parallel to the distal lunula, typically affecting all 20 nails [2]. Muehrcke's lines may be more prominent in the second, third, and fourth fingernails [6]. In transverse true leukonychia and transverse pseudoleukonychia, the white bands move distally with nail growth [2]. In transverse apparent leukonychia, white bands do not move distally with nail growth [2]. Transverse leukonychia limited to a few nails is likely secondary to trauma, whereas involvement of all nails is suggestive of a systemic etiology [6]. Leukonychia is typically asymptomatic [6].

42.5 Clinical Features in Skin of Color

Distinct clinical presentations of transverse leukonychia in skin of color have not been characterized. White discoloration may be more difficult to visualize in patients with higher Fitzpatrick skin types. Longitudinal melanonychia may be present, particularly in adult patients.

42.6 Requirements for Diagnosis

Transverse leukonychia is a clinical diagnosis. Dermoscopy may aid in visualization of the white bands. Disappearance of white discoloration upon pressure is suggestive of apparent leukonychia, whereas persistence of white discoloration upon pressure is suggestive of true leukonychia or pseudoleukonychia, which can aid in determination of etiology. A history of systemic disease or chemotherapy is a supportive feature.

42.7 Cases

Figures 42.1, 42.2, 42.3, 42.4, 42.5, 42.6, 42.7, and 42.8 demonstrate the presentation of transverse leukonychia in a clinical setting.

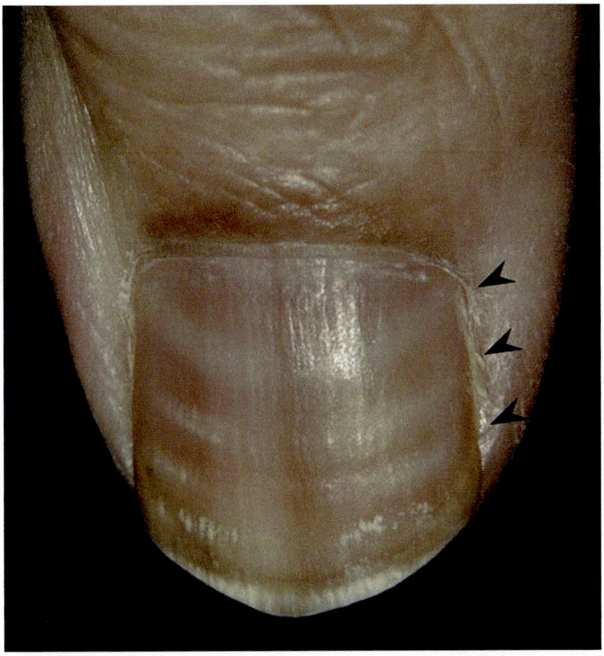

Fig. 42.1 62-Year-old female, Fitzpatrick type I, transverse leukonychia (Mees' lines (arrowheads)) of the thumbnail (*from* Song and Lee [17]; *with permission*)

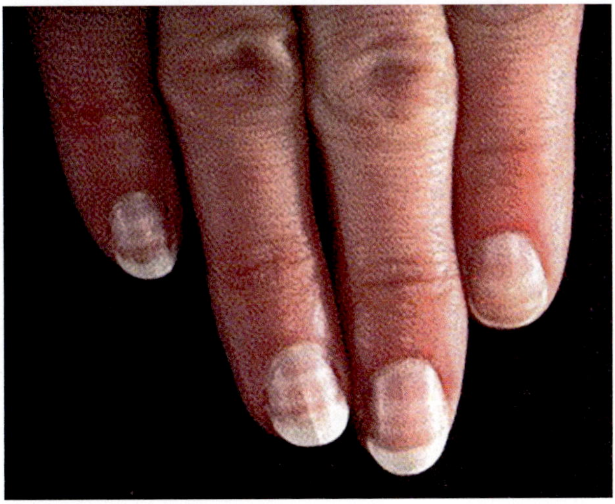

Fig. 42.2 28-Year-old female, Fitzpatrick type II, transverse leukonychia (Muehrcke's nails) (*from* Skoog and Boardman [18]; *with permission*)

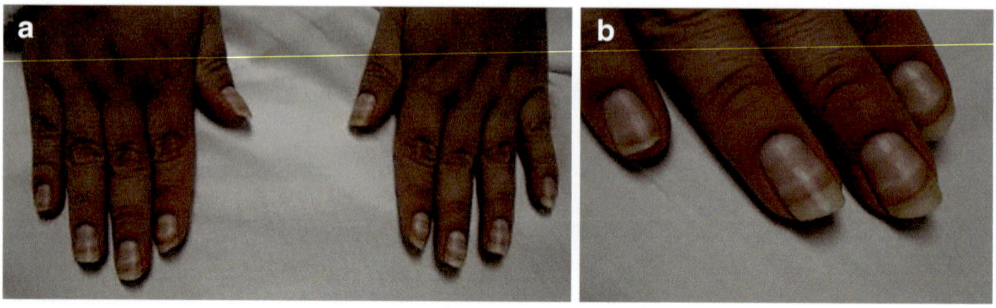

Fig. 42.3 (**a**) 29-Year-old female, Fitzpatrick type II, transverse leukonychia (Muehrcke's lines), patient with nephrotic syndrome and hypoalbuminemia. (**b**) 29-year-old female, Fitzpatrick type II, transverse leukonychia (Muehrcke's lines) (*from* Short and Shah [19]; *with permission*)

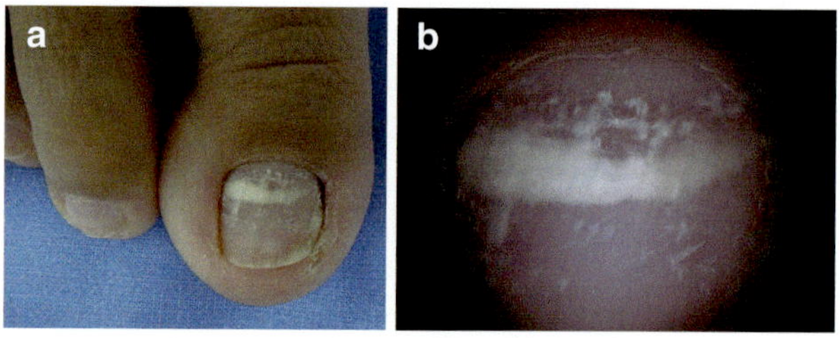

Fig. 42.4 (**a**) Adult patient, Fitzpatrick type III, transverse leukonychia, with white transverse band of the right great toenail. (**b**) Adult patient, Fitzpatrick type III, transverse leukonychia, with white transverse band of the right great toenail. Dermoscopy of (**a**). (*courtesy of* Dr. Nilton Gioia Di Chiacchio, MD, PhD)

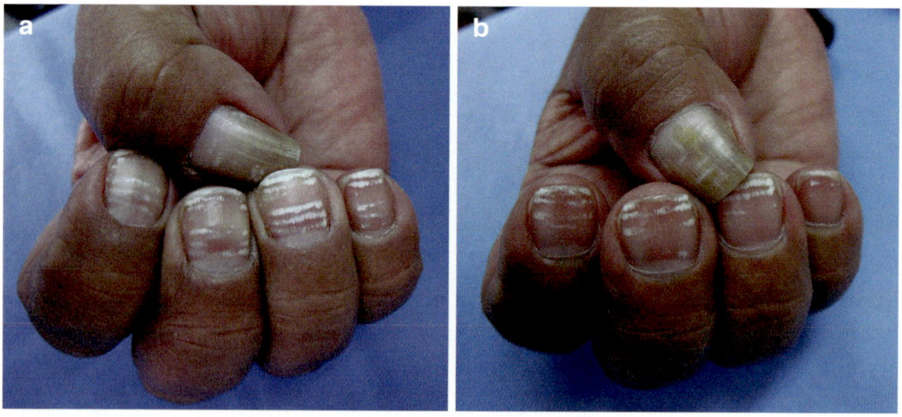

Fig. 42.5 (**a**) Adult patient, Fitzpatrick type IV, transverse leukonychia, with transverse white bands of the fingernails. (**b**) Adult patient, Fitzpatrick type IV, transverse leukonychia, with transverse white bands of the fingernails. Same patient as (**a**), 3 months later, demonstrating distal movement of transverse bands with nail growth. (*courtesy of* Dr. Nilton Gioia Di Chiacchio, MD, PhD)

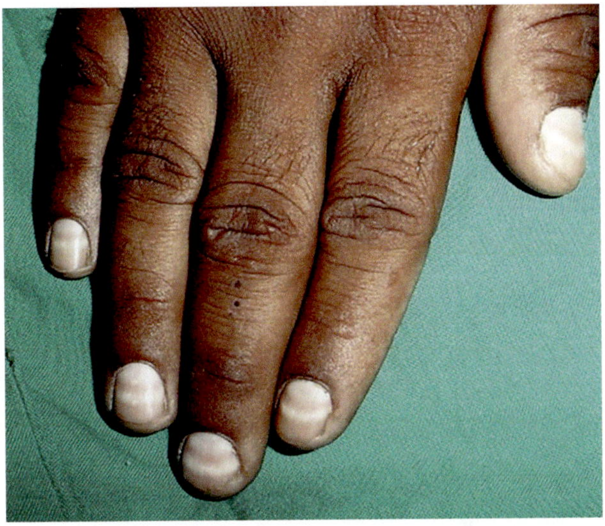

Fig. 42.6 19-Year-old male, Fitzpatrick type V, Mees' lines, with transverse white bands clearly visible on the nails (*from* Chauhan et al. [20]; *with permission*)

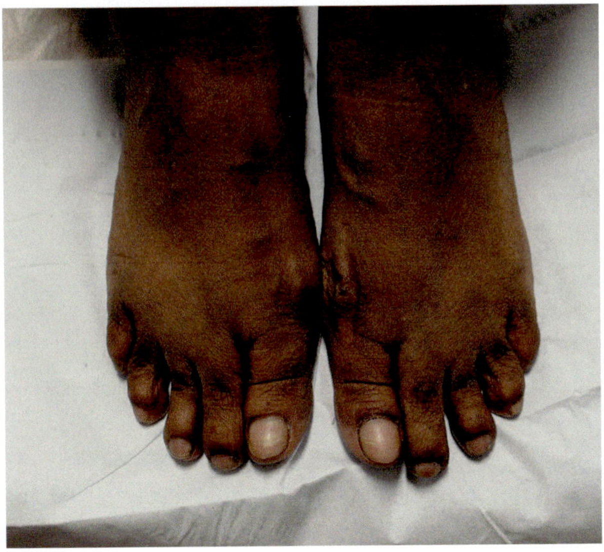

Fig. 42.7 53-Year-old female, Fitzpatrick type V, transverse leukonychia, with transverse white bands of the bilateral great toenails and right third toenail

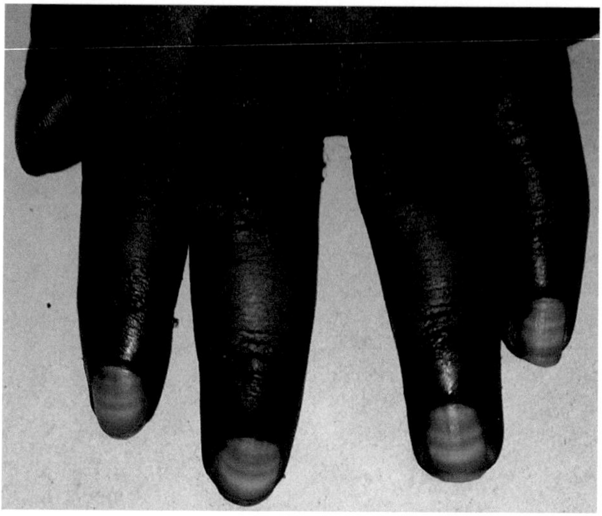

Fig. 42.8 7-Month-old infant, Fitzpatrick type VI, Mees' lines, with transverse white bands clearly visible on the nails (*from* Williams and Jayashree [15]; *with permission*)

References

1. Fernandez-Nieto D, Jimenez-Cauhe J, Ortega-Quijano D, Diaz-Guimaraens B, Dominguez-Santas M, Martinez-Rubio J. Transverse leukonychia (Mees' lines) nail alterations in a COVID-19 patient. Dermatol Ther. 2020;33(6):e13863.
2. Lipner SR, Scher RK. Evaluation of nail lines: color and shape hold clues. Cleve Clin J Med. 2016;83(5):385–91.
3. Baran R, Perrin C. Transverse leukonychia of toenails due to repeated microtrauma. Br J Dermatol. 1995;133(2):267–9.
4. Howard SR, Siegfried EC. A case of leukonychia. J Pediatr. 2013;163(3):914–5.
5. Maino KL, Stashower ME. Traumatic transverse leukonychia. Skinmed. 2004;3(1):53–5.
6. Iorizzo M, Starace M, Pasch MC. Leukonychia: what can white nails tell us? Am J Clin Dermatol. 2022;23(2):177–93.
7. Follows AM, Follows GA. Transverse leukonychia (Mees' lines). N Engl J Med. 2023;389(22):e48.
8. Robert C, Sibaud V, Mateus C, et al. Nail toxicities induced by systemic anticancer treatments. Lancet Oncol. 2015;16(4):e181–9.
9. Sharma S, Gupta A, Deshmukh A, Puri V. Arsenic poisoning and Mees' lines. QJM. 2016;109(8):565–6.
10. Assadi F. Leukonychia associated with increased blood strontium level. Clin Pediatr (Phila). 2005;44(6):531–3.
11. Zhao G, Ding M, Zhang B, et al. Clinical manifestations and management of acute thallium poisoning. Eur Neurol. 2008;60(6):292–7.
12. Lu CI, Huang CC, Chang YC, et al. Short-term thallium intoxication: dermatological findings correlated with thallium concentration. Arch Dermatol. 2007;143(1):93–8.
13. Kibby T, Ring DS. Nail injury and diquat exposure: forgotten but not gone. Dermatitis. 2012;23(4):176–8.
14. Samman PD, Johnston EN. Nail damage associated with handling of paraquat and diquat. Br Med J. 1969;1(5647):818–9.

15. Williams V, Jayashree M. Muehrcke Lines in an Infant. J Pediatr. 2017;189:234.
16. Gupta AK, Baran R, Summerbell RC. Fusarium infections of the skin. Curr Opin Infect Dis. 2000;13(2):121–8.
17. Song IC, Lee HJ. Transverse lines of the nails. Am J Med. 2017;130(6):e259–60.
18. Skoog S, Boardman L. Image of the month. Muehrcke's nails in Peutz-Jeghers syndrome with hepatic adenoma. Clin Gastroenterol Hepatol. 2004;2(s):xxiv.
19. Short N, Shah C. Muehrcke's lines. Am J Med. 2010;123(11):991–2.
20. Chauhan S, D'Cruz S, Singh R, Sachdev A. Mees' lines. Lancet. 2008;372(9647):1410.

Longitudinal Leukonychia

43

Kaya L. Curtis and Shari R. Lipner

43.1 Description of Disease

Longitudinal leukonychia is defined as a longitudinal white band extending the length of the nail plate. Pathogenesis of longitudinal true leukonychia is a disturbance in the nail matrix, which results in focal parakeratosis and keratin filament disorganization [1]. Pathogenesis of longitudinal apparent leukonychia is vascular bed abnormalities [2].

43.2 Epidemiology

Longitudinal leukonychia can affect patients of all ages. Patients with Darier disease typically develop onychodystrophies, including longitudinal leukonychia, during childhood [3].

43.3 Risk Factors

Patients with Darier disease frequently present with longitudinal true leukonychia in association with longitudinal erythronychia. Darier disease (also known as keratosis follicularis or Darier-White disease) is an autosomal dominant keratinization disorder characterized by hyperkeratotic papules and plaques in seborrheic regions [4]. In Darier disease, epithelial hyperplasia of the matrix results in white lines, while matrix disease results in thin nails which present as red lines [1]. These alternating red and white bands are referred to as candy cane nails. Longitudinal true leukonychia may also be observed in patients with Hailey-Hailey disease, an autosomal dominant keratinization disorder characterized by grouped, erythematous, flaccid vesicles in flexural regions [5]. Approximately 70% of patients with Hailey-Hailey disease have longitudinal leukonychia [6]. Other etiologies of longitudinal

S. R. Lipner, *Atlas of Nail Disorders Across All Skin Colors*,
https://doi.org/10.1007/978-3-031-74272-9_43

true leukonychia include tuberous sclerosis, onychomatricoma, lichen planus, and trauma [1, 7, 8]. Longitudinal apparent leukonychia etiologies include onychopapilloma, squamous cell carcinoma, and longitudinal subungual acanthoma [9, 10]. Longitudinal pseudoleukonychia may be observed in patients with white superficial onychomycosis or proximal subungual onychomycosis [11].

43.4 Clinical Features

Longitudinal true leukonychia secondary to Darier disease presents together with longitudinal erythronychia as alternating red and white bands (candy cane nails) in multiple nails, often associated with a distal wedge-shaped notch [12], which are present in 92–95% of Darier disease patients [3, 13]. Patients with Hailey-Hailey disease present with isolated longitudinal white bands [14]. Longitudinal leukonychia is present in approximately 70% of Hailey-Hailey disease patients [6]. Longitudinal true leukonychia secondary to onychopapilloma presents with a longitudinal white band originating in the distal lunula with a subungual hyperkeratotic papule at the hyponychium seen with end on dermoscopy [15, 16]. Longitudinal pseudoleukonychia secondary to onychomycosis presents as irregular longitudinal white bands, which may show "spikes" with dermoscopy and is highly suggestive of a dermatophytoma, which is a collection of densely packed hyphae [2]. Though leukonychia is typically asymptomatic, patients with longitudinal leukonychia secondary to onychopapilloma may complain of an associated nail split, which may catch on fibers [1].

43.5 Clinical Features in Skin of Color

Distinct clinical presentations of longitudinal leukonychia in skin of color have not been characterized. White discoloration may be more difficult to visualize in patients with higher Fitzpatrick skin types. Longitudinal melanonychia may also be present, particularly in adult skin of color patients.

43.6 Requirements for Diagnosis

Longitudinal leukonychia is a clinical diagnosis. Disappearance of white discoloration with pressure is suggestive of apparent leukonychia, whereas persistence of white discoloration upon pressure is suggestive of true leukonychia or pseudoleukonychia. A history of a genodermatosis or concurrent cutaneous involvement suggestive of Darier disease or Hailey-Hailey disease is a supportive feature. Dermoscopy may aid in the visualization of white bands. In Hailey-Hailey disease, dermoscopy demonstrates multiple parallel longitudinal white bands of varying width originating in the lunula, potentially associated with splinter hemorrhages or distal notch [14]. In Darier disease, dermoscopy demonstrates alternating longitudinal red and white bands, potentially associated with subungual hyperkeratosis, splinter hemorrhages, or distal wedge-shaped notch [17]. Patients with longitudinal leukonychia secondary to a genodermatosis may endorse a positive family history of nail changes.

43.7 Cases

Figures 43.1, 43.2, 43.3, 43.4, 43.5, 43.6, and 43.7 demonstrate the presentation of longitudinal leukonychia in a clinical setting.

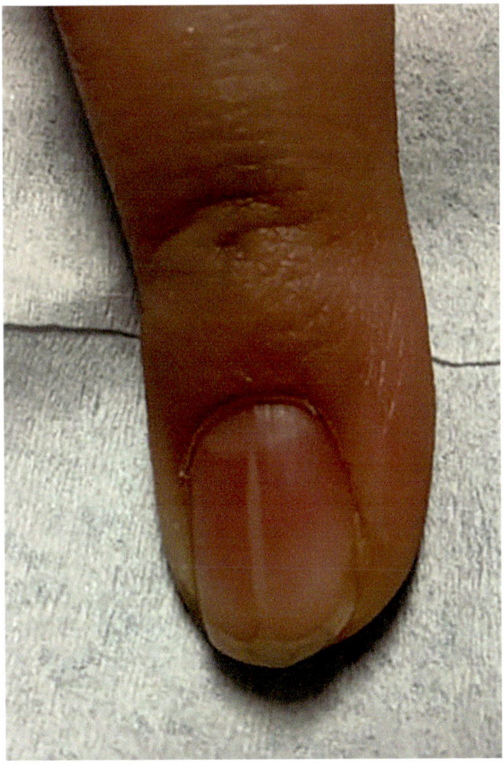

Fig. 43.1 10-Year-old female, Fitzpatrick type I, longitudinal leukonychia secondary to onychopapilloma, with longitudinal white band of the right second fingernail originating in the distal lunula

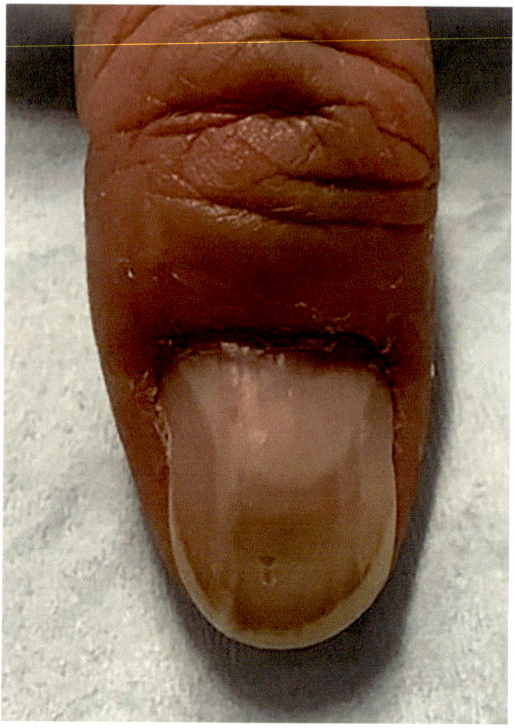

Fig. 43.2 64-Year-old female, Fitzpatrick type II, longitudinal leukonychia secondary to onychopapilloma, with longitudinal white band of the left thumbnail

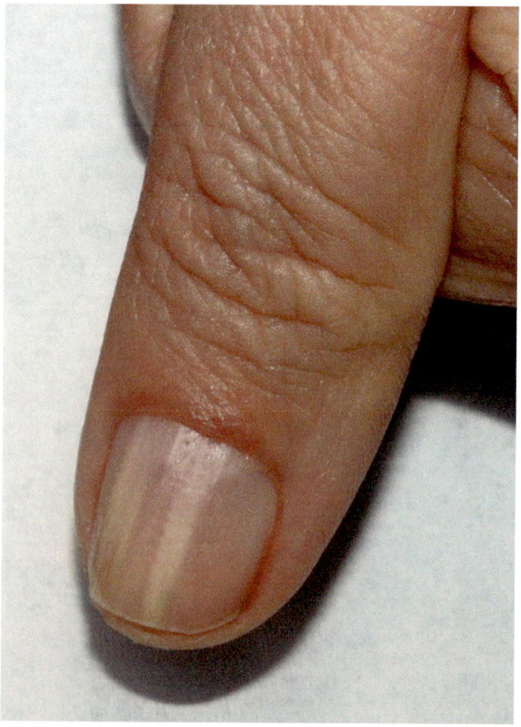

Fig. 43.3 40-Year-old female, Fitzpatrick type II, longitudinal leukonychia of unknown etiology, with longitudinal white bands of the left thumbnail

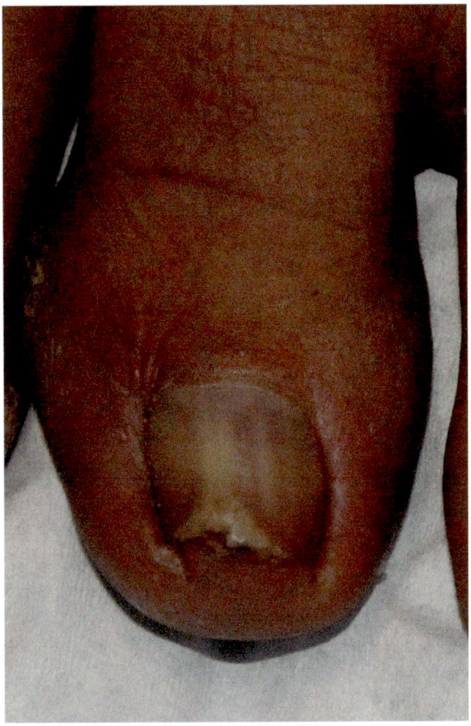

Fig. 43.4 40-Year-old female, Fitzpatrick type II, longitudinal leukonychia of unknown etiology, with longitudinal white bands of the left great toenail

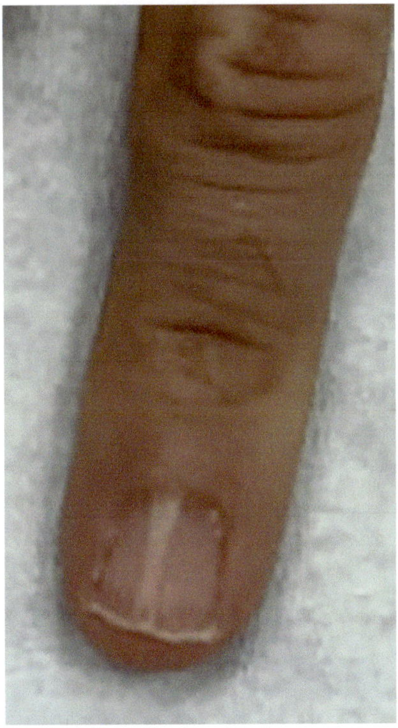

Fig. 43.5 53-Year-old male, Fitzpatrick type III, longitudinal leukonychia secondary to onychotillomania, with longitudinal white band and ridge of the left fifth fingernail

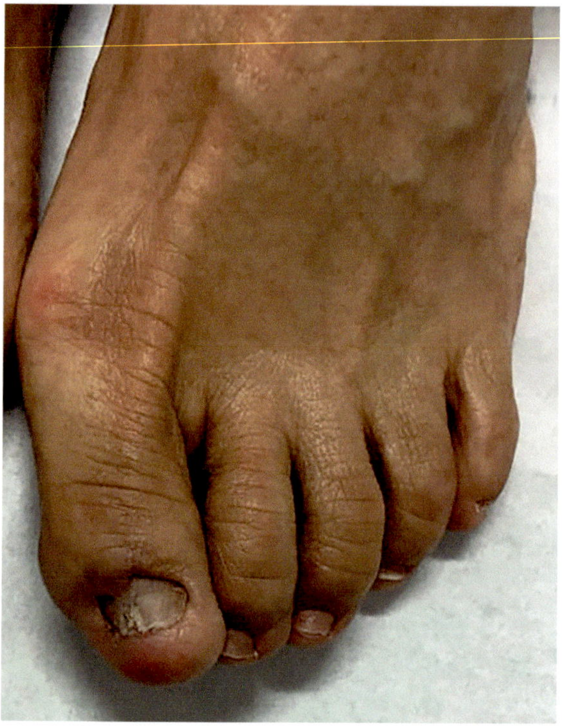

Fig. 43.6 74-Year-old female, Fitzpatrick type III, longitudinal leukonychia secondary to nail biopsy, with pterygium and longitudinal white band of the left great toenail

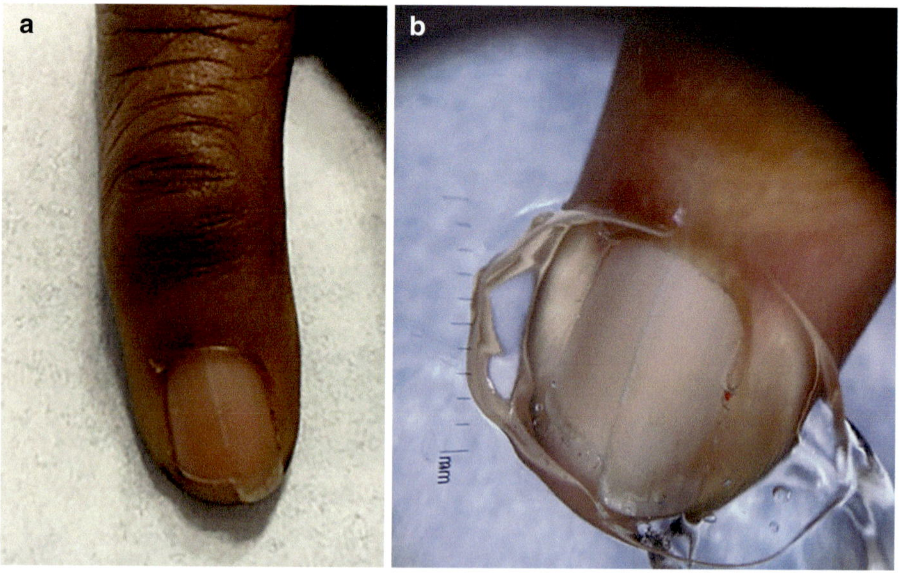

Fig. 43.7 (**a**) 57-Year-old female, Fitzpatrick type V, longitudinal leukonychia secondary to onychopapilloma, with longitudinal ridge and longitudinal white band of the right fifth fingernail. (**b**) 57-year-old female, Fitzpatrick type V, longitudinal leukonychia secondary to onychopapilloma, with longitudinal ridge and longitudinal white band of the right fifth fingernail. Dermoscopy of (**a**)

References

1. Iorizzo M, Starace M, Pasch MC. Leukonychia: what can white nails tell us? Am J Clin Dermatol. 2022;23(2):177–93.
2. Lipner SR, Scher RK. Evaluation of nail lines: color and shape hold clues. Cleve Clin J Med. 2016;83(5):385–91.
3. Burge SM, Wilkinson JD. Darier-White disease: a review of the clinical features of 163 patients. J Am Acad Dermatol. 1992;27:40–50.
4. Takagi A, Kamijo M, Ikeda S. Darier disease. J Dermatol. 2016;43(3):275–9.
5. Ben Lagha I, Ashack K, Khachemoune A. Hailey-Hailey disease: an update review with a focus on treatment data. Am J Clin Dermatol. 2020;21(1):49–68.
6. Kostaki D, Castillo JC, Ruzicka T, Sárdy M. Longitudinal leuconychia striata: is it a common sign in Hailey-Hailey and Darier disease? J Eur Acad Dermatol Venereol. 2014;28(1):126–7.
7. Lesort C, Debarbieux S, Duru G, Dalle S, Poulhalon N, Thomas L. Dermoscopic features of onychomatricoma: a study of 34 cases. Dermatology. 2015;231(2):177–83.
8. Aldrich CS, Hong CH, Groves L, Olsen C, Moss J, Darling TN. Acral lesions in tuberous sclerosis complex: insights into pathogenesis. J Am Acad Dermatol. 2010;63(2):244–51.
9. Halteh P, Magro C, Scher RK, Lipner SR. Onychopapilloma presenting as leukonychia: case report and review of the literature. Skin Appendage Disord. 2017;2(3–4):89–91.
10. de Berker DA, Perrin C, Baran R. Localized longitudinal erythronychia: diagnostic significance and physical explanation. Arch Dermatol. 2004;140(10):1253–7.
11. Conway J, Lipner SR. Onychomycosis presenting as longitudinal leukonychia. J Cutan Med Surg. 2023;27(3):298.
12. Jellinek NJ. Longitudinal erythronychia: suggestions for evaluation and management. J Am Acad Dermatol. 2011;64:167.e1–167.e11.
13. Munro CS. The phenotype of Darier's disease: penetrance and expressivity in adults and children. Br J Dermatol. 1992;127:126–30.
14. Bel B, Soudry-Faure A, Vabres P. Diagnostic value of nail examination in Hailey-Hailey disease. Eur J Dermatol. 2014;24(5):628–9.
15. Kim TR, Bae KN, Son JH, et al. Onychopapilloma: its clinical, dermoscopic and pathologic features. J Eur Acad Dermatol Venereol. 2022;36(11):2235–40.
16. Tosti A, Schneider SL, Ramirez-Quizon MN, Zaiac M, Miteva M. Clinical, dermoscopic, and pathologic features of onychopapilloma: a review of 47 cases. J Am Acad Dermatol. 2016;74(3):521–6.
17. Sánchez-Bernal J, Álvarez-Salafranca M, Ara-Martín M. Candy-cane nails. Actas Dermosifiliogr (Engl Ed). 2021; https://doi.org/10.1016/j.adengl.2021.06.001.

Partial Leukonychia

44

Kaya L. Curtis and Shari R. Lipner

44.1 Description of Disease

Partial leukonychia is characterized by incomplete white discoloration of the nail(s). Partial apparent leukonychia, including Terry's nails and half-and-half nails, is most frequently associated with systemic diseases.

44.2 Epidemiology

Epidemiologic studies on partial leukonychia have not been conducted. However, because common etiologies of partial leukonychia are systemic diseases, partial leukonychia is likely more prevalent among adult patients.

44.3 Risk Factors

Partial leukonychia is most frequently acquired in association with systemic diseases. Half-and-half nails (also known as Lindsay's nails) are a type of partial apparent leukonychia that are estimated to occur in 10–30% of patients with chronic renal disease [1–3], and may resolve with kidney transplantation [2]. Other comorbidities associated with half-and-half nails include Kawasaki disease, Crohn's disease, and zinc deficiency [4]. Terry's nails are a type of partial apparent leukonychia that are associated with hepatic cirrhosis (typically alcoholic), Reiter syndrome, heart failure, type 2 diabetes mellitus, hematologic disease, and peripheral vascular disease [5–7]. Rarely, partial leukonychia may be inherited. In Pakornphadungsit et al.'s literature review [8] of 43 inherited leukonychia cases, 15 patients (34.9%) had partial leukonychia, and 28 patients (65.1%) had total leukonychia. Partial pseudoleukonychia may be associated with onychomycosis or onycholysis [9].

S. R. Lipner, *Atlas of Nail Disorders Across All Skin Colors*,
https://doi.org/10.1007/978-3-031-74272-9_44

44.4 Clinical Features

Half-and-half nails are characterized by sharply demarcated white discoloration proximally (20–60% of the nail length) and pink or red-brown discoloration distally [4]. Terry's nails are characterized by apparent leukonychia involving >80% of the nail length proximally, with accompanying red-brown discoloration distally [4]. The lunula is frequently not visible in half-and-half nails and Terry's nails [9]. All nails are typically involved in partial leukonychia [9].

44.5 Clinical Features in Skin of Color

Distinct clinical presentations of inherited total leukonychia in skin of color have not been characterized. White discoloration may be more difficult to visualize in patients with higher Fitzpatrick skin types.

44.6 Requirements for Diagnosis

Partial leukonychia is a clinical diagnosis. Disappearance of white discoloration with pressure is suggestive of apparent leukonychia, whereas persistence of white discoloration with pressure is suggestive of true leukonychia or pseudoleukonychia. Terry's nails and half-and-half nails are characterized as partial apparent leukonychias [4], and therefore discoloration will disappear with pressure. In patients with partial pseudoleukonychia, a nail clipping may be performed to evaluate for onychomycosis.

44.7 Cases

Figures 44.1, 44.2, 44.3, 44.4, 44.5, 44.6, 44.7, and 44.8 demonstrate the presentation of partial leukonychia in a clinical setting.

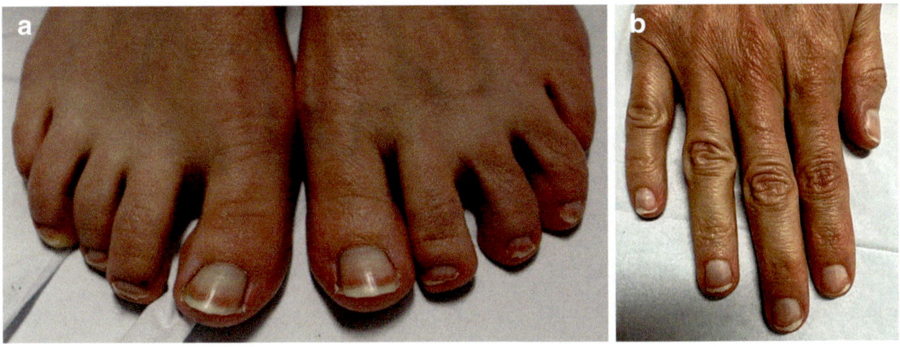

Fig. 44.1 (**a**) 54-Year-old female, Fitzpatrick type II, partial leukonychia (Terry's nails), with toenails with white discoloration involving 80% of the nail plates and associated distal pink-brown transverse brown bands. (**b**) 54-Year-old female, Fitzpatrick type II, partial leukonychia (Terry's nails), with fingernails with white discoloration involving 80% of the nail plates and associated distal pink-brown transverse brown bands

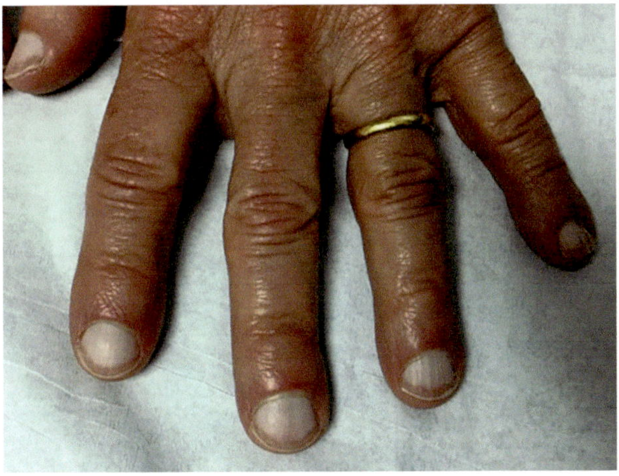

Fig. 44.2 75-Year-old male, Fitzpatrick type II, partial leukonychia (Terry's nails), with fingernails with white discoloration involving 80% of the nail plates and associated distal pink-brown transverse brown bands

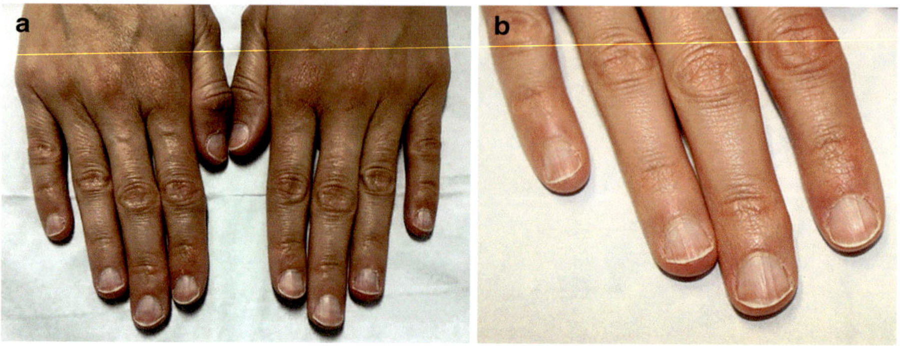

Fig. 44.3 (**a**) 32-Year-old female, Fitzpatrick type III, partial leukonychia (Terry's nails), with white discoloration involving 80% of the nail plates and associated distal pink-brown transverse brown bands. (**b**) 32-Year-old female, Fitzpatrick type III, partial leukonychia (Terry's nails), with white discoloration involving 80% of the nail plates and associated distal pink-brown transverse brown bands

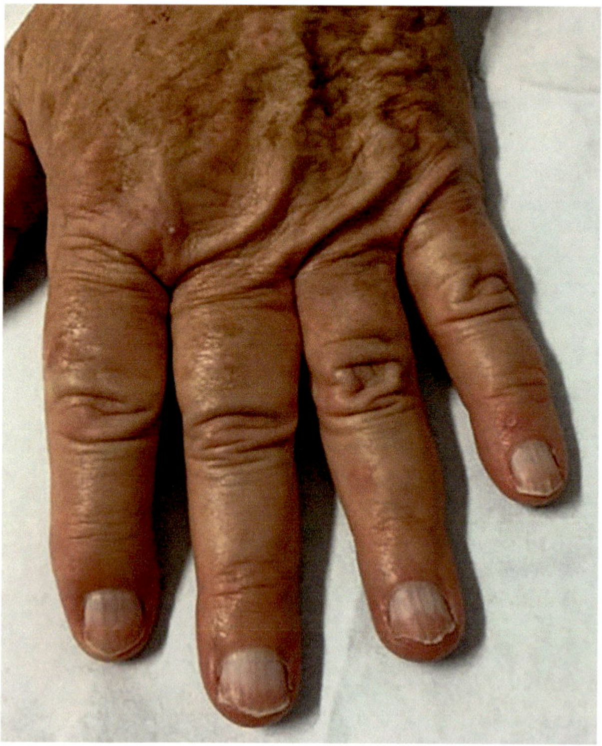

Fig. 44.4 86-Year-old male, Fitzpatrick type III, partial true leukonychia, with fingernails with white discoloration of the proximal nail plates. The white color did not blanch with pressure. The patient had underlying brittle nail syndrome

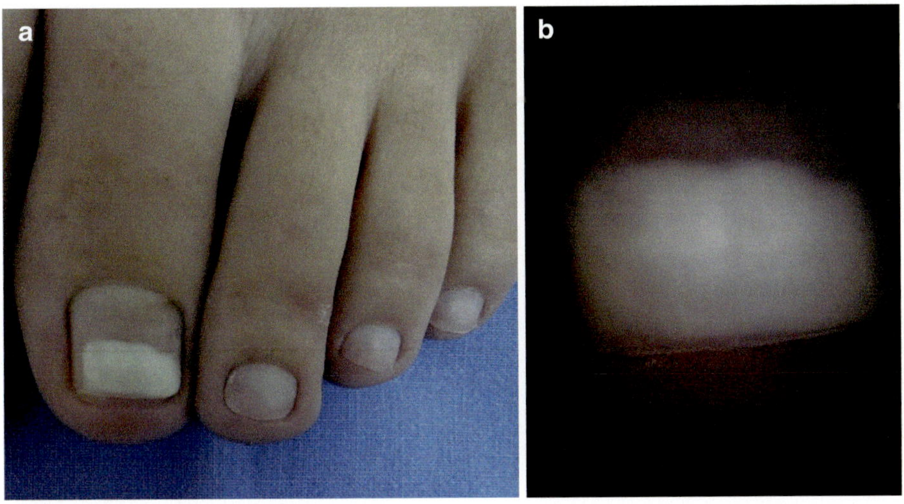

Fig. 44.5 (**a**) Adult patient, Fitzpatrick type IV, partial leukonychia, with white discoloration of the distal half of the nail plate of the left great toenail. The white color did not blanch with pressure. (**b**) Adult patient, Fitzpatrick type IV, partial leukonychia, with white discoloration of the distal half of the nail plate of the left great toenail. Dermo scopy of (**a**). The white color did not blanch with pressure

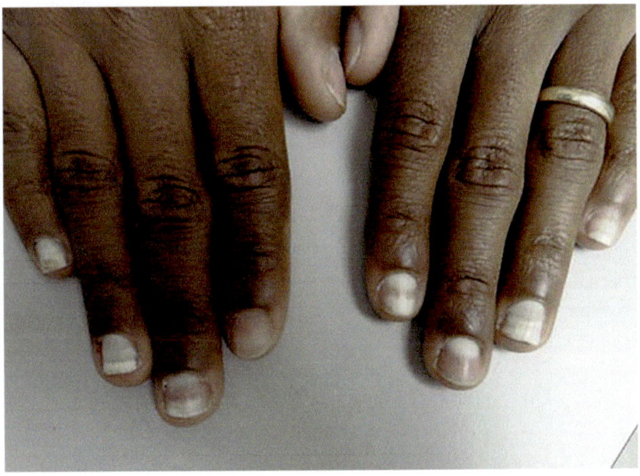

Fig. 44.6 25-Year-old male, Fitzpatrick type V, idiopathic total (leukonychia totalis) and partial (leukonychia partialis) whitening of seven fingernails (*from* Canavan et al. [10]; *with permission*)

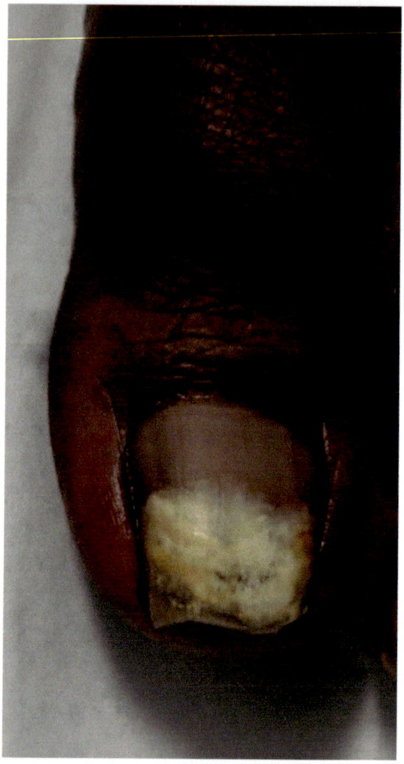

Fig. 44.7 56-Year-old female, Fitzpatrick type VI, partial leukonychia, with white discoloration of the distal half of the nail plate of the left great toenail, likely secondary to trauma from pedicures

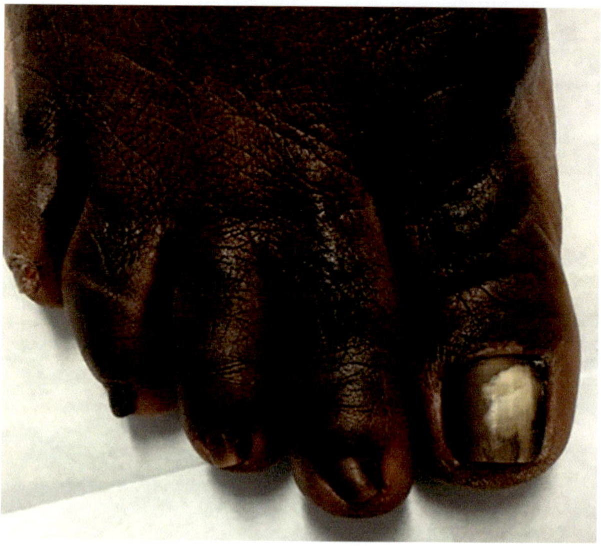

Fig. 44.8 57-Year-old female, Fitzpatrick type VI, partial leukonychia, with partial white discoloration of the nail plate of the right great toenail secondary to trauma

References

1. Saray Y, Seckin D, Gulec AT, Akgun S, Haberal M. Nail disorders in hemodialysis patients and renal transplant recipients: a case-control study. J Am Acad Dermatol. 2004;50(2):197–202.
2. Lubach D, Strubbe J, Schmidt J. The "half and half nail" phenomenon in chronic hemodialysis patients. Dermatologica. 1982;164(5):350–3.
3. Masmoudi A, Hajjaji Darouiche M, Ben Salah H, Ben Hmida M, Turki H. Cutaneous abnormalities in patients with end stage renal failure on chronic hemodialysis: a study of 458 patients. J Dermatol Case Rep. 2014;8(4):86–94.
4. Lipner SR, Scher RK. Evaluation of nail lines: color and shape hold clues. Cleve Clin J Med. 2016;83(5):385–91.
5. Jemec GB, Kollerup G, Jensen LB, Mogensen S. Nail abnormalities in nondermatologic patients: prevalence and possible role as diagnostic aids. J Am Acad Dermatol. 1995;32(6):977–81.
6. Terry R. White nails in hepatic cirrhosis. Lancet. 1954;266:757–9.
7. Coskun BK, Saral Y, Ozturk P, Coskun N. Reiter syndrome accompanied by Terry nail. J Eur Acad Dermatol Venereol. 2005;19(1):87–9.
8. Pakornphadungsit K, Suchonwanit P, Sriphojanart T, Chayavichitsilp P. Hereditary leukonychia totalis: a case report and review of the literature. Case Rep Dermatol. 2018;10(1):82–8.
9. Iorizzo M, Starace M, Pasch MC. Leukonychia: what can white nails tell us? Am J Clin Dermatol. 2022;23(2):177–93.
10. Canavan T, Tosti A, Mallory H, McKay K, Cantrell W, Elewski B. An idiopathic leukonychia totalis and leukonychia partialis case report and review of the literature. Skin Appendage Disord. 2015;1(1):38–42.

Total Leukonychia

45

Kaya L. Curtis and Shari R. Lipner

45.1 Description of Disease

Total leukonychia is characterized by complete whiteness of all nails. The pathogenesis for inherited total leukonychia is a mutation in phospholipase C delta-1 (*PLCD1*) gene, which encodes a phosphoinositide-specific PLCD1 subunit, an enzyme involved in phosphoinositide metabolism [1]. Pathogenesis in acquired total leukonychia has been hypothesized to be neurovascular deterioration and edema of the fingers causing chronic trauma to the nail matrix [2].

45.2 Epidemiology

Inherited total leukonychia is rare. Inherited total leukonychia has a male predilection, but the reasons are unknown, and Y-chromosomal inheritance with variable penetrance has been hypothesized [3]. Acquired total leukonychia is more common than inherited total leukonychia [3].

45.3 Risk Factors

Total leukonychia may be acquired or inherited. In Pakornphadungsit et al.'s literature review [1] of 43 congenital leukonychia cases, family history was reported in 79% of cases. Inherited leukonychia is typically inherited in an autosomal dominant manner [1], though there have been few case reports [4] of an autosomal recessive inherited pattern. Acquired total apparent leukonychia has many etiologies, including lymphedema and selenium deficiency [3]. Total pseudoleukonychia may be caused by onychomycosis or onycholysis [3]. Idiopathic acquired total leukonychia cases have also been reported [5–9].

S. R. Lipner, *Atlas of Nail Disorders Across All Skin Colors*,
https://doi.org/10.1007/978-3-031-74272-9_45

45.4 Clinical Features

Inherited total leukonychia is characterized by milky, chalky, or porcelain white nails. All of the nails are typically involved. In isolated hereditary total leukonychia, there are no associated non-nail clinical features. However, total leukonychia has been reported with hereditary syndromes, including acrokeratosis verruciformis of Hopf, palmoplantar keratoderma with deafness, and keratoderma-hypotrichosis-leukonychia totalis syndrome [3]. In Pakornphadungsit et al.'s literature review [1] of 43 inherited leukonychia cases, 28 patients (65.1%) had total leukonychia, while 15 patients (34.9%) had partial leukonychia.

45.5 Clinical Features in Skin of Color

Distinct clinical presentations of inherited total leukonychia in skin of color have not been characterized. White discoloration may be more difficult to visualize in patients with darker Fitzpatrick skin types.

45.6 Requirements for Diagnosis

Total leukonychia is a clinical diagnosis. Disappearance of white discoloration with pressure is suggestive of apparent leukonychia, whereas persistence of white discoloration upon pressure is suggestive of true leukonychia or pseudoleukonychia. In patients with total pseudoleukonychia of a few nails, a nail clipping may be conducted to evaluate for onychomycosis.

45.7 Cases

Figures 45.1, 45.2, 45.3, 45.4, 45.5, and 45.6 demonstrate the presentation of total leukonychia in a clinical setting.

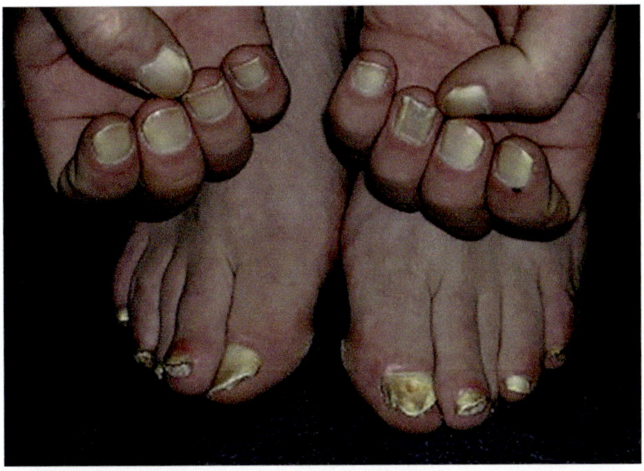

Fig. 45.1 Adult male patient, Fitzpatrick type I, leukonychia totalis (*from* Le Corre et al. [10]; *with permission*)

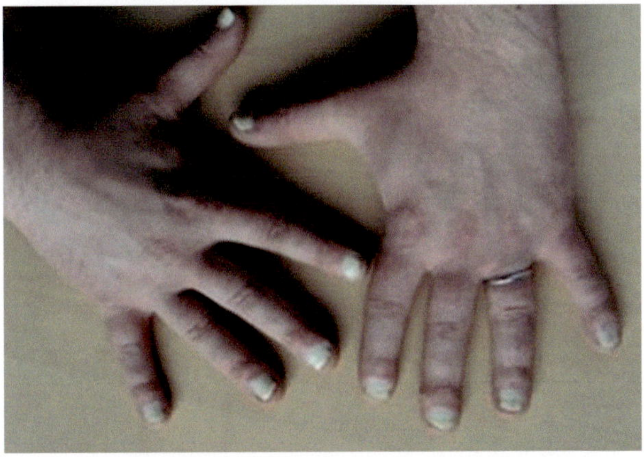

Fig. 45.2 29-Year-old male, Fitzpatrick type II, with leukonychia (hands) (*from* Boulé et al. [11]; *with permission*)

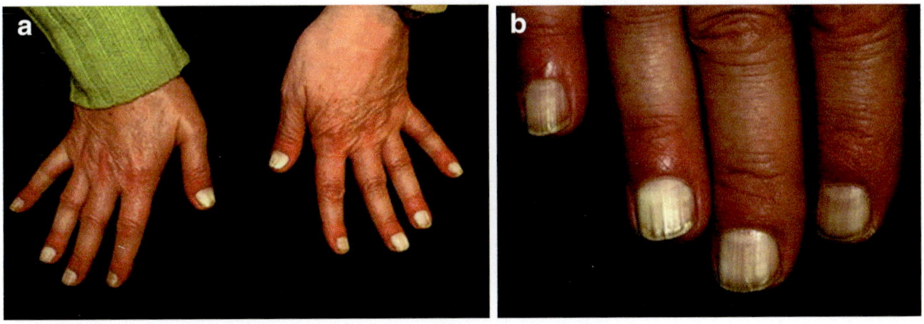

Fig. 45.3 (**a**) 59-Year-old male, Fitzpatrick type III, total leukonychia, with complete whitening of all ten nail plates on the hands. (**b**) 59-year-old male, Fitzpatrick type III, total leukonychia, with detail showing true leukonychia at closer range (*from* Pielasinski-Rodríguez et al. [9]; *with permission*)

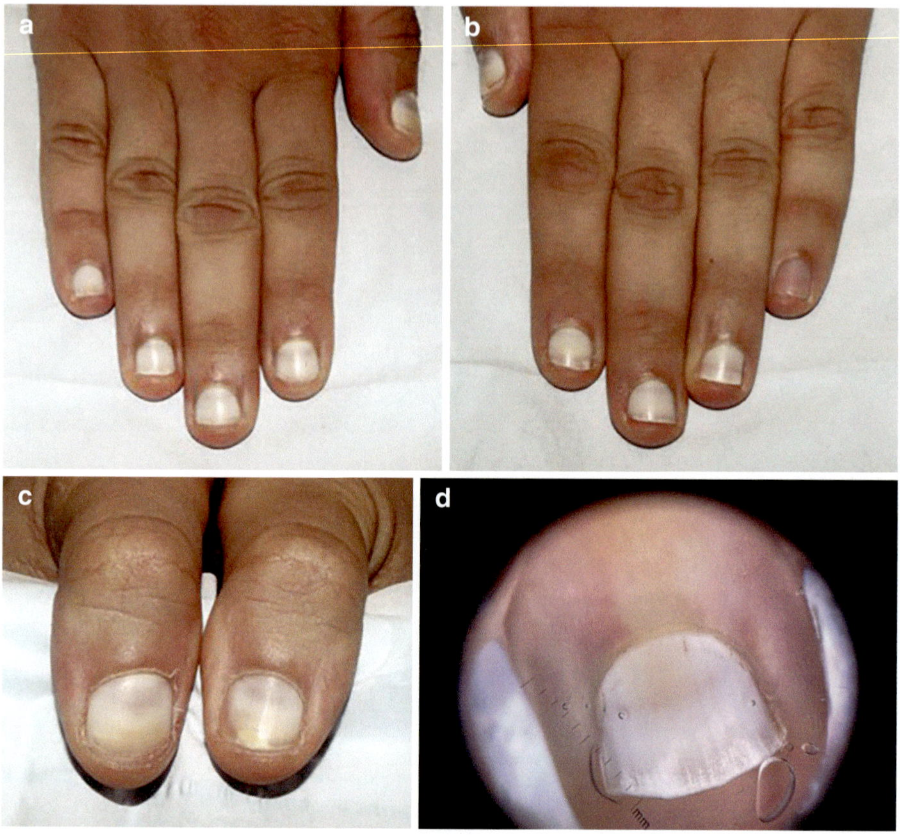

Fig. 45.4 (**a**) 40-Year-old male, Fitzpatrick type IV, total leukonychia, with complete white discoloration of all right fingernails. (**b**) 40-year-old male, Fitzpatrick type IV, total leukonychia, with complete white discoloration of left first, second, third, and fourth fingernails. (**c**) 40-year-old male, Fitzpatrick type IV, total leukonychia, with complete white discoloration of bilateral thumbnails. (**d**) 40-year-old male, Fitzpatrick type IV, total leukonychia, with complete white discoloration of fingernail. Dermoscopy of (**c**)

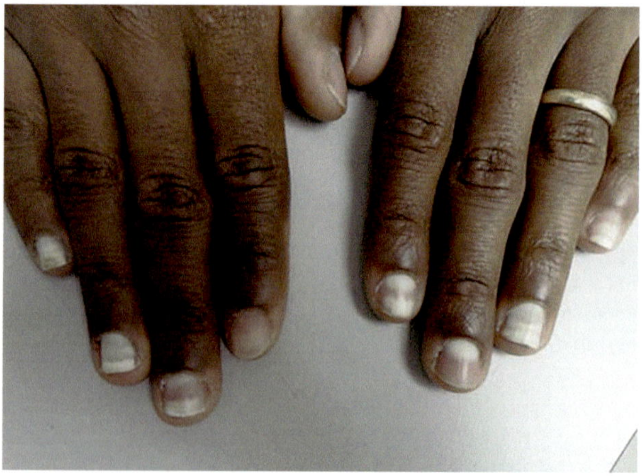

Fig. 45.5 25-Year-old male, Fitzpatrick type V, idiopathic total (leukonychia totalis) and partial (leukonychia partialis) whitening of seven fingernails (*from* Canavan et al. [12]; *with permission*)

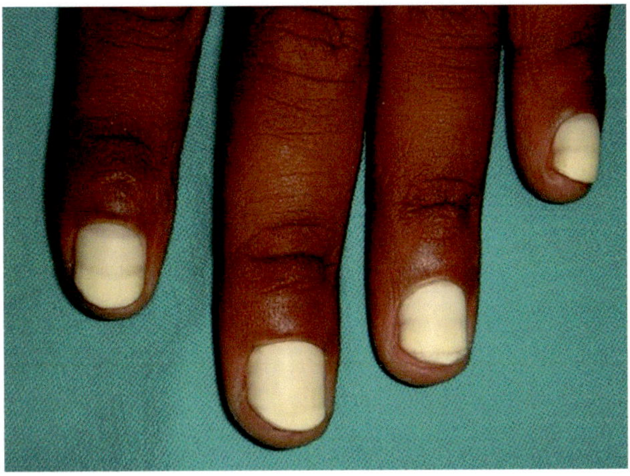

Fig. 45.6 20-Year-old male, Fitzpatrick type VI, total leukonychia, with clinical examination showing total leukonychia in all fingernails (*from* Dlova and Tosti [8]; *with permission*)

References

1. Pakornphadungsit K, Suchonwanit P, Sriphojanart T, Chayavichitsilp P. Hereditary leukonychia totalis: a case report and review of the literature. Case Rep Dermatol. 2018;10(1):82–8.
2. Vanhooteghem O, Andre J, Halkin V, Song M. Leuconychia in reflex sympathetic dystrophy: a chance association? Br J Dermatol. 1998;139(2):355–6.
3. Iorizzo M, Starace M, Pasch MC. Leukonychia: what can white nails tell us? Am J Clin Dermatol. 2022;23(2):177–93.
4. Frydman M, Cohen HA. Leukonychia totalis in two sibs. Am J Med Genet. 1993;47(4):540–1.
5. Das A, Bandyopadhyay D, Podder I. Idiopathic acquired true leukonychia totalis. Indian J Dermatol. 2016;61(1):127.
6. Bakry OA, Attia AM, Shehata WA. Idiopathic acquired true leukonychia totalis. Pediatr Dermatol. 2014;31:404–5.
7. Claudel CD, Zic JA, Boyd AS. Idiopathic leukonychia totalis and partialis in a 12-year-old patient. J Am Acad Dermatol. 2001;44:379–80.
8. Dlova NC, Tosti A. Idiopathic acquired true total and subtotal leukonychia: report of two cases. Int J Dermatol. 2014;53:e261–3.
9. Pielasinski-Rodríguez Ú, Machan S, Fariña-Sabaris MC, Requena-Caballero L. Acquired total leukonychia in a patient with human immunodeficiency virus infection. Actas Dermosifiliogr. 2012;103(10):934–5.
10. Le Corre Y, Steff M, Croue A, Filmon R, Verret JL, Le Clech C. Hereditary leukonychia totalis, acanthosis-nigricans-like lesions and hair dysplasia: a new syndrome? Eur J Med Genet. 2009;52(4):229–33.
11. Boulé S, Fressart V, Laux D, et al. Expanding the phenotype associated with a desmoplakin dominant mutation: Carvajal/Naxos syndrome associated with leukonychia and oligodontia. Int J Cardiol. 2012;161(1):50–2.
12. Canavan T, Tosti A, Mallory H, McKay K, Cantrell W, Elewski B. An idiopathic leukonychia totalis and leukonychia partialis case report and review of the literature. Skin Appendage Disord. 2015;1(1):38–42.

Part X

Nail Disorders Caused by Medications and Toxins

Nail Dystrophies Secondary to Chemotherapies

46

Eden Axler and Shari R. Lipner

46.1 Description of Disease

Nail toxicity is an underrecognized side effect associated with chemotherapy [1, 2]. The cytotoxic effects of antineoplastic medications, particularly those with antimitotic activity, are thought to disrupt the normal growth of nail matrix cells, triggering nail changes [2, 3]. As a result, nail toxicities commonly involve multiple nails and occur in conjunction with drug administration [4].

46.2 Epidemiology

Chemotherapy-induced nail changes are common, and nail findings may vary significantly depending on the type of drug administered during cancer treatment. In a cross-sectional study of 500 chemotherapy patients, 37.6% experienced nail changes [5]. Patients undergoing prolonged chemotherapy courses or receiving higher doses of medications may be more likely to experience nail toxicity.

46.2.1 Taxanes

Taxanes, including paclitaxel and docetaxel, are commonly associated with nail toxicity. In a prospective study of 84 patients undergoing docetaxel treatment, 26% exhibited nail changes, with an association between incidence of nail changes with weekly administration (OR = 0.232; 95% CI: 0.067–0.805; $P < 0.02$) and number of chemotherapy cycles (OR = 0.084; 95% CI: 0.014–0.510; $P < 0.01$) [6].

S. R. Lipner, *Atlas of Nail Disorders Across All Skin Colors*,
https://doi.org/10.1007/978-3-031-74272-9_46

46.2.2 Anthracyclines

In a prospective study of 407 patients who received liposomal doxorubicin, nail and periungual changes occurred in 13% of patients [7].

46.2.3 Targeted Therapies

In a prospective study of 66 patients taking ibrutinib for chronic lymphoid leukemia, 66.6% reported nail changes within 6.5 months of starting treatment [8]. In a retrospective study of 2107 patients who received treatment with EGFR inhibitors, the overall incidence of all-grade nail toxicity was 17.2% [9].

46.3 Risk Factors

46.3.1 Type of Chemotherapy

Certain chemotherapy drugs, particularly taxanes (such as paclitaxel and docetaxel) and anthracyclines (such as doxorubicin), are commonly associated with nail changes. Higher doses of chemotherapy and prolonged treatment durations increase the likelihood of nail adverse effects [6]. The frequency and intensity of chemotherapy cycles also impact the severity of nail changes. More frequent or higher dosage treatment schedules may lead to cumulative damage to the nail matrix and bed, resulting in more severe nail toxicity [3, 10].

46.3.2 Nail Care Practices

Improper nail care during chemotherapy can exacerbate nail toxicity. Trauma to the nail bed or cuticles, such as aggressive trimming or picking at the nails, can increase susceptibility to nail damage and infection. Patients are advised to maintain gentle nail care practices and avoid activities that may cause trauma to the nails [11].

46.4 Clinical Features

46.4.1 Pigmentation Changes

Melanonychia arises from agents stimulating nail matrix melanocytes, appearing as diffuse black or dark gray pigmentation, or longitudinal brown/black bands [12]. Transverse melanonychia typically emerges one to two months after beginning treatment, presenting as distinct transverse bands that correlate with chemotherapy cycles [3]. Transverse leukonychia is another presentation associated with chemotherapy, presenting as transverse white bands parallel to the lunula [12].

46.4.2 Onycholysis

Onycholysis refers to the separation of the nail plate from the nail bed and may occur in isolation or in conjunction with subungual abscesses or purpura. Taxanes sometimes trigger a distinct type of hand-foot syndrome (HFS) known as "periarticular thenar erythema with onycholysis," characterized by reddish-purple erythema and concurrent onycholysis [5]. Onycholysis may become complicated by *Pseudomonas aeruginosa* colonization, leading to green discoloration and/or pus formation under the nail plate [13].

46.4.3 Nail Growth Disorders

Chemotherapy drugs can lead to altered nail growth, including Beau's lines and onychomadesis. Beau's lines are transverse grooves in the nail plate that result from a temporary halt in epithelial cell growth. The depth of these grooves reflects the severity of damage to matrix keratinocytes, while their width indicates the duration of the injury [10]. Generally, each groove corresponds to a single systemic insult [10]. Onychomadesis is a more severe condition on this spectrum, characterized by the complete detachment of the proximal and distal nail plates, leading to eventual shedding of the nail plate [11].

46.4.4 Nail Infections

Chemotherapy-induced acute paronychia (CAP) is characterized by inflammation of the proximal and/or lateral nail folds, presenting with pain and erythema. Secondary infections may occur, potentially affecting the nail matrix and resulting in onychodystrophy [4]. The prevalence of CAP varies, affecting between 10% and 30% of patients treated with EGFR inhibitors [1].

46.4.5 Vascular Disorders

Pyogenic granuloma (PG) is a benign vascular proliferation commonly associated with chemotherapy or secondary to paronychia [14]. It typically presents as a rapidly expanding reddish or purplish nodule on the skin or mucous membranes. Drug-induced PGs occur on the lateral nail folds and can extend into the subungual space and nail bed [15]. Possible complications of PG include ulceration and bleeding, and therefore treatment is necessary [14].

46.5 Requirements for Diagnosis

Diagnosing chemotherapy-induced nail toxicity requires a thorough assessment of nail changes. The evaluation begins with obtaining a detailed medical history, focusing on the types of chemotherapy drugs administered, their dosages, and the duration of treatment. The nails are inspected for signs of leukonychia, melanonychia, onycholysis, Beau's lines, or any other characteristic alterations. In some cases, nail changes associated with chemotherapy may appear similarly to nail dystrophy related to onychomycosis or nail psoriasis, and a nail clipping may be required for definitive diagnosis. In most cases, a nail biopsy is not required. Patients are reassured that nail changes associated with chemotherapy are not indicative of their cancer but are instead a consequence of their medication.

46.6 Cases

Figures 46.1, 46.2, 46.3, 46.4, 46.5, 46.6, 46.7, and 46.8 demonstrate the presentation of nail dystrophies secondary to chemotherapies in a clinical setting.

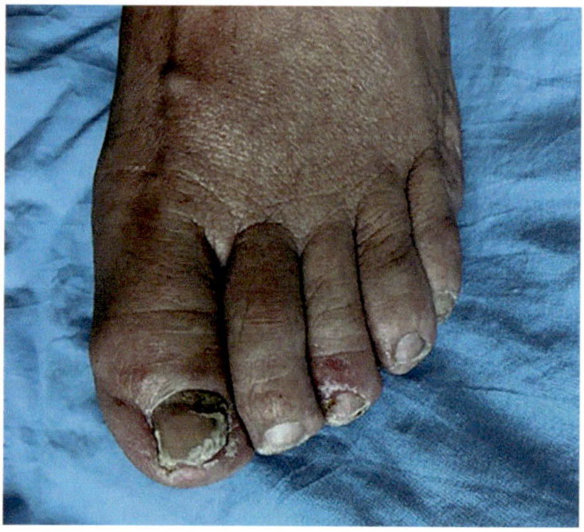

Fig. 46.1 A 71-year-old male, Fitzpatrick type II, chemotherapy-associated paronychia. Patient is on afatinib for stage IV lung adenocarcinoma with mild erythema of nail folds of the left great toenail and left third toenail. There is yellowing and crumbling of the toenails and granulation tissue present on the nail fold of the left third toe (*courtesy of* Dr. Beth N. McLellan; *From* Gupta and Lipner [1]; *with permission*)

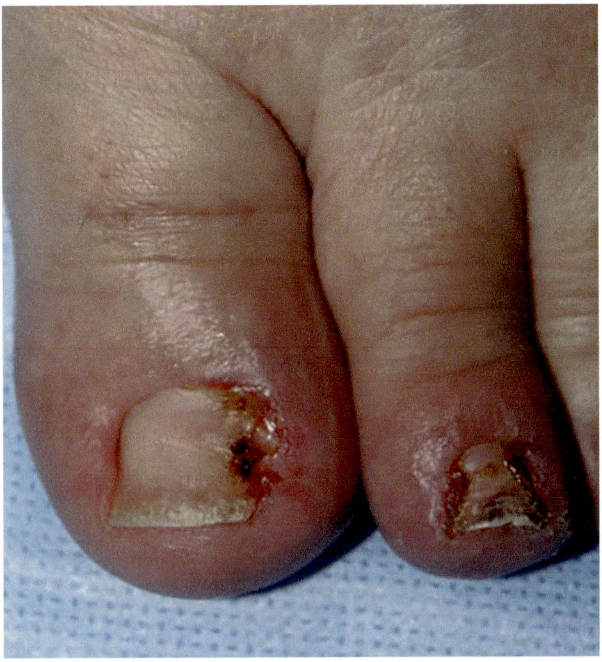

Fig. 46.2 A 68-year-old female, Fitzpatrick type II, on osimertinib for non-small cell lung cancer with paronychia of the right first and second toes (*courtesy of* Dr. Mario Lacouture; *From* Gupta and Lipner [1]; *with permission*)

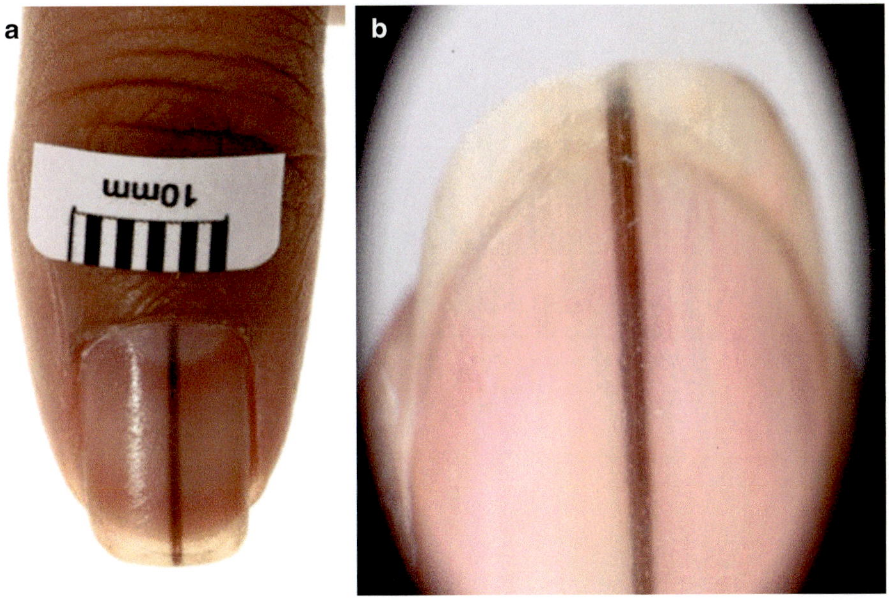

Fig. 46.3 (**a**) A 36-year-old female, Fitzpatrick type IV, with longitudinal melanonychia of the left thumbnail after two courses of 5-fluorouracil, epirubicin, cyclophosphamide, and docetaxel chemotherapy. (**b**) Dermoscopy with a 1 mm brown-gray band with regular lines (*from* Hussain et al. [16]; CC-BY 4.0, https://creativecommons.org/licenses/by/4.0)

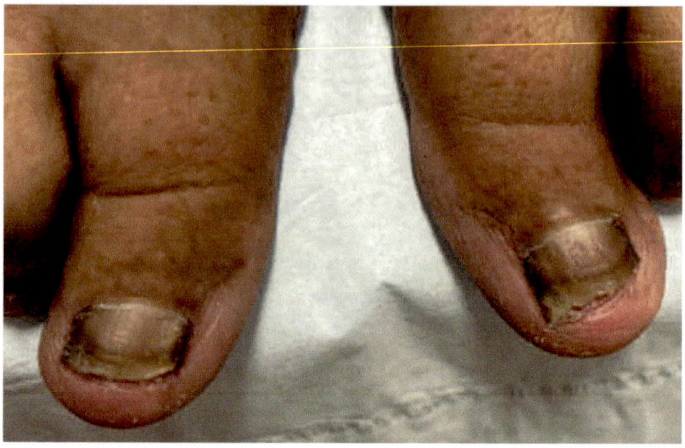

Fig. 46.4 A 74-year-old female, Fitzpatrick type IV, transverse melanonychia after treatment with capecitabine chemotherapy for colorectal cancer

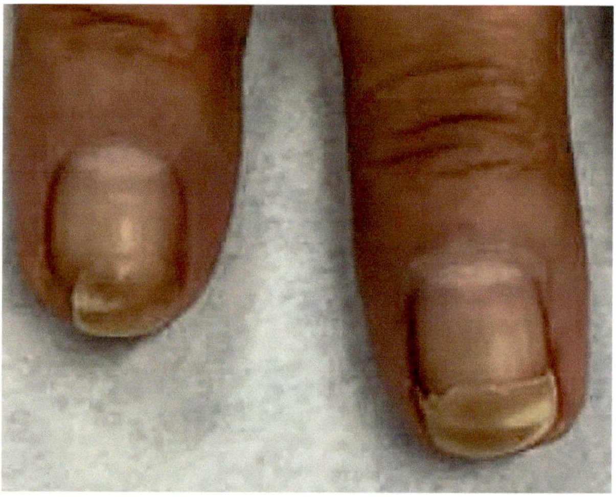

Fig. 46.5 A 78-year-old female, Fitzpatrick type IV, with onychomadesis secondary to decitabine for acute myeloid leukemia. Left second and third fingernails some with distal detachment of nail plate

Fig. 46.6 A 49-year-old female, Fitzpatrick type V, with longitudinal melanonychia secondary to doxorubicin for treatment of breast cancer. Left second fingernail with brown longitudinal band 4 mm proximally, 3 mm distally

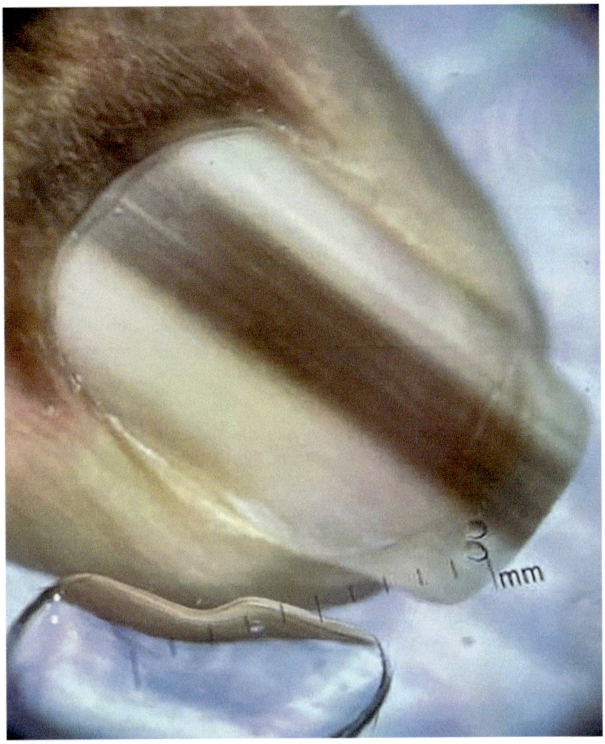

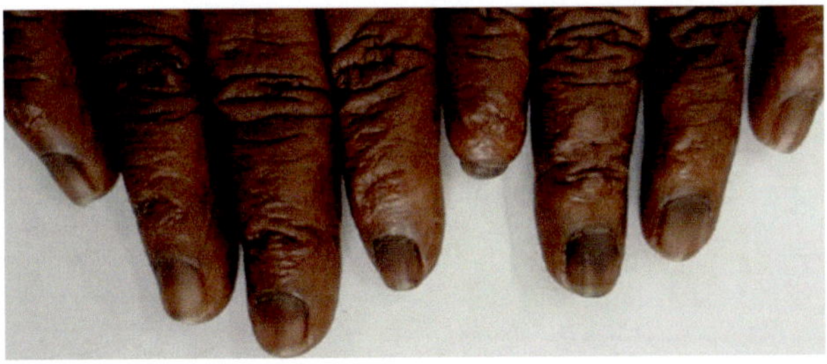

Fig. 46.7 Female, Fitzpatrick type V, with diffuse melanonychia of all fingernails due to cisplatin and paclitaxel combination chemotherapy

Fig. 46.8 Female, Fitzpatrick type V, presenting with Beau's lines and melanonychia in both thumbnails due to paclitaxel, 5 fluorouracil, doxorubicin, cyclophosphamide, and trastuzumab combination chemotherapy

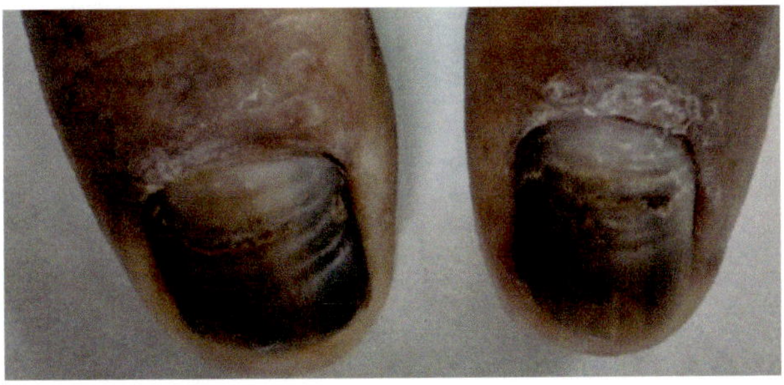

References

1. Gupta MK, Lipner SR. Review of chemotherapy-associated paronychia. Int J Dermatol. 2022;61(4):410–5. Epub 2021/07/10. https://doi.org/10.1111/ijd.15740.
2. Gilbar P, Hain A, Peereboom VM. Nail toxicity induced by cancer chemotherapy. J Oncol Pharm Pract. 2009;15(3):143–55. Epub 2009/01/28. https://doi.org/10.1177/1078155208100450.
3. Hinds G, Thomas VD. Malignancy and cancer treatment-related hair and nail changes. Dermatol Clin. 2008;26(1):59–68, viii. Epub 2007/11/21. https://doi.org/10.1016/j.det.2007.08.003.
4. Piraccini BM, Iorizzo M. Drug reactions affecting the nail unit: diagnosis and management. Dermatol Clin. 2007;25(2):215–21, vii. Epub 2007/04/14. https://doi.org/10.1016/j.det.2007.01.006.
5. Trivedi M, Mehta RD, Kumar HS, Ghiya BC, Soni P, et al. Nail changes caused by chemotherapy among cancer patients: a cross-sectional study of Northwest Rajasthan. Indian Dermatol Online J. 2020;11(6):953–8. Epub 2020/12/22. https://doi.org/10.4103/idoj.IDOJ_84_20.
6. Hong J, Park SH, Choi SJ, Lee SH, Lee KC, Lee JI, Kyung SY, An CH, Lee SP, Park JW, Jeong SH, Nam E, Bang SM, Cho EK, Shin DB, Lee JH. Nail toxicity after treatment with docetaxel: a prospective analysis in patients with advanced non-small cell lung cancer. Jpn J Clin Oncol. 2007;37(6):424–8. Epub 2007/06/23. https://doi.org/10.1093/jjco/hym042.
7. Vaccaro M, Barbuzza O, Guarneri F, Guarneri B. Nail and periungual toxicity following capecitabine therapy. Br J Clin Pharmacol. 2008;66(2):325–6. Epub 2008/04/04. https://doi.org/10.1111/j.1365-2125.2008.03174.x.
8. Bitar C, Farooqui MZ, Valdez J, Saba NS, Soto S, Bray A, Marti G, Wiestner A, Cowen EW. Hair and nail changes during long-term therapy with ibrutinib for chronic lymphocytic leukemia. JAMA Dermatol. 2016;152(6):698–701. Epub 2016/03/17. https://doi.org/10.1001/jamadermatol.2016.0225.
9. Garden BC, Wu S, Lacouture ME. The risk of nail changes with epidermal growth factor receptor inhibitors: a systematic review of the literature and meta-analysis. J Am Acad Dermatol. 2012;67(3):400–8. Epub 2011/11/18. https://doi.org/10.1016/j.jaad.2011.10.009.
10. Minisini AM, Tosti A, Sobrero AF, Mansutti M, Piraccini BM, Sacco C, Puglisi F. Taxane-induced nail changes: incidence, clinical presentation and outcome. Ann Oncol. 2003;14(2):333–7. Epub 2003/02/04. https://doi.org/10.1093/annonc/mdg050.
11. Robert C, Sibaud V, Mateus C, Verschoore M, Charles C, Lanoy E, Baran R. Nail toxicities induced by systemic anticancer treatments. Lancet Oncol. 2015;16(4):e181–9. Epub 2015/04/08. https://doi.org/10.1016/s1470-2045(14)71133-7.
12. Iorizzo M, Starace M, Pasch MC. Leukonychia: what can white nails tell us? Am J Clin Dermatol. 2022;23(2):177–93. Epub 2022/02/04. https://doi.org/10.1007/s40257-022-00671-6.
13. Iorizzo M. Tips to treat the 5 most common nail disorders: brittle nails, onycholysis, paronychia, psoriasis, onychomycosis. Dermatol Clin. 2015;33(2):175–83. Epub 2015/04/02. https://doi.org/10.1016/j.det.2014.12.001.
14. Wollina U. Systemic drug-induced chronic paronychia and periungual pyogenic granuloma. Indian Dermatol Online J. 2018;9(5):293–8. Epub 2018/09/28. https://doi.org/10.4103/idoj.IDOJ_133_18.
15. Piraccini BM, Iorizzo M, Starace M, Tosti A. Drug-induced nail diseases. Dermatol Clin. 2006;24(3):387–91. Epub 2006/06/27. https://doi.org/10.1016/j.det.2006.03.004.
16. Hussain F, Gnanappiragasam D, Shaffrali F. Chemotherapy-related striate melanonychia: a case report. J Med Case Rep. 2021;15(1):27. Epub 2021/01/31. https://doi.org/10.1186/s13256-020-02612-5.

Nail Dystrophies Secondary to Medications Other Than Chemotherapies

47

Eden Axler and Shari R. Lipner

47.1 Description of Disease

Drug-induced nail toxicity is defined as nail manifestations triggered by medications that are administered systemically, topically, or intralesionally [1]. These changes commonly involve multiple nails and align with the timing of drug intake [2]. They may affect any part of the nail unit, including the nail matrix, nail bed, nail plate, and/or periungual tissue [3, 4]. Additionally, drug deposition at the dermal level may contribute to nail plate pigmentation, often coinciding with skin or mucous membrane pigmentation [4]. While chemotherapeutic agent nail toxicities (discussed in Chap. 48) have been well documented, non-chemotherapeutic agent-induced nail toxicities are likely underreported, and existing literature is mainly limited to case reports and case series. These nail changes may cause cosmetic concerns, discomfort, or functional limitations [3]. In this chapter, we review non-chemotherapy-induced nail changes.

47.2 Epidemiology

The epidemiology of drug-induced nail toxicity varies depending on the classes of drugs administered, with certain medications being more commonly associated with nail findings than others. The prevalence is difficult to ascertain due to under-reporting and variability in clinical recognition. However, it is known that certain drug classes are often associated with nail changes.

47.2.1 Antibiotics

Antibiotics, especially tetracyclines and fluoroquinolones, have been associated with nail toxicities [5–8]. These antibiotics are commonly used to treat a wide range

S. R. Lipner, *Atlas of Nail Disorders Across All Skin Colors*,
https://doi.org/10.1007/978-3-031-74272-9_47

of bacterial infections, including respiratory tract infections, urinary tract infections, and skin infections. Antibiotics are prescribed for all age groups, therefore it is important to monitor patients of all ages taking these medications for nail changes.

47.2.2 Retinoids

Retinoids are primarily prescribed for acne, as well as inflammatory skin diseases. Retinoids, including isotretinoin and acitretin, may exhibit a range of nail toxicities due to their effects on keratinization [9, 10]. Retinoid-induced nail changes may occur in younger patients since they are more often treated for acne than adults. In patients with psoriasis, it may be difficult to differentiate drug-induced nail changes from psoriatic nail disease.

47.2.3 Anticonvulsants

Several anticonvulsants, including carbamazepine, valproic acid, and trimethadione, have been associated with nail toxicity [11]. Patients with epilepsy who are prescribed anti-seizure medications should be assessed for nail changes.

47.2.4 Antimalarials

Antimalarials, including chloroquine and hydroxychloroquine, have been linked to nail toxicity due to drug deposition in the dermis [4, 12]. While these drugs are used as both prophylaxis and treatment for malaria, they are also used to treat autoimmune diseases, including systemic lupus erythematosus and rheumatoid arthritis. Therefore, patients from malaria endemic regions and travelers to these countries, and patients with autoimmune disease, may develop nail changes from use of these medications.

47.2.5 Antiretrovirals

Lamivudine, azidothymidine, and indinavir have been associated with various nail toxicities [13]. Patients with human immunodeficiency virus (HIV) should be monitored for nail changes while taking antiretroviral therapy.

47.2.6 Beta Blockers

Beta blockers are commonly prescribed for cardiovascular conditions, including hypertension, arrhythmias, and heart failure, and may impair digital perfusion, leading to various nail manifestations [14].

47.2.7 Psoralens

Individuals undergoing treatment with psoralens and UVA radiation sometimes experience nail toxicity as a result of a photo-mediated toxic or allergic reaction to the medication [4]. Many patients with psoriasis may undergo phototherapy. Therefore, patients with psoriasis may develop more drug-induced nail changes.

47.3 Risk Factors

Risk factors for drug induced nail changes and correlation between drug dose and duration with nail toxicity have not been well studied. Similarly, data is needed to quantify the risk of patients taking more than one medication that can cause nail toxicity, and the role of underlying comorbidities.

47.4 Clinical Features

47.4.1 Nail Disorders Induced by Toxicity to the Nail Matrix

47.4.1.1 Beau's Lines

Beau's lines are depressions in the nail caused by the transient arrest in mitotic activity of keratinocytes in the nail matrix due to drug toxicity. Due to the subtle and transient nature of this nail finding, cases may be underreported in the literature. One case report describes a 45-year-old man who developed Beau's lines during a 30-day course of moxifloxacin 400 mg/daily for pneumonia [15]. Another case describes a 61-year-old man who developed Beau's lines after a three month course of itraconazole 200 mg daily for onychomycosis [16]. Retinoids have also been associated with Beau's lines [1, 4]. Beau's lines grow out with nail growth after cessation of the causative medication.

47.4.1.2 Onychomadesis

Onychomadesis presents with a complete separation of the proximal and distal nail plate with eventual nail plate shedding. Onychomadesis is a more severe manifestation of Beau's lines characterized by complete arrest of nail growth [17]. Description of drug-induced onychomadesis is limited to case reports. One case report describes a 31-year-old male with partial seizure disorder who developed shedding of all 20 fingernails after treatment with 100 mg of carbamazepine twice daily, increased to 200 mg three times a day over three weeks [18]. Another case report describes a three-year-old who developed onychomadesis of the right great toenail after treatment with valproic acid monotherapy 20 mg/kg for myoclonic jerks. Nail growth returned to normal after medication termination [19].

47.4.1.3 Nail Thinning and Fragility

Drug-induced toxicity to nail matrix keratinocytes can lead to increased nail fragility, known as brittle nail syndrome, manifesting as onychoschizia, nail splitting, onychorrhexis, and nail ridging. It is common in patients treated with retinoids. One case describes a 23-year-old female who developed nail fragility after isotretinoin 40 mg/day treatment for acne [20].

47.4.2 Nail Disorders Due to Toxicity to Nail Bed Keratinocytes

47.4.2.1 Photo-Onycholysis

Photo-onycholysis refers to separation of the nail plate from the nail bed induced by ultraviolet radiation. Tetracyclines and psoralens are the most common culprits of drug-induced photo-onycholysis. Photo-onycholysis may occur with drug administration in conjunction with natural sunlight or any exposure that mimics UV radiation exposure, including tanning beds, phototherapy, or UV lamps or bulbs [4]. One study reports that of 28 patients who had photosensitivity reactions to the tetracycline demeclocycline hydrochloride, seven experienced onycholysis [21]. Other medications associated with photo-onycholysis in case reports include quinolones, diclofenac, psychotropics, and diuretics [4, 5, 22, 23].

47.4.3 Drug-Induced Nail Pigmentation

Drug-induced nail pigmentation refers to changes in nail color caused by medications. These pigmentation alterations can manifest as various hues, including brown, blue, or yellow, and may affect one or multiple nails. The mechanism may be related to drug-induced stimulation of matrix melanocytes or drug metabolite deposition in the dermis.

47.4.3.1 Brown Discoloration

Certain medications can trigger activation of nail matrix melanocytes, leading to melanin production and the subsequent appearance of a melanonychia band or multiple longitudinal or transverse bands. These bands can vary in color from light brown to black. For example, a 63-year-old woman developed brownish-gray transverse hyperpigmentation of her thumbnails after undergoing two months of PUVA phototherapy for psoriasis [24]. Similar brown nail discoloration has also been described in case reports in association with hydroxychloroquine, zidovudine, clofazimine, and lithium [2, 4, 25–28].

47.4.3.2 Blue Discoloration

Blue nail discoloration can manifest as a diffuse bluish hue, longitudinal bands, or patches affecting parts of the nail, and may be caused by antibiotics (such as minocycline and sparfloxacin), antimalarials (like amodiaquine, hydroxychloroquine, and quinacrine), antiretrovirals (zidovudine), and anticonvulsants (ezogabine and retigabine) [29, 30]. A literature review of 943 cases of blue nail discoloration identified minocycline as the cause in 29 cases of polydactylic blue nail discoloration [30]. Additionally, zidovudine was associated with blue nail discoloration in 17 cases, with an average patient age of 31.4 years, predominantly affecting males (75.6%) [30].

47.4.4 Drug-Induced Nail Fold Damage

47.4.4.1 Paronychia

Acute paronychia refers to erythema and swelling of the nail fold, which may progress to purulence and abscess formation. Implicated drugs include zidovudine, lamivudine, indinavir, and isotretinoin [4, 31]. Acute paronychia has been associated with use of antiretrovirals [32]. One case series describes 12 patients with HIV taking lamivudine who all presented with acute paronychia [33].

47.4.4.2 Pyogenic Granuloma

Pyogenic granuloma, a benign overgrowth of blood vessels on the skin and mucous membranes, typically develops following minor injuries or paronychia [34, 35]. Pyogenic granulomas present as red or purplish nodules that bleed or ulcerate, sometimes resembling warts [36]. Retinoids are associated with pyogenic granuloma formation [37]. One case describes an 18-year-old male who developed two pyogenic granulomas on his left and right third digits after one month of treatment with isotretinoin 60 mg/day [38]. Retinoids are thought to potentially induce localized exfoliative dermatitis within the nail matrix, leading to the buildup of scales and debris in the nail folds that triggers a foreign body reaction and granulation tissue formation [38].

47.5 Clinical Features in Skin of Color

Nail changes induced by drugs may share similarities across different skin types. In individuals with darker Fitzpatrick skin types, it is important to differentiate longitudinal melanonychia from drug-induced pigmentation versus physiologic melanocytic activation.

47.6 Requirements for Diagnosis

Diagnosing drug-induced nail changes requires a clinical assessment, including a detailed medical history and nail examination. Essential aspects include identifying medications the patient has been exposed to, noting the onset of nail findings in relation to drug initiation or discontinuation, and observing the pattern of nail involvement. It is crucial to exclude other potential causes of onychodystrophies, such as dermatologic conditions or systemic diseases. Additionally, resolution of nail changes following discontinuation of the suspected medication supports the likelihood of a drug-induced etiology. In some cases, drug-induced nail changes may appear similarly to onychomycosis or nail psoriasis, and histopathological diagnosis may be required via nail clipping. Nail biopsy is not typically required to diagnose drug-induced nail changes.

47.7 Cases

Figures 47.1, 47.2, 47.3, 47.4, 47.5, and 47.6 depict the clinical presentation of nail dystrophies secondary to medications other than chemotherapies.

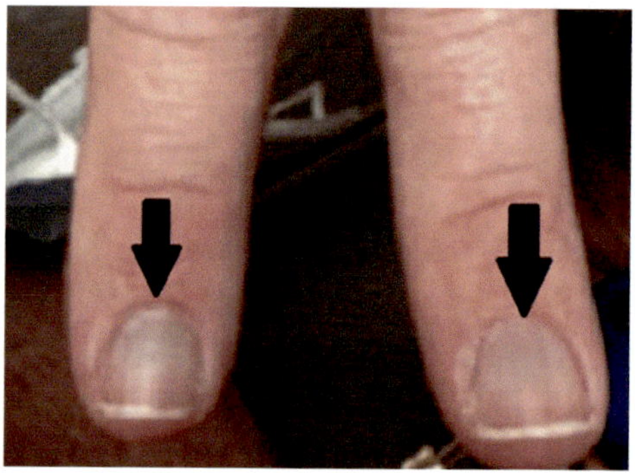

Fig. 47.1 66-Year-old male, Fitzpatrick type II, blue-gray hyperpigmentation of the fingernails is seen in the left second and third fingernails (*from* Varghese et al. [39]; CC-BY 4.0, https://creativecommons.org/licenses/by/4.0)

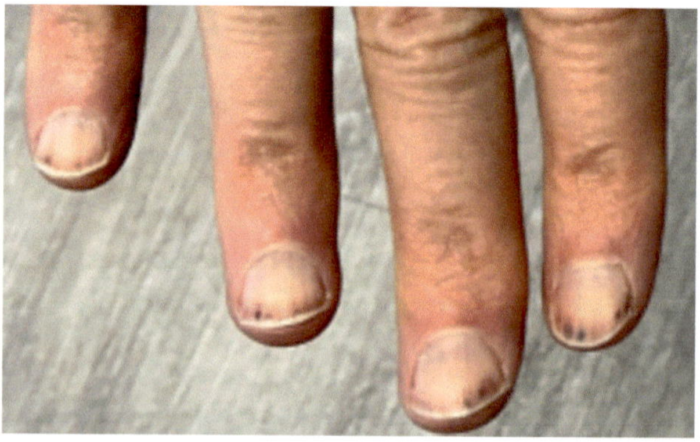

Fig. 47.2 59-Year-old female, Fitzpatrick type II, splinter hemorrhages after a short course of nitrofurantoin for a UTI. Thin reddish-brown lines or streaks located under the nail on distal nail plates (*from* Acosta et al. [40]; CC-BY 4.0, https://creativecommons.org/licenses/by/4.0)

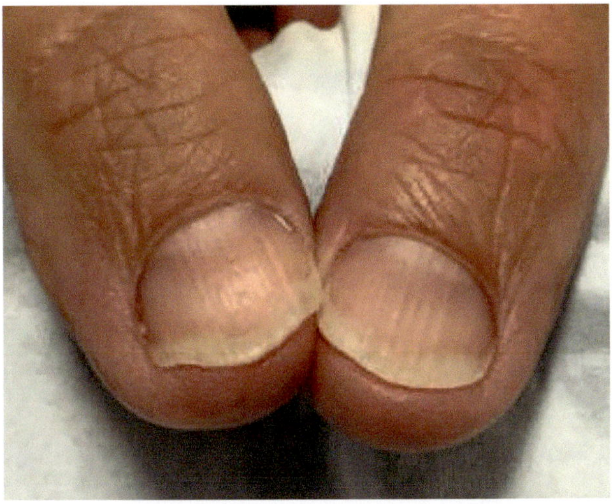

Fig. 47.3 57-Year-old female, Fitzpatrick type III, photo-onycholysis due to doxycycline, with onycholysis and increased ridging involving the bilateral thumbnails

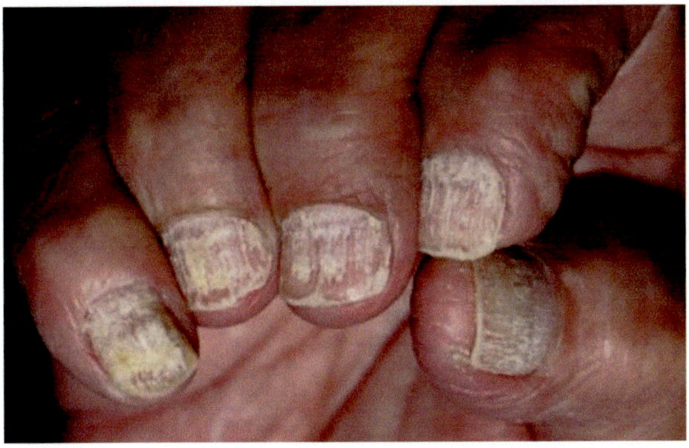

Fig. 47.4 65-Year-old male, Fitzpatrick type IV, acitretin-induced trachyonychia, with hyperkeratosis, rough texture, and increased ridging of the fingernails (*from* Thieman et al. [41]; CC-BY 4.0, https://creativecommons.org/licenses/by/4.0)

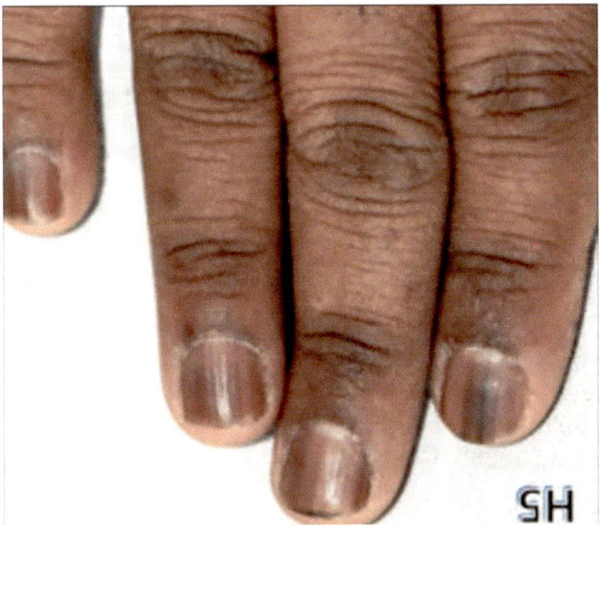

Fig. 47.5 Fitzpatrick type V, longitudinal melanonychia induced by zidovudine was seen in a patient with HIV undergoing HAART (*from* Satasia and Sutaria [42]; CC-BY 4.0, https://creativecommons.org/licenses/by/4.0)

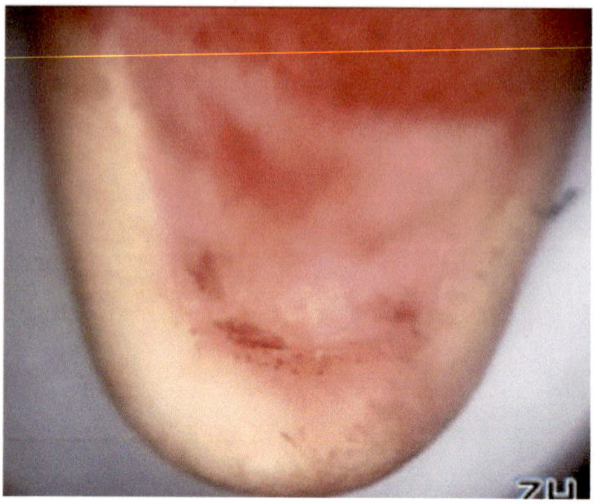

Fig. 47.6 Fitzpatrick type V, capecitabine-induced anonychia. On dermoscopy, nail plate atrophy is appreciated (*from* Satasia and Sutaria [42]; CC-BY 4.0, https://creativecommons.org/licenses/by/4.0)

References

1. Piraccini BM, Iorizzo M. Drug reactions affecting the nail unit: diagnosis and management. Dermatol Clin. 2007;25(2):215–21, vii. https://doi.org/10.1016/j.det.2007.01.006.
2. Piraccini BM, Iorizzo M, Starace M, Tosti A. Drug-induced nail diseases. Dermatol Clin. 2006;24(3):387–91. https://doi.org/10.1016/j.det.2006.03.004.
3. Piraccini BM, Tosti A. Drug-induced nail disorders: incidence, management and prognosis. Drug Saf. 1999;21(3):187–201. https://doi.org/10.2165/00002018-199921030-00004.
4. Piraccini BM, Alessandrini A. Drug-related nail disease. Clin Dermatol. 2013;31(5):618–26. https://doi.org/10.1016/j.clindermatol.2013.06.013.
5. Lasser AE, Steiner MM. Tetracycline photo-onycholysis. Pediatrics. 1978;61(1):98–9.
6. Rabar D, Combemale P, Peyron F. Doxycycline-induced photo-onycholysis. J Travel Med. 2004;11(6):386–7. https://doi.org/10.2310/7060.2004.19210.
7. Ricardo JW, Shah K, Minkis K, Lipner SR. Blue skin, nail, and scleral pigmentation associated with minocycline. Case Rep Dermatol. 2022;14(2):239–42. https://doi.org/10.1159/000526067.
8. Kestel JL Jr. Photo-onycholysis from minocycline. Side effects of minocycline therapy. Cutis. 1981;28(1):53–4.
9. Özçelik S, Kılıç FA. Effects of ısotretinoin on the growth rate and thickness of the nail plate. Int J Dermatol. 2021;60(10):1258–62. https://doi.org/10.1111/ijd.15635.
10. Allegue F, González-Vilas D, Zulaica A. Isotretinoin-induced elkonyxis. Actas Dermosifiliogr. 2017;108(2):166–7. https://doi.org/10.1016/j.ad.2016.08.007.
11. Drug-induced nail disorders. Prescrire Int. 2014;23(151):180–2.
12. Horta-Baas G. Chloroquine-induced oral mucosal hyperpigmentation and nail dyschromia. Reumatol Clin (Engl Ed). 2018;14(3):177–8. https://doi.org/10.1016/j.reuma.2017.06.003.
13. Gupta A, Kuchana SK, Guleria S, Suri D. Azathioprine-induced melanonychia. J Clin Rheumatol. 2020;26(6):e162–3. https://doi.org/10.1097/rhu.0000000000001031.
14. Bostanci S, Ekmekci P, Akyol A, Peksari Y, Gürgey E. Pincer nail deformity: inherited and caused by a beta-blocker. Int J Dermatol. 2004;43(4):316–8. https://doi.org/10.1111/j.1365-4632.2004.01666.x.
15. Burkhardt O, Allewelt M, Pletz MW, Welte T, Lode H. Beau's lines in a patient treated with moxifloxacin for anaerobic pulmonary infection. Scand J Infect Dis. 2003;35(8):516–8. https://doi.org/10.1080/00365540310012398.

16. Chen HH, Liao YH. Beau's lines associated with itraconazole. Acta Derm Venereol. 2002;82(5):398. https://doi.org/10.1080/000155502320624276.
17. Hardin J, Haber RM. Onychomadesis: literature review. Br J Dermatol. 2015;172(3):592–6. https://doi.org/10.1111/bjd.13339.
18. Mishra D, Singh G, Pandey SS. Possible carbamazepine-induced reversible onychomadesis. Int J Dermatol. 1989;28(7):460–1. https://doi.org/10.1111/j.1365-4362.1989.tb02507.x.
19. Poretti A, Lips U, Belvedere M, Schmitt B. Onychomadesis: a rare side-effect of valproic acid medication? Pediatr Dermatol. 2009;26(6):749–50. https://doi.org/10.1111/j.1525-1470.2009.00867.x.
20. Onder M, Oztaş MO, Oztaş P. Isotretinoin-induced nail fragility and onycholysis. J Dermatol Treat. 2001;12(2):115–6. https://doi.org/10.1080/095466301317085426.
21. Orentreich N, Harber L, Tromovitch TA. Photosensitivity and photo-onycholysis due to demethylchlortetracycline. Arch Dermatol. 1961;83:730–7. https://doi.org/10.1001/archderm.1961.01580110018003.
22. Al-Kathiri L, Al-Asmaili A. Diclofenac-induced photo-onycholysis. Oman Med J. 2016;31(1):65–8. https://doi.org/10.5001/omj.2016.12.
23. Bentabet Dorbani I, Badri T, Benmously R, Fenniche S, Mokhtar I. Griseofulvin-induced photo-onycholysis. Presse Med. 2012;41(9 Pt 1):879–81. https://doi.org/10.1016/j.lpm.2011.11.014.
24. Ledbetter LS, Hsu S. Melanonychia associated with PUVA therapy. J Am Acad Dermatol. 2003;48(2 Suppl):S31–2. https://doi.org/10.1067/mjd.2003.117.
25. Ricardo JW, Chikeka I, Silvers DN, Lipner SR. Longitudinal melanonychia and skin hyperpigmentation associated with hydroxychloroquine therapy. JAAD Case Rep. 2021;7:23–5. https://doi.org/10.1016/j.jdcr.2020.10.030.
26. Buontempo MG, Chaudhry ZS, Raval RS, et al. Hydroxyurea-induced melanonychia. JAAD Case Rep. 2023;42:91–4. https://doi.org/10.1016/j.jdcr.2023.09.027.
27. Clark A, Ambur A, Nathoo R. Isolated nail pigmentation induced by minocycline: a case report. Innov Pharm. 2022;13(1) https://doi.org/10.24926/iip.v13i1.4493.
28. Lipner SR, Scher RK. Dermatologic manifestations of hydroxychloroquine therapy: a closer look at the nails. J Am Acad Dermatol. 2020;83(4):e291–2. https://doi.org/10.1016/j.jaad.2020.04.177.
29. Eisen D, Hakim MD. Minocycline-induced pigmentation. Incidence, prevention and management. Drug Saf. 1998;18(6):431–40. https://doi.org/10.2165/00002018-199818060-00004.
30. Hwang JK, Lipner SR. Blue nail discoloration: literature review and diagnostic algorithms. Am J Clin Dermatol. 2023;24(3):419–41. https://doi.org/10.1007/s40257-023-00768-6.
31. Figueiras Dde A, Ramos TB, Marinho AK, Bezerra MS, Cauas RC. Paronychia and granulation tissue formation during treatment with isotretinoin. An Bras Dermatol. 2016;91(2):223–5. https://doi.org/10.1590/abd1806-4841.20163817.
32. Tosti A, Piraccini BM, D'Antuono A, Marzaduri S, Bettoli V. Paronychia associated with antiretroviral therapy. Br J Dermatol. 1999;140(6):1165–8. https://doi.org/10.1046/j.1365-2133.1999.02883.x.
33. Sibel S, Macher A, Goosby E. Paronychia in patients receiving antiretroviral therapy for human immunodeficiency virus infection. J Am Podiatr Med Assoc. 2000;90(2):98–100. https://doi.org/10.7547/87507315-90-2-98.
34. Wollina U. Systemic drug-induced chronic paronychia and periungual pyogenic granuloma. Indian Dermatol Online J. 2018;9(5):293–8. https://doi.org/10.4103/idoj.IDOJ_133_18.
35. Thomas M, Shon W, Truong AK. Acitretin-induced periungual pyogenic granulomas and review. Dermatol Online J. 2021;27(7) https://doi.org/10.5070/d327754369.
36. Sarwal P, Lapumnuaypol K. Pyogenic granuloma. In: StatPearls. StatPearls Publishing; 2024.
37. Badri T, Hawilo AM, Benmously R, Fenniche S, Mokhtar I. Acitretin-induced pyogenic granuloma. Acta Dermatovenerol Alp Pannonica Adriat. 2011;20(4):217–8.
38. Benedetto C, Crasto D, Ettefagh L, Nami N. Development of periungual pyogenic granuloma with associated paronychia following isotretinoin therapy: a case report and a review of the literature. J Clin Aesthet Dermatol. 2019;12(4):32–6.

39. Varghese K, Dykstra J, Bisbee E. Minocycline-induced hyperpigmentation of nails. Cureus. 2023;15(5):e38640. https://doi.org/10.7759/cureus.38640.
40. Acosta AS, Jafri Z, Khalil K, Kerdel F. Nitrofurantoin-induced splinter hemorrhages: a forgotten culprit. JAAD Case Rep. 2024;47:38–40. https://doi.org/10.1016/j.jdcr.2024.02.031.
41. Thieman T, Clarey D, Johnson RA, Trowbridge RM. Trachyonychia secondary to acitretin usage. Cureus. 2020;12(1):e6703. https://doi.org/10.7759/cureus.6703.
42. Satasia M, Sutaria AH. Nail whispers revealing dermatological and systemic secrets: an analysis of nail disorders associated with diverse dermatological and systemic conditions. Cureus. 2023;15(9):e45007. https://doi.org/10.7759/cureus.45007.

Part XI

Pediatric Nail Disorders

Congenital Nail Malalignment

48

Kaya L. Curtis and Shari R. Lipner

48.1 Description of Disease

Congenital nail malalignment is characterized by lateral deviation of the nail plate relative to the phalanx [1]. It may be inherited in some cases, and the etiology remains idiopathic. Pathophysiologically, there may be lateral rotation of the underlying nail matrix [2] due to inherited nail matrix or ligamental abnormalities, or external factors such as abnormal in utero fetal positioning.

48.2 Epidemiology

Congenital nail malalignment typically presents in infancy or childhood. Estimated prevalence is 1–2% in pediatric patients [3], though underdiagnosis is likely [4]. Late onset is uncommon, though patients may present at a later age due to complications such as retronychia or onychomycosis [4]. In Catalfo et al.'s literature review [4] of 33 patients from articles published 1950–2016, age of onset was at birth in 25 cases, during the first 2 years in 2 cases, and during adolescence (15 and 16 years) in 2 cases. Female-to-male ratio was 1.1:1.

48.3 Risk Factors

Some cases of congenital malalignment are likely inherited with an autosomal dominant inheritance pattern with variable expressivity. There have been multiple case reports of affected family members [5–7], including multiple generations of single families, as well as occurrence in monozygotic and dizygotic twins. In Catalfo et al.'s literature review [4] of 33 patients, a family history of congenital nail malalignment was confirmed in 5 cases and likely in 2 cases. In this review, three sets of monozygotic twins, two sets of dizygotic twins, and two triplets were

S. R. Lipner, *Atlas of Nail Disorders Across All Skin Colors*,
https://doi.org/10.1007/978-3-031-74272-9_48

affected. Extrinsic factors may be causative, including abnormal fetal positioning in utero [6, 8], toe constriction by amniotic bands, increased intrauterine pressure, or fetal vascular abnormalities, but have not been formally studied [9]. An abnormality in the ligament connecting the distal phalanx periosteum to the nail matrix has also been hypothesized as an etiology [10]. The onychodystrophy presentation may be due to a combination of inherited toenail malalignment and accumulated effects of postnatal trauma [7, 11].

48.4 Clinical Features

Congenital nail malalignment frequently affects the bilateral great toenails. In Catalfo et al.'s literature review [4] of 33 patients, the bilateral great toenails were affected in 29 cases, and one toenail was affected in 1 case. Physical examination is notable for lateral deviation of the nail plate relative to the phalanx, accompanied by nail thickening and brown–gray discoloration [12]. Medial deviation has only been reported in three cases [13]. The toenail may have a triangular or trapezoidal shape [4]. Congenital nail malalignment may persist into adulthood, and spontaneous resolution has been suggested in up to 50% [1, 14, 15]. Onycholysis and lateral impingement of the nail fold resulting in onychogryphosis may develop over time [12, 14]. The lateral deviation of the nail plate also subjects the nail to trauma, which may result in transverse ridging [6, 16], paronychia, onychomadesis, retronychia, and onychomycosis [4, 17, 18]. Chronic onycholysis may result in epithelization of part of the nail bed, termed 'the disappearing nail bed' [19, 20]. Patients may complain of ambulation-associated pain [15]. Associated systemic findings have not been reported in patients with congenital nail malalignment [4].

48.5 Clinical Features in Skin of Color

Distinct clinical presentations of congenital nail malalignment in skin of color have not been characterized. Longitudinal melanonychia may be present, particularly in adult patients.

48.6 Requirements for Diagnosis

Congenital nail malalignment is a clinical diagnosis. Nail involvement since birth or childhood is an important historical feature. Family history of congenital nail malalignment is supportive. The bilateral great toenails are most frequently affected. Nail clipping may aid in diagnosis by ruling out other nail diseases such as onychomycosis.

48.7 Cases

Figures 48.1, 48.2, 48.3, 48.4, 48.5, and 48.6 demonstrate the presentation of congenital nail malalignment in a clinical setting.

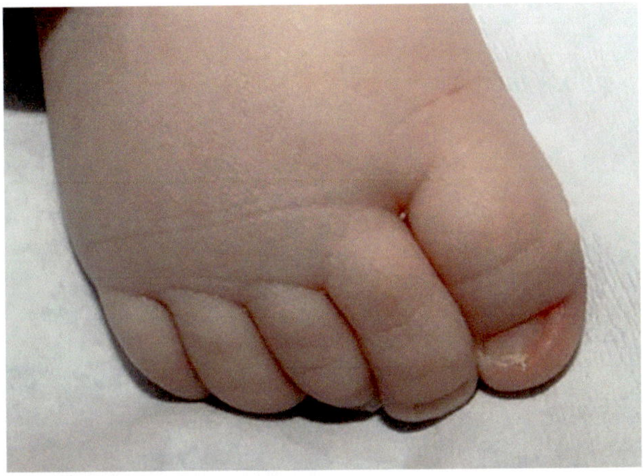

Fig. 48.1 3-Month-old female, Fitzpatrick type I, congenital nail malalignment, with lateral deviation of the right great toenail

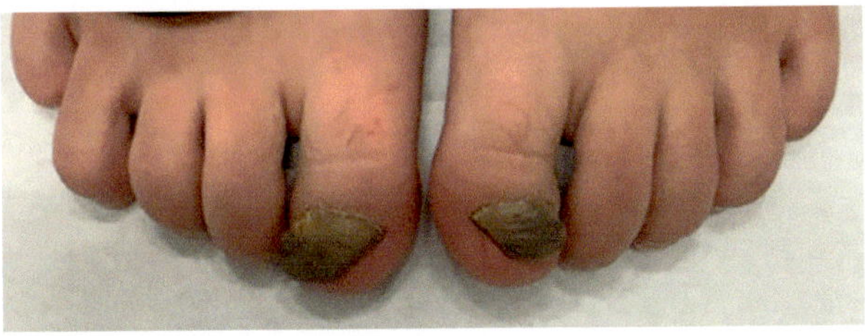

Fig. 48.2 20-Year-old female, Fitzpatrick type II, congenital nail malalignment, with lateral deviation and brown-grey discoloration of the bilateral great toenails

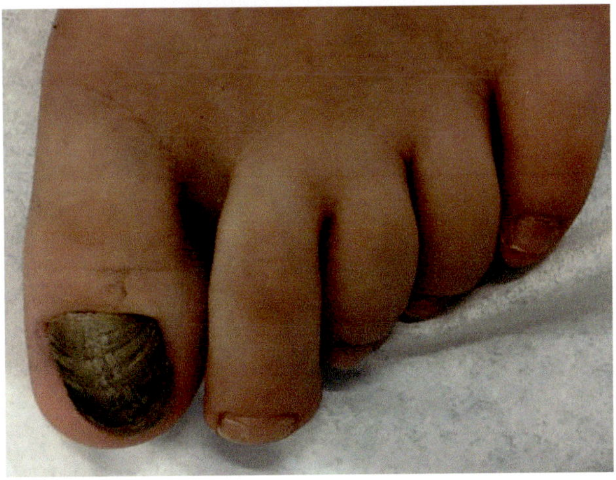

Fig. 48.3 8-Year-old male, Fitzpatrick type II, congenital nail malalignment, with lateral deviation, layering, and brown-gray discoloration of the left great toenail, present since birth

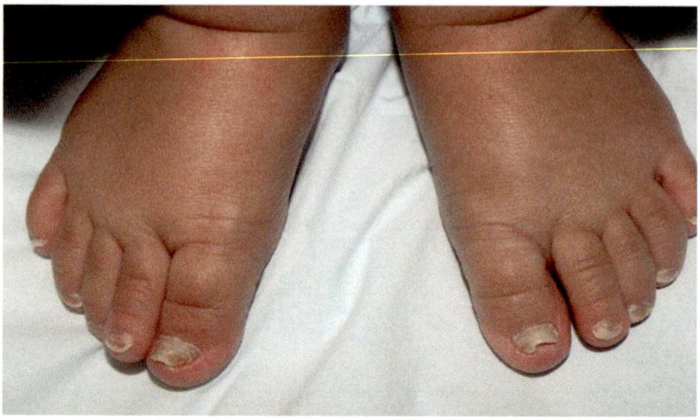

Fig. 48.4 Pediatric patient, Fitzpatrick type III, congenital nail malalignment, with lateral deviation of the bilateral great toenails

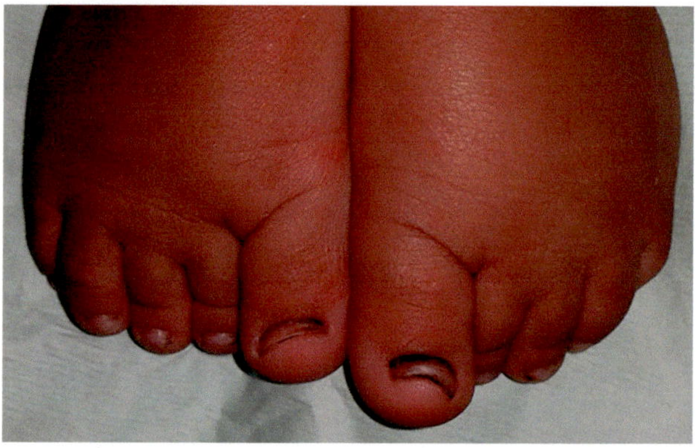

Fig. 48.5 Infant, Fitzpatrick type IV, congenital bilateral great toenail malalignment, with bilateral clubfoot using braces (*from* Agarwal et al. [21]; *with permission*)

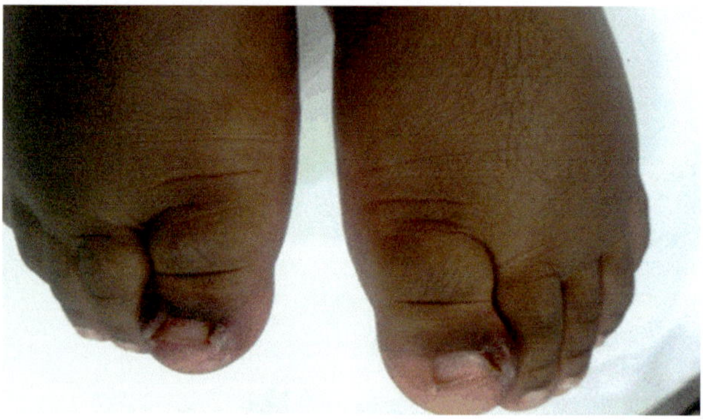

Fig. 48.6 2-Year-old male, Fitzpatrick type V, with bilateral infantile ingrown toenails (*from* Kobe et al. [22]; CC-BY 4.0, https://creativecommons.org/licenses/by/4.0)

References

1. Samman PD. Great toe nail dystrophy. Clin Exp Dermatol. 1978;3(1):81–2.
2. Harper KJ, Beer WE. Congenital malalignment of the great toe-nails—an inherited condition. Clin Exp Dermatol. 1986;11(5):514–6.
3. Perlis CS, Telang GH. Congenital malalignment of the great toenails mimicking onycho mycosis. J Pediatr. 2005;146:575.
4. Catalfo P, Musumeci ML, Lacarrubba F, Dinotta F, Micali G. Congenital malalignment of the great toenails: a review. Skin Appendage Disord. 2018;4(4):230–5.
5. Dawson TA. An inherited nail dystrophy principally affecting the great toe nails. Clin Exp Dermatol. 1979;4(3):309–13.
6. Cohen JL, Scher RK, Pappert AS. Congenital malalignment of the great toenails. Pediatr Dermatol. 1991;8(1):40–2.
7. Barth JH, Dawber RP, Ashton RE, Baran R. Congenital malalignment of great toenails in two sets of monozygotic twins. Arch Dermatol. 1986;122(4):379–80.
8. Hendricks WM. Congenital ingrown toenails. Cutis. 1979;24(4):393–4.
9. Baden HP, Mizner R. Association of congenital malalignment of the nail and a constricting band of the digit. Birth Defects Res A Clin Mol Teratol. 2003;67:202.
10. Guero S, Guichard S, Fraitag S. Ligamentary structure of the base of the nail. Surg Radiol Anat. 1994;16:47–52.
11. Kim M, Kang JH, Cho BK, Song CH, Ock SM, Park HJ. Great toenail dystrophy: a single-center experience and review of the literature. Korean J Fam Med. 2015;36:113–20.
12. Bellet JS. Pediatric nail disorders. Dermatol Clin. 2021;39(2):231–43.
13. Baran R, Bureau H. Congenital malalignment of the big toenail: a new subtype. Arch Dermatol. 1987;123:437.
14. Wulkan AJ, Tosti A. Pediatric nail conditions. Clin Dermatol. 2013;31(5):564–72.
15. Handfield-Jones SE, Harman RR. Spontaneous improvement of congenital malalignment of the great toe nails. Br J Dermatol. 1988;118:305–6.
16. Kus S, Tahmaz E, Gurunluoglu R, Candan I, Uygur T. Congenital malalignment of the great toenails in dizygotic twins. Pediatr Dermatol. 2005;22(5):434–5.
17. Wagner G, Sachse MM. Congenital malalignment of the big toe nail. J Dtsch Dermatol Ges. 2012;10(5):326–30.
18. Braswell MA, Daniel CR 3rd, Brodell RT. Beau lines, onychomadesis, and retronychia: a unifying hypothesis. J Am Acad Dermatol. 2015;73(5):849–55.
19. Daniel CR 3rd, Tosti A, Iorizzo M, Piraccini BM. The disappearing nail bed: a possible outcome of onycholysis. Cutis. 2005;76:325–7.
20. Buttars B, Scott SG, Glinka D, Daniel CR, Brodell RT, Braswell MA. Congenital malalignment of the great toenail, the disappearing nail bed, and distal phalanx deviation: a review. Skin Appendage Disord. 2022;8(1):8–12.
21. Agarwal A, Kumar A, Khanna D, Shaharyar A, Bhat MS, Mishra M. Nail changes in casted and braced clubfoot: a preliminary study. Foot Ankle Surg. 2016;22(4):229–32.
22. Kobe IO, Khamalla NW. Infantile bilateral ingrown toe nails: a case report from sub-Saharan Africa. Int J Case Rep Images. 2018;9:100899Z01IK2018.

Lichen Striatus

49

Kaya L. Curtis and Shari R. Lipner

49.1 Description of Disease

Lichen striatus is a benign, self-limiting linear dermatosis that develops along the lines of Blaschko (lines corresponding to developmental growth patterns during embryogenesis) [1]. Lichen striatus is frequently asymptomatic, though cutaneous lesions may be associated with mild pruritus [2]. Lichen striatus presents acutely and self-resolves. Lichen striatus rarely affects the nail unit and is characterized by longitudinal fissuring and onycholysis, typically limited to the lateral portion of the nail plate [1]. There is often concurrent cutaneous involvement with nail changes, or cutaneous lesions may occur before or after nail involvement [1]. Though less frequent, nail dystrophy without skin involvement may occur. Etiology is thought to be cutaneous mosaicism, in which somatic mutations result in abnormal keratinocyte clones that remain silent until a triggering event occurs [3]. A trigger interrupts immunologic tolerance and induces expression of novel membrane antigens, resulting in a self-limited autoimmune CD8+ T lymphocyte-mediated response [4, 5]. Multiple triggers have been hypothesized to play a role, including trauma, viral infections, vaccines, pregnancy, and hypersensitivity reactions [6–11]. Pathophysiologically, there is an inflammatory process in the nail matrix resulting in abnormal keratin synthesis [12].

49.2 Epidemiology

Lichen striatus typically presents in infants and children, though adults may also be affected [2]. Lichen striatus has been reported in all ethnic groups; there may be a female predilection [6, 13, 14]. In Kim et al.'s case series [1] of seven patients with nail lichen striatus, median age was 11 years (range: 4–33 years) with male:female ratio of 4:3. In Tosti et al.'s case series [15] of 5 patients, mean age was 17 years (range: 17–28) with a male:female ratio of 1:4.

S. R. Lipner, *Atlas of Nail Disorders Across All Skin Colors*,
https://doi.org/10.1007/978-3-031-74272-9_49

49.3 Risk Factors

Risk factors for lichen striatus are unknown, though genetic, environmental, and infectious factors may be involved [16]. Atopy may be a predisposing risk factor. A personal or family history of asthma, atopic dermatitis, or allergic rhinitis has been reported in 60–85% of patients with lichen striatus [6, 17, 18]. A case of lichen striatus with nail involvement following trauma to the hand was reported [19]. However, in Iorizzo et al.'s case series [2] of five patients, there was no history of trauma preceding development of nail lichen striatus in any patients. Only one patient had a history of atopy, while the remaining four patients did not have other dermatologic disorders. Lichen striatus eruptions associated with COVID-19 infection have been reported [20, 21]. Co-occurrence of cases in multiple family members has also been reported, suggesting a genetic component [7, 22–25].

49.4 Clinical Features

Cutaneous lichen striatus presents as a 1–3 mm wide continuous or interrupted linear band composed of pink or flesh-color papules [1]. In a review [6] of 115 pediatric patients with lichen striatus, only three patients (2.6%) had nail dystrophy. However, prevalence may be higher, due to under-recognition of nail symptoms and underdiagnosis [16]. Nail changes are typically limited to one side of the nail plate, though central nail plate involvement cases have also been reported [1, 2, 19]. In Kim et al.'s case series [1] of seven patients, the most common nail findings were longitudinal fissuring ($n = 4$), onychorrhexis ($n = 2$), onycholysis ($n = 2$), subungual hyperkeratosis ($n = 2$), fraying ($n = 2$), splitting ($n = 2$), partial loss of nail plate ($n = 2$), and transverse grooves ($n = 1$). Patients with isolated nail involvement were excluded from this series. Six cases had paronychial skin involvement. A single digit was affected in five patients and two digits in two patients. The fingernail(s) were affected in five patients and the toenail(s) in two patients. Nail changes occurred before ($n = 1$), after ($n = 3$), and concurrently ($n = 3$) with cutaneous lesions. Nail involvement duration was on average 6.4 months. Six patients had asymptomatic, skin-colored clusters of papules on the extremities occurring along lines of Blaschko, and one patient had pruritic, erythematous scaly patches of the lower extremity. In Tosti et al.'s case series [15] of five patients, the most common nail abnormalities were nail thinning with longitudinal ridging and splitting. Nail changes were isolated to the lateral nail in three patients and the medial nail in two patients. Mean duration of nail involvement was 14 months. One finger was involved in four patients and one toe in one patient. Two of five patients had concurrent skin lesions, while three patients presented with only nail findings.

49.5 Clinical Features in Skin of Color

In darker skin tones, cutaneous lichen striatus lesions may be initially hypopigmented [26]. Distinct clinical presentations of nail lichen striatus in skin of color have not been characterized.

49.6 Requirements for Diagnosis

Isolated lateral nail involvement of a single nail in a child or young adult should raise suspicion for nail lichen striatus [15]. Dermoscopy may enhance characteristic nail findings, including longitudinal nail fissures involving only a single portion of the nail plate, red spots in the lunula, and subungual hyperkeratosis [2]. A physical examination assessing for accompanying cutaneous lesions is recommended. The cutaneous lesions of lichen planus are usually pruritic, while cutaneous lesions in lichen striatus are asymptomatic [2]. Additionally, nail dystrophy in lichen planus is typically more severe and progressive and involves the entirety of the nail plate, whereas nail lichen striatus is often isolated to a single portion of the nail unit [2]. The diagnosis is usually clinical, and skin biopsies are generally avoided in children. In equivocal cases, where diagnosis would influence treatment, a biopsy can be considered. Skin biopsy of lichen striatus lesions demonstrates dense band-like lymphohistiocytic infiltrate in the papillary dermis and an inflammatory cell infiltrate around the hair follicles and eccrine glands in the reticular dermis, with spongiosis with exocytosis of lymphocytes and focal parakeratosis [1]. Nail biopsy demonstrates band-like lymphocytic infiltrate in the superficial dermis of the distal nail matrix, with exocytosis, spongiosis, focal hypergranulosis, and dyskeratotic cells on nail matrix epithelium [1]. However, nail biopsy is invasive and is generally considered unnecessary for this self-limited and benign condition, especially in children.

49.7 Cases

Figures 49.1, 49.2, 49.3, 49.4, 49.5, 49.6, and 49.7 demonstrate the presentation of nail lichen striatus in a clinical setting.

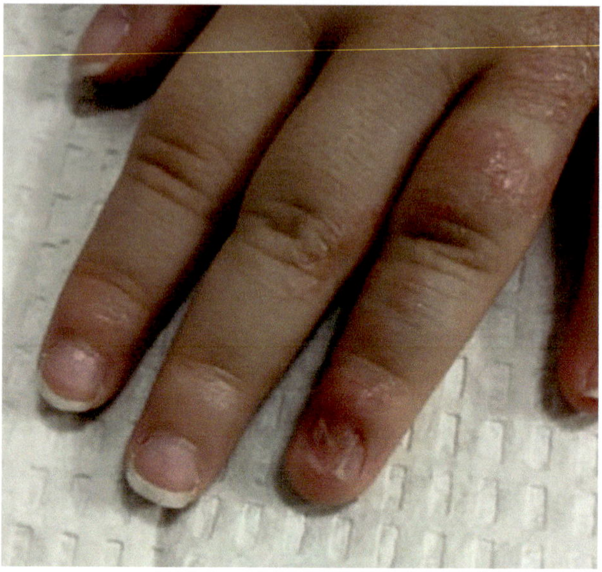

Fig. 49.1 4-Year-old female, Fitzpatrick type II, nail lichen striatus, with left fourth digit with erythematous papules coalescing into linear plaque and left fourth fingernail with atrophy, ridges, and grooves

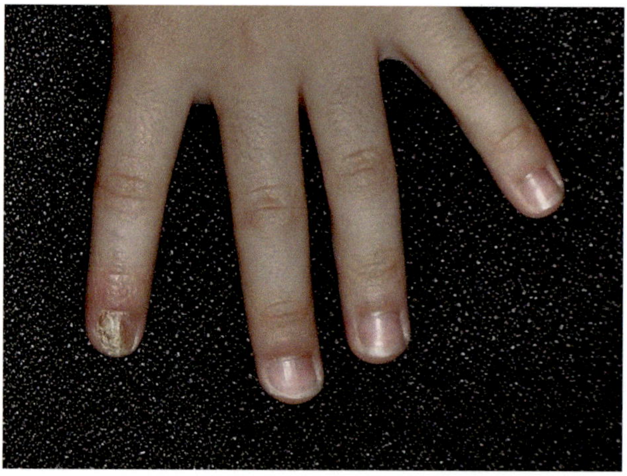

Fig. 49.2 6-Year-old male, Fitzpatrick type II, nail lichen striatus, with multiple minute skin-colored papules in a linear distribution on the left index finger, mild erythema of the proximal nail fold, and onychodystrophy (hard to appreciate ridging in the image) and subungual hyperkeratosis in the nail (*from* Leung et al. [27]; CC-BY 4.0, https://creativecommons.org/licenses/by/4.0)

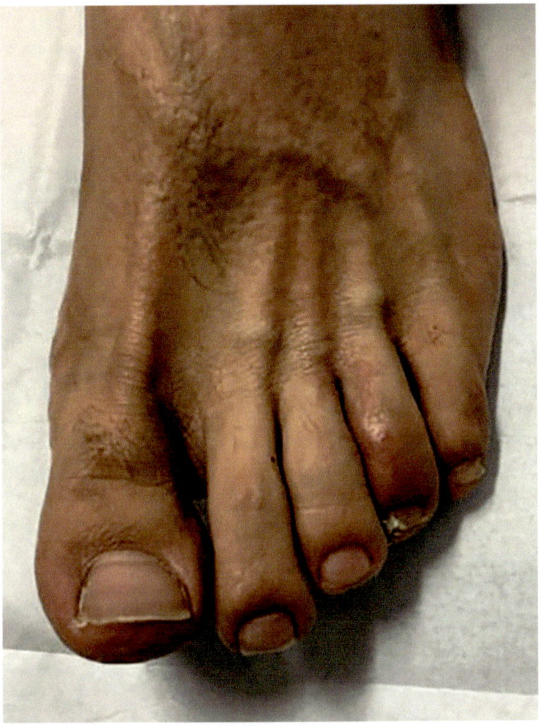

Fig. 49.3 39-Year-old male, Fitzpatrick type III, nail lichen striatus, with left fourth toe with erythematous patch contiguous with onycholysis and ridge of the left fourth toenail

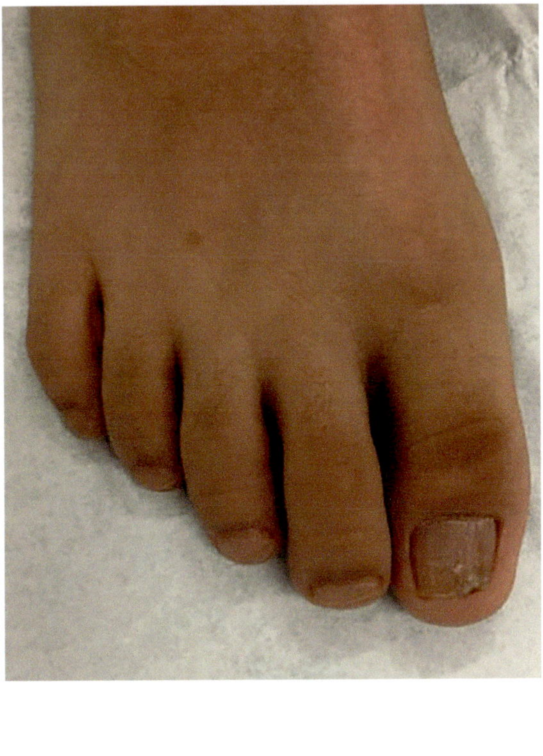

Fig. 49.4 9-Year-old female, Fitzpatrick type IV, nail lichen striatus, with right great toenail with onycholysis and longitudinal grooves involving majority of nail

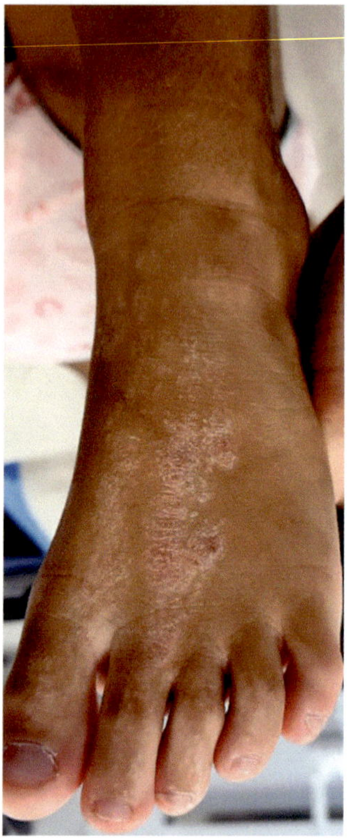

Fig. 49.5 Pediatric patient, Fitzpatrick type IV, nail lichen striatus, with flat-topped erythematous papules forming a continuous thick band along Blaschko lines on the patient's shin, dorsum of the foot, and first three toes, also involving the nail of the third toe, causing longitudinal ridging (nail lichen striatus) (*from* Herzum et al. [28]; *with permission*)

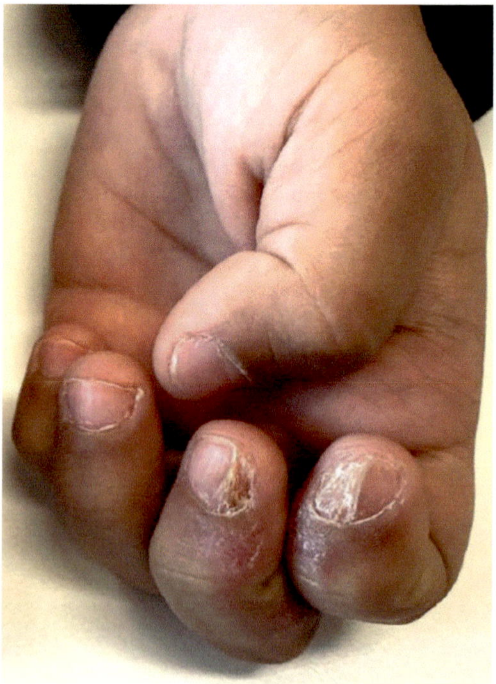

Fig. 49.6 5-Year-old male, Fitzpatrick type IV, nail lichen striatus, with multiple pinkish papules with blaschkoid distribution, affecting the left index and medium finger with partial involvement of the two adjacent nail plates (*from* Gnesotto et al. [29]; *with permission*)

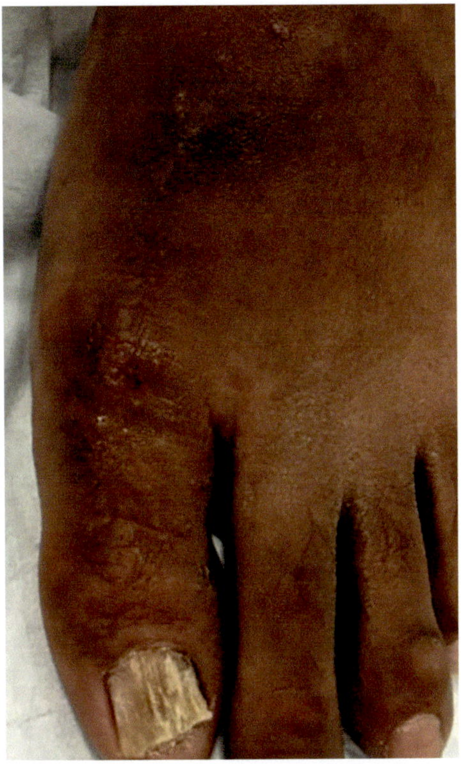

Fig. 49.7 38-Year-old female, Fitzpatrick type V, nail lichen striatus, with left dorsal foot and left great toe with linear plaque of violaceous flat-topped papules extending to left great toenail, which is dystrophic with yellowing and onychorrhexis

References

1. Kim M, Jung HY, Eun YS, Cho BK, Park HJ. Nail lichen striatus: report of seven cases and review of the literature. Int J Dermatol. 2015;54(11):1255–60.
2. Iorizzo M, Rubin AI, Starace M. Nail lichen striatus: is dermoscopy useful for the diagnosis? Pediatr Dermatol. 2019;36(6):859–63.
3. Taieb A, El Youbi A, Grosshans E, Maleville J. Lichen striatus: a Blaschko linear acquired inflammatory skin eruption. J Am Acad Dermatol. 1991;25:637–42.
4. Shepherd V, Lun K, Strutton G. Lichen striatus in adult following trauma. Australas J Dermatol. 2005;46:25–8.
5. Gianotti R, Restano L, Grimalt R, Berti E, Alessi E, Caputo R. Lichen striatus—a chameleon: an histopathological and immunohistological study of forty-one cases. J Cutan Pathol. 1995;22(1):18–22.
6. Patrizi A, Neri I, Fiorentini C, Bonci A, Ricci G. Lichen striatus: clinical and laboratory features of 115 children. Pediatr Dermatol. 2004;21(3):197–204.
7. Racette AJ, Adams AD, Kessler SE. Simultaneous lichen striatus in siblings along the same Blaschko line. Pediatr Dermatol. 2009;26(1):50–4.
8. Dragos V, Mervic L, Zgavec B. Lichen striatus in a child after immunization. A case report. Acta Dermatovenerol Alp Pannonica Adriat. 2006;15(4):178–80.
9. Karakaş M, Durdu M, Uzun S, Karakaş P, Tuncer I, Cevlik F. Lichen striatus following HBV vaccination. J Dermatol. 2005;32(6):506–8.

10. Brennand S, Khan S, Chong AH. Lichen striatus in a pregnant woman. Australas J Dermatol. 2005;46(3):184–6.
11. Hwang SM, Ahn SK, Lee SH, Choi EH. Lichen striatus following BCG vaccination. Clin Exp Dermatol. 1996;21(5):393–4.
12. Zhang Y, McNutt NS, Lichen striatus. Histological, immunohistochemical, and ultrastructural study of 37 cases. J Cutan Pathol. 2001;28:65–71.
13. Kennedy D, Rogers M. Lichen striatus. Pediatr Dermatol. 1996;13(2):95–9.
14. Hofer T. Lichen striatus in adults or 'adult blaschkitis'? There is no need for a new naming. Dermatology. 2003;207(1):89–92.
15. Tosti A, Peluso AM, Misciali C, Cameli N. Nail lichen striatus: clinical features and long-term follow-up of five patients. J Am Acad Dermatol. 1997;36(6 Pt 1):908–13.
16. Palleschi GM, D'Erme AM, Lotti T. Lichen striatus and nail involvement: truly rare or question of time? Int J Dermatol. 2012;51(6):749–50.
17. Toda K, Okamoto H, Horio T. Lichen striatus. Int J Dermatol. 1986;25(9):584–5.
18. García-Briz MI, Santos-Alarcón S, Fuertes-Prosper MD, Mateu-Puchades A. Lichen striatus in childhood: is it associated with atopic dermatitis? Actas Dermosifiliogr. 2017;108(9):882–4. English, Spanish.
19. Coto-Segura P, Costa-Romero M, Gonzalvo P, Mallo-García S, Curto-Iglesias JR, Santos-Juanes J. Lichen striatus in an adult following trauma with central nail plate involvement and its dermoscopy features. Int J Dermatol. 2008;47(12):1324–5.
20. Conforti C, Dianzani C, Agozzino M, et al. Cutaneous manifestations in confirmed COVID-19 patients: a systematic review. Biology (Basel). 2020;9(12):449.
21. Chersi F, Conforti C, Zalaudek I, di Meo N. Lichen striatus post-COVID-19 infection: clinical and dermoscopic presentations. Dermatol Pract Concept. 2023;13(1):e2023006.
22. Patrizi A, Neri I, Fiorentini C, Chieregato C, Bonci A. Simultaneous occurrence of lichen striatus in siblings. Pediatr Dermatol. 1997;14(4):293–5.
23. Kanegaye JT, Frieden IJ. Lichen striatus: simultaneous occurrence in siblings. Pediatrics. 1992;90(1 Pt 1):104–6.
24. Yaosaka M, Sawamura D, Iitoyo M, Shibaki A, Shimizu H. Lichen striatus affecting a mother and her son. J Am Acad Dermatol. 2005;53(2):352–3.
25. Tripathy T, Singh BSTP, Kar BR. Co-occurrence of lichen striatus in twins. Indian J Dermatol Venereol Leprol. 2019;85(6):632–4.
26. Leung AKC, Lam JM, Barankin B, Leong KF. Lichen striatus: an updated review. Curr Pediatr Rev. 2024; https://doi.org/10.2174/0115733963273945240101042423.
27. Leung AKC, Leong KF, Barankin B. Lichen striatus with nail involvement in a 6-year-old boy. Case Rep Pediatr. 2020;2020:1494760.
28. Herzum A, Viglizzo G, Gariazzo L, Ferro J, Vellone VG, Occella C. Lichen striatus after COVID-19. Clin Dermatol. 2022;40(6):744–6.
29. Gnesotto L, Mioso G, Starace M, Piraccini BM, Naldi L, Sechi A. Nail lichen striatus affecting adjacent nails: a sign of Blaschko lines. Dermatol Pract Concept. 2023;13(4):e2023208.

50 Darier Disease

Kaya L. Curtis and Shari R. Lipner

50.1 Description of Disease

Darier disease (also known as keratosis follicularis or Darier-White disease) is a rare, autosomal dominant keratinization disorder characterized by greasy, hyperkeratotic papules and plaques involving seborrheic regions, including the face, chest, back, and flexural regions [1, 2]. Almost all patients have nail involvement [2]. The pathognomonic nail finding is alternating red and white longitudinal streaks in a "candy-cane" pattern with distal V-shaped notching [3]. There is oral involvement in 15–50% of cases [3, 4], including white papules of the gingiva (cobblestoning), gingival hypertrophy, and obstructive sialadenitis [5]. Darier disease is due to a mutation in *ATP2A2*, a gene encoding sarcoplasmic/endoplasmic reticulum ATPase type 2 (SERCA2), an endoplasmic reticulum calcium pump. It is hypothesized that the dysfunctional SERCA2 pump causes accumulation of calcium in the cytosol, leading to reduced calcium in the keratinocyte endoplasmic reticulum [6]. Deficiency of calcium in the keratinocyte endoplasmic reticulum interferes with protein trafficking and causes acantholysis [6].

50.2 Epidemiology

Estimated prevalence of Darier disease is 1/36,000–1/100,000 [7–9]. Darier disease typically presents in adolescents and young adults [10], and affects men and women equally [2]. In Burge et al.'s cross-sectional study [3] of 163 Darier disease cases, 92% had nail involvement, and many patients recalled nail abnormalities during childhood. In Munro et al.'s cross-sectional study [9] of 75 cases, nail abnormalities were present in 99% of patients.

S. R. Lipner, *Atlas of Nail Disorders Across All Skin Colors*,
https://doi.org/10.1007/978-3-031-74272-9_50

50.3 Risk Factors

Darier disease is inherited in an autosomal dominant fashion with high penetrance and variable expressivity [9]. Over 270 *ATP2A2* mutations associated with Darier disease have been identified [11, 12]. However, phenotype-genotype correlations remain unclear, except for two subtypes of Darier disease (acral hemorrhagic and acrokeratotis verruciformis of Hopf) [6]. Heat, friction, mechanical trauma, infection, stress, sweating, and ultraviolet B irradiation may exacerbate Darier disease manifestations [10, 13–15].

50.4 Clinical Features

Patients with Darier disease have nails that classically show alternating red and white linear streaks (referred to as "candy-cane" nails), often accompanied by subungual keratosis or a distal V-shaped or wedge-shaped notch [16]. Other nail findings include nail plate ridging, splitting, and sandpaper texture [17]. Due to variable expressivity, some patients may only develop limited features of Darier disease, such as nail abnormalities or acrodermatitis verruciformis [2]. In Burge et al.'s cross-sectional study [3] of 163 patients, most patients had involvement of 2–3 nails, while a minority of patients had involvement of all nails. Toenails were less frequently and less severely affected than fingernails. Involved skin may be malodorous, pruritic, and/or painful [18]. Extracutaneous associations of Darier disease include neuropsychiatric disorders and type I diabetes mellitus [10].

50.5 Clinical Features in Skin of Color

Patients with darker skin types may present with hypopigmented macules in seborrheic regions [19]. Distinct clinical presentations of nail abnormalities in Darier disease in skin of color have not been characterized. Since longitudinal melanonychia due to melanocyte activation is common in skin of color patients, theoretically, darker-skinned patients with Darier disease may have white bands admixed with red and gray-brown longitudinal bands, resembling peppermint bark.

50.6 Requirements for Diagnosis

A thorough physical examination is performed to assess for characteristic cutaneous findings. Diagnosis is confirmed by skin biopsy, which demonstrates suprabasal clefts with acantholysis extending throughout all epidermis layers with papillated epidermal hyperplasia [20–22]. Histopathologic confirmation is required to distinguish Darier disease from other acantholytic dyskeratoses, including Hailey-Hailey disease and Grover disease [2]. Though nail biopsy is typically unnecessary, nail histopathology demonstrates suprabasilar clefts with acantholytic and dyskeratotic cells in the nail matrix [23]. Patients may report nail changes prior to cutaneous findings [3]. A family history of Darier disease is supportive in making the diagnosis. However, a negative familial history does not rule out Darier disease given variable expressivity. Some patients may deny a family history of Darier disease, but mild features may be found in relatives on physical examination [9]. Personal or family history of neuropsychiatric disorders may be supportive features. Other differential diagnoses for patients presenting with polydactylous longitudinal erythronychia include lichen planus, amyloidosis, graft-versus-host disease, or acantholytic epidermolysis bullosa [16]. Polydactylous longitudinal leukonychia may be seen in Hailey-Hailey disease [24]. The presence of both longitudinal erythronychia and longitudinal leukonychia would increase likelihood of Darier disease.

50.7 Cases

Figures 50.1, 50.2, 50.3, 50.4, 50.5, 50.6, and 50.7 demonstrate the presentation of Darier disease in a clinical setting.

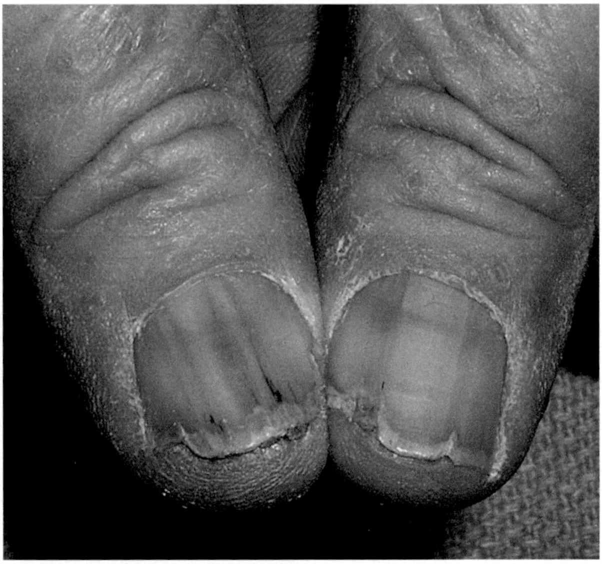

Fig. 50.1 Adult patient, Fitzpatrick type I, Darier disease, with nails with "candy-cane" polydactylous longitudinal erythronychia, distal onycholysis, splinter hemorrhages, and hyperkeratosis of hyponychium distal to red bands (*from* Jellinek et al. [16]; *with permission*)

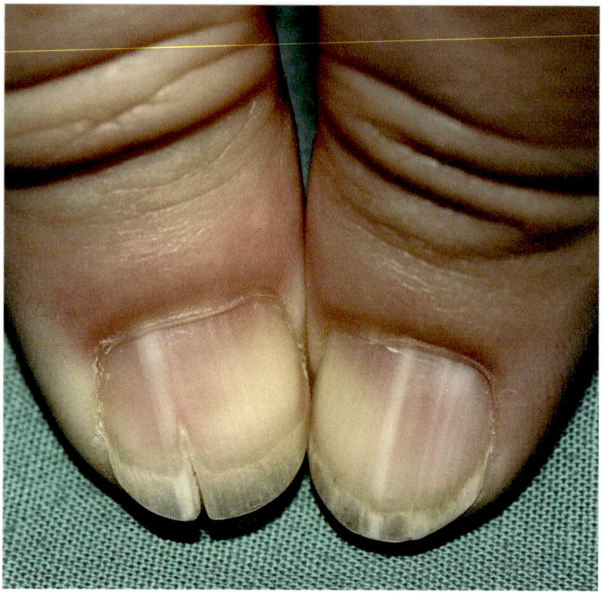

Fig. 50.2 Adult patient, Fitzpatrick type II, Darier disease, with characteristic V-shaped notch on the distal end of the nail plate (*from* Engin et al. [14]; *with permission*)

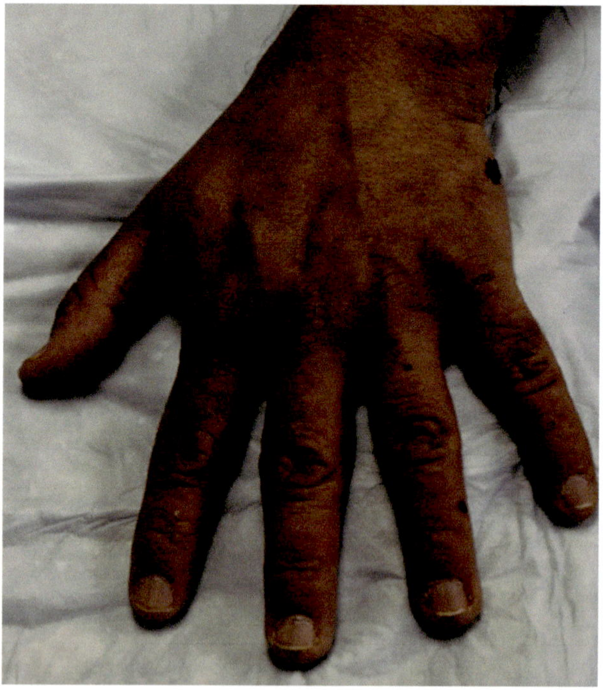

Fig. 50.3 41-Year-old male, Fitzpatrick type IV, acral hemorrhagic Darier disease, with dorsal aspects of the hands of the patient (*from* Hong et al. [25]; *with permission*)

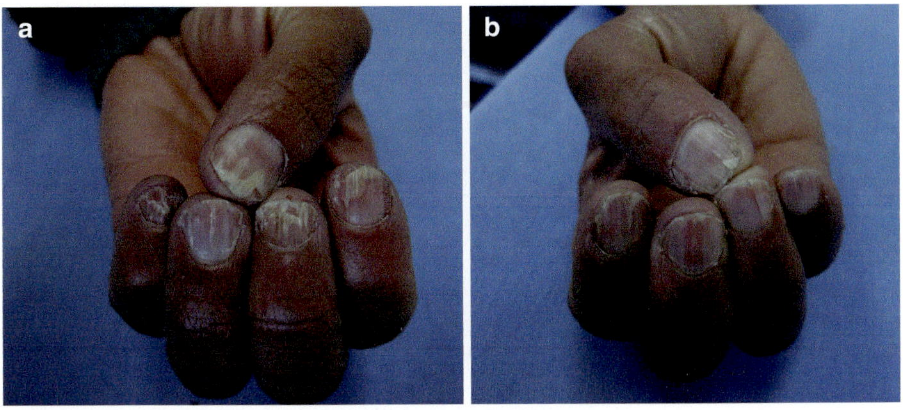

Fig. 50.4 (**a**) Adult patient, Fitzpatrick type IV, Darier disease, with alternating longitudinal erythronychia and longitudinal leukonychia (candy-cane nails), onycholysis, splitting, and distal V-shaped notching of the left fingernails. (**b**) Adult patient, Fitzpatrick type IV, Darier disease, with alternating longitudinal erythronychia and longitudinal leukonychia (candy-cane nails), onycholysis, splitting, and distal V-shaped notching of the right fingernails. (*courtesy of* Dr. Nilton Gioia Di Chiacchio, MD, PhD)

Fig. 50.5 Adult Indian patient, Fitzpatrick type V, Darier disease, with longitudinal erythronychia and distal V-shaped notching (*courtesy of* Dr. Chander Grover, MD, DNB)

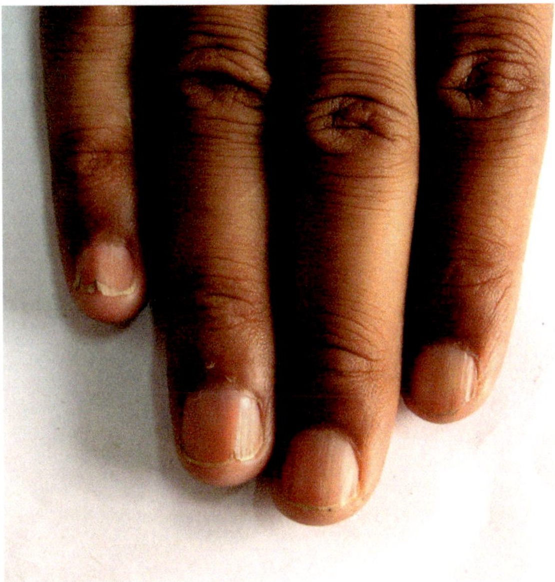

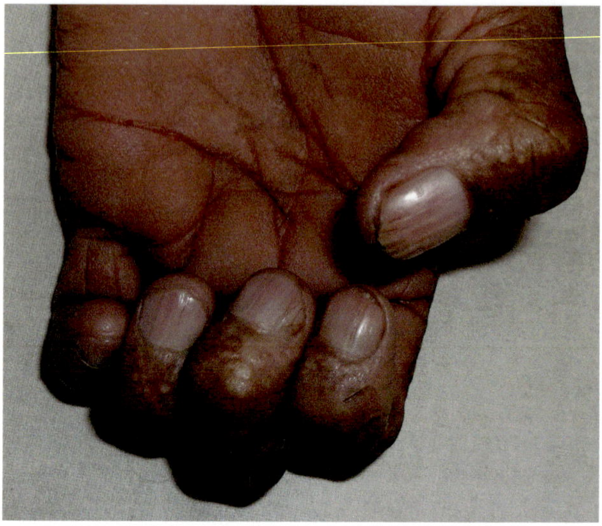

Fig. 50.6 Adult Indian patient, Fitzpatrick type V, Darier disease, with alternating longitudinal erythronychia and longitudinal leukonychia (candy-cane nails) and distal V-shaped notching (*courtesy of* Dr. Chander Grover, MD, DNB)

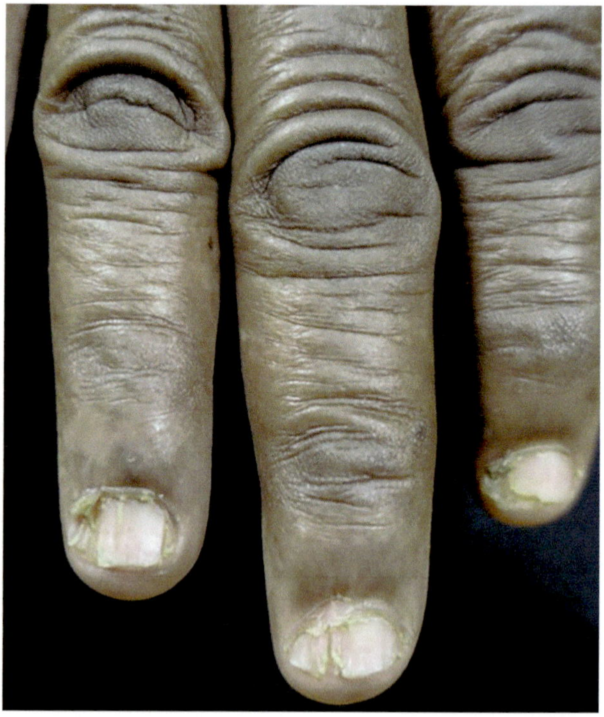

Fig. 50.7 55-Year-old male, Fitzpatrick type VI, Darier disease, with subungual hyperkeratosis and V-shaped scalloping of the fingernails (*from* Harb et al. [26]; *with permission*)

References

1. Takagi A, Kamijo M, Ikeda S. Darier disease. J Dermatol. 2016;43(3):275–9.
2. Cooper SM, Burge SM. Darier's disease: epidemiology, pathophysiology, and management. Am J Clin Dermatol. 2003;4(2):97–105.
3. Burge SM, Wilkinson JD. Darier-White disease: a review of the clinical features in 163 patients. J Am Acad Dermatol. 1992;27(1):40–50.
4. Macleod RI, Munro CS. The incidence and distribution of oral lesions in patients with Darier's disease. Br Dent J. 1991;171:133–6.
5. Shwetha V, Sujatha S, Yashoda Devi BK, et al. Spectrum of features in Darier's disease: a case report with emphasis on differential diagnosis. J Oral Biol Craniofac Res. 2019;9:215–20.
6. Hohl D. Darier disease and Hailey-Hailey disease. Saunders Elsevier; 2012. p. 887–97.
7. Svendson IB, Albrectsen B. The prevalence of dyskeratosis follicularis (Darier's disease) in Denmark. Acta Derm Venereol. 1959;39:256–9.
8. Wilkinson JD, Marsden RA, Dawber RPR. Review of Darier's disease in the Oxford region. Br J Dermatol. 1977;97(Suppl. 15):15–6.
9. Munro CS. The phenotype of Darier's disease: penetrance and expressivity in adults and children. Br J Dermatol. 1992;127:126–30.
10. Bachar-Wikström E, Wikström JD. Darier disease—a multi-organ condition? Acta Derm Venereol. 2021;101(4):adv00430.
11. Prasad V, Lorenz JN, Lasko VM, Nieman ML, Huang W, Wang Y, Wieczorek DW, Shull GE. SERCA2 haploinsufficiency in a mouse model of Darier disease causes a selective predisposition to heart failure. Biomed Res Int. 2015;2015:251598.
12. Nellen RG, Steijlen PM, van Steensel MA, Vreeburg M, European Professional Contributors, Frank J, et al. Mendelian disorders of cornification caused by defects in intracellular calcium pumps: mutation update and database for variants in ATP2A2 and ATP2C1 associated with Darier disease and Hailey-Hailey disease. Hum Mutat. 2017;38:343–56.
13. Suryawanshi H, Dhobley A, Sharma A, Kumar P. Darier disease: a rare genodermatosis. J Oral Maxillofac Pathol. 2017;21(2):321.
14. Engin B, Kutlubay Z, Erkan E, Tüzün Y. Darier disease: a fold (intertriginous) dermatosis. Clin Dermatol. 2015;33(4):448–51.
15. Godic A, Miljkovic J, Kansky A, Vidmar G. Epidemiology of Darier's disease in Slovenia. Acta Dermatovenerol Alp Pannonica Adriat. 2005;14(2):43–8.
16. Jellinek NJ. Longitudinal erythronychia: suggestions for evaluation and management. J Am Acad Dermatol. 2011;64(1):167.e1–11.
17. Sehgal VN, Chatterjee K, Chaudhuri A, Verma P, Sharma S. Twenty-nail dystrophy and Darier's (Darier-White) disease. Skinmed. 2015;13(4):313–5.
18. Patel TS, Herrera-Martinez M. Darier disease. Mayo Clin Proc. 2021;96(3):688–9.
19. Berth-Jones J, Hutchinson PE. Darier's disease with perifollicular depigmentation. Br J Dermatol. 1989;120:827–30.
20. See SHC, Peternel S, Adams D, North JP. Distinguishing histopathologic features of acantholytic dermatoses and the pattern of acantholytic hypergranulosis. J Cutan Pathol. 2019;46:6–15.
21. Kositkuljorn C, Suchonwanit P. Darier's disease: report of a case with facial involvement. Case Rep Dermatol. 2019;11:327–33.
22. Gupta LK, Garg A, Khare AK, Mittal A. A case of zosteriform Darier's disease with seasonal recurrence. Indian Dermatol Online J. 2013;4:219–21.
23. Zaias N, Ackerman AB. The nail in Darier-White disease. Arch Dermatol. 1973;107(2):193–9.
24. Schneider SL, Tosti A. Tips to diagnose uncommon nail disorders. Dermatol Clin. 2015;33(2):197–205.
25. Hong E, Hu R, Posligua A, Choate K, Durkin JR. Acral hemorrhagic Darier disease: a case report of a rare presentation and literature review. JAAD Case Rep. 2022;31:93–6.
26. Harb JN, Motaparthi K. Clinicopathologic findings of guttate leukoderma in Darier disease: a helpful diagnostic feature. JAAD Case Rep. 2018;4(3):262–6.

Pachyonychia Congenita

51

Kaya L. Curtis and Shari R. Lipner

51.1 Description of Disease

Pachyonychia congenita is a group of autosomal dominant inherited keratinization disorders characterized by a clinical triad of palmoplantar keratoderma, plantar pain, and hypertrophic nail dystrophy [1]. Pachyonychia congenita is classified into five subtypes based on keratin gene mutations. Clinical features, age of onset, and severity of clinical findings differ by subtype [2].

51.2 Epidemiology

Pachyonychia congenita is rare. Number of total cases is 1,000–10,000 patients worldwide, though actual prevalence is likely higher given underdiagnosis, especially of milder subtypes [3]. Male and female patients are equally affected, and there is no difference in prevalence between racial and ethnic groups [3]. Patients typically present during childhood by age 10 years [1].

51.3 Risk Factors

Pachyonychia congenita is inherited in an autosomal dominant manner. Genetic mutations in five keratin genes have been identified, including *KRT6A*, *KRT6B*, *KRT6C*, *KRT16*, and *KRT17* [1]. Each genetic mutation is associated with a distinct phenotype. De novo mutations are responsible for approximately 30% of cases [4].

S. R. Lipner, *Atlas of Nail Disorders Across All Skin Colors*,
https://doi.org/10.1007/978-3-031-74272-9_51

51.4 Clinical Features

Nail dystrophy is typically the initial presenting symptom of pachyonychia congenita and occurs during the first months of life [1]. There are two main nail phenotypes [5]. In the first nail phenotype, nails grow full length at an upward slant with increased curvature due to prominent distal hyperkeratosis [5]. In the second nail phenotype, nails have a premature nail plate termination with a distal hyperkeratotic sloping region and exposed distal region [5]. Splinter hemorrhages, increased transverse curvature, and paronychia, may also be observed [1, 6]. Both the fingernails and toenails may be involved. There is typically involvement of all nails, though fewer nail involvement is also possible depending on genetic mutation [2, 6]. Genetic variants may serve as predictors of clinical manifestations [7]. In a phenotype review [2] of 254 patients with genetically confirmed pachyonychia congenita, toenail thickening was the most frequently reported clinical finding (98%). Average number of toenails affected was 8.8 toenails, and median age of toenail dystrophy onset was 1 month [2]. Average age of toenail dystrophy onset for patients with *KRT6A*, *KRT17*, *KRT16*, and *KRT6B* mutations was 0.35, 0.9, 6.8, and 9.5 years, respectively [2]. Fingernail thickening was reported in 87% (220/254). Patients with *KRT6B* mutations had fewer fingernails affected compared with those with other keratin gene mutations [2]. In Shah et al.'s cross-sectional survey study [4] of 101 patients with genetically confirmed pachyonychia congenita, there was later onset and less frequent occurrence of nail dystrophy and keratoderma in patients with *KRT6B*, *KRT6C*, and *KRT16* mutations. Patients were *KRT6A* and *KRT17* mutations were more likely to have concurrent fingernail and toenail thickening [4]. Highly visible nail dystrophy and painful plantar thickening can impair mobility and profoundly affect quality of life [4]. Other clinical features include pruritus, follicular hyperkeratosis, pilosebaceous cysts, natal teeth, oral leukokeratosis, and hyperhidrosis [1].

51.5 Clinical Features in Skin of Color

Distinct clinical presentations of pachyonychia congenita in skin of color have not been characterized. Nail discoloration may be gray to brown in darker skin tones, compared to xanthonychia in lighter skin tones. Longitudinal melanonychia may also be present in darker skin types.

51.6 Requirements for Diagnosis

Thickening of multiple nails in early childhood is suggestive of pachyonychia congenita. This disorder is frequently misdiagnosed. In Shah et al.'s cross-sectional survey study [4] of 101 patients, the diagnosis of pachyonychia congenita was made by a physician before 1 year of age in only 27 patients (26.7%), despite the presence of toenail and fingernail dystrophy and positive family history in 60% and 44%, respectively. Diagnosis is based on presence of the clinical triad of palmoplantar keratoderma, plantar pain, and nail dystrophy, which are common clinical findings among all pachyonychia congenita subtypes [2]. Identification of genetic mutation in one of the five implicated keratin genes via molecular testing is required for definitive diagnosis [1]. Free genetic testing is available for patients through an expert genetics team at the Pachyonychia Congenita Project (https://www.pachyonychia.org). A positive family history of pachyonychia congenita is a supportive feature, though not necessary, given that a third of cases are caused by de novo genetic mutations [4]. In a study assessing histopathologic features of nail plates ($n = 56$) in 19 patients with genetically confirmed pachyonychia congenita, no specific histopathological features were identified [8].

51.7 Cases

Figures 51.1, 51.2, 51.3, 51.4, 51.5, 51.6, 51.7, 51.8, 51.9, 51.10, and 51.11 demonstrate the presentation of pachyonychia congenita in a clinical setting.

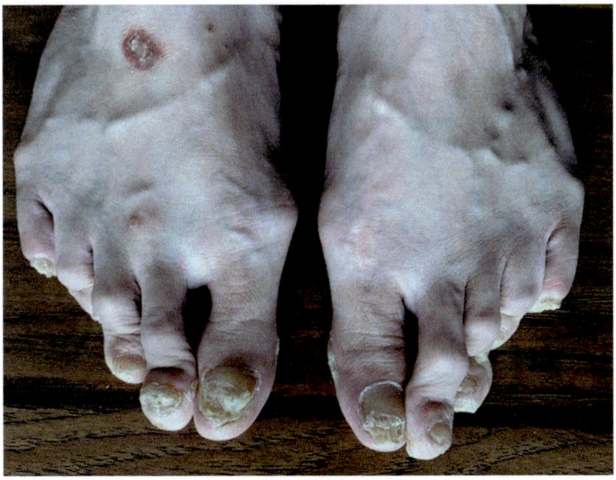

Fig. 51.1 47-Year-old female, Fitzpatrick type I, pachyonychia congenita secondary to *KRT6A* mutation, with thickening and xanthonychia of the toenails (*courtesy of* the Pachyonychia Congenita Project)

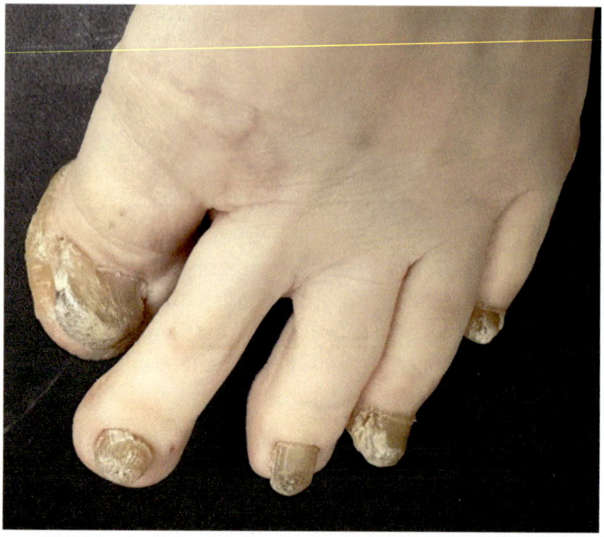

Fig. 51.2 49-Year-old female, Fitzpatrick type I, pachyonychia congenita secondary to *KRT6A* mutation, with xanthonychia and thickening of the toenails (*courtesy of* the Pachyonychia Congenita Project)

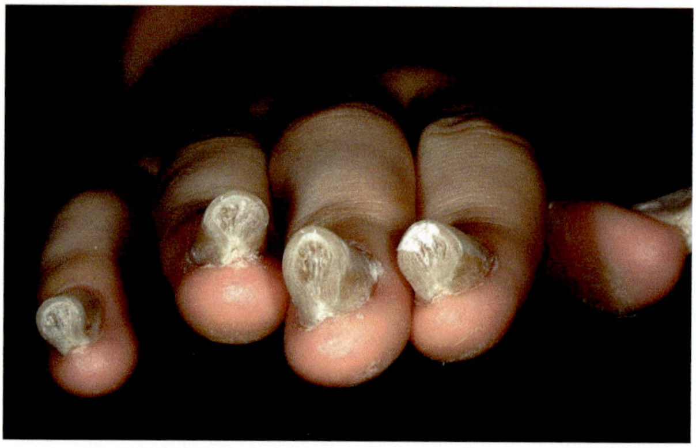

Fig. 51.3 29-Year-old female, Fitzpatrick type I, pachyonychia congenita secondary to *KRT16* mutation, with increased curvature and upward slanted growth of fingernails secondary to distal hyperkeratosis (*courtesy of* the Pachyonychia Congenita Project)

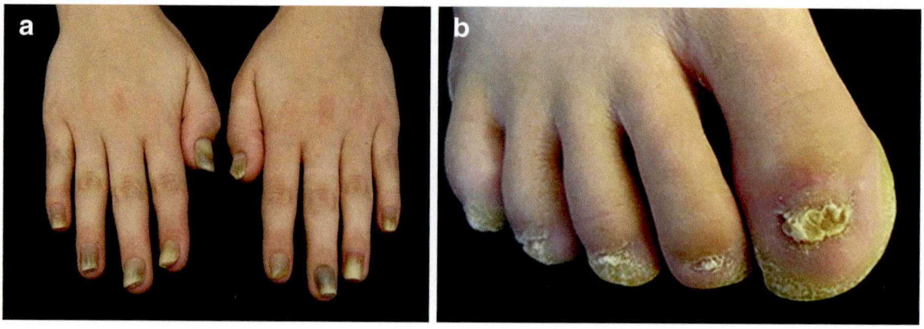

Fig. 51.4 (**a**) 40-Year-old female, Fitzpatrick type II, pachyonychia congenita secondary to *KRT6A* mutation, with xanthonychia, subungual hyperkeratosis, and thickening of the fingernails. (**b**) 40-Year-old female, Fitzpatrick type II, pachyonychia congenita secondary to *KRT6A* mutation, with xanthonychia and dystrophy of the toenails. There is premature nail plate termination of the toenails exposing the distal region (*courtesy of* the Pachyonychia Congenita Project)

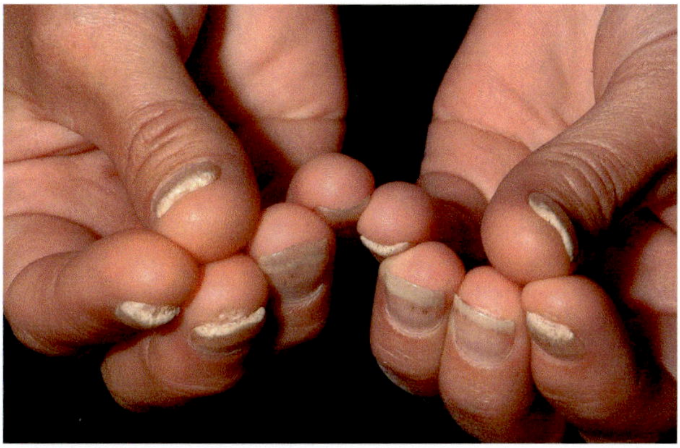

Fig. 51.5 59-Year-old female, Fitzpatrick type III, pachyonychia congenita secondary to *KRT17* mutation, with thickening, splinter hemorrhages, and subungual hyperkeratosis of the fingernails (*courtesy of* the Pachyonychia Congenita Project)

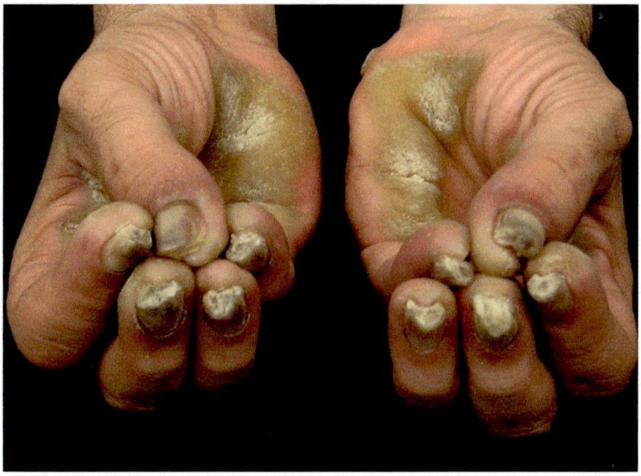

Fig. 51.6 58-Year-old male, Fitzpatrick type III, pachyonychia congenita secondary to *KRT16* mutation, with xanthonychia, thickening, and subungual hyperkeratosis of the fingernails. There is palmar keratoderma (*courtesy of* the Pachyonychia Congenita Project)

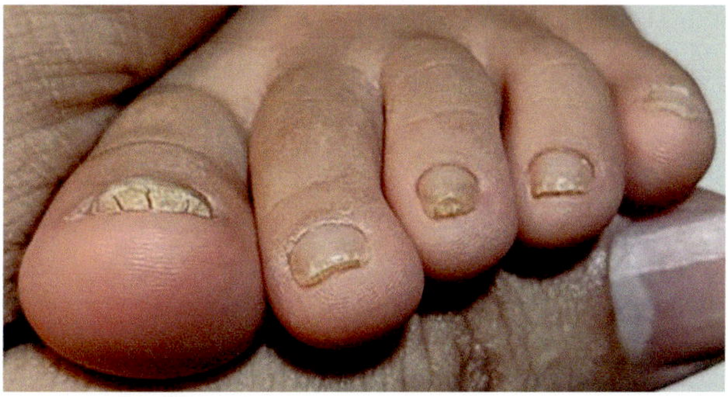

Fig. 51.7 2-Year-old male, Fitzpatrick type III, pachyonychia congenita secondary to *KRT17* mutation, with thickening of the toenails (*courtesy of* the Pachyonychia Congenita Project)

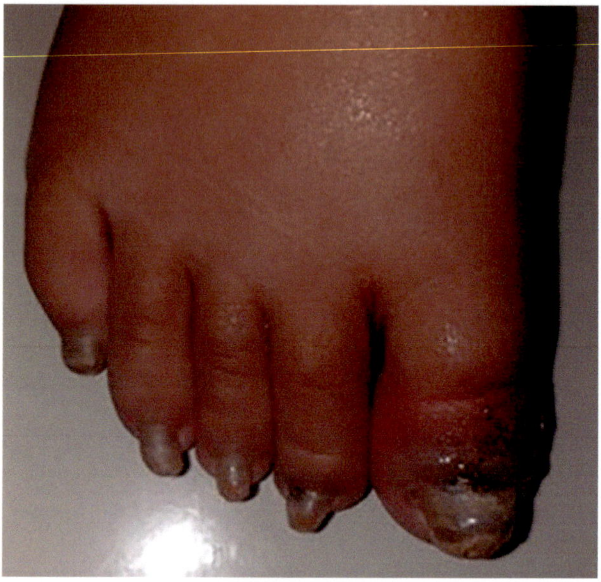

Fig. 51.8 6-Year-old female, Fitzpatrick type IV, pachyonychia congenita secondary to *KRT6A* mutation, with thickening and dystrophy of the toenails. There is paronychia of the right great toenail (*courtesy of* the Pachyonychia Congenita Project)

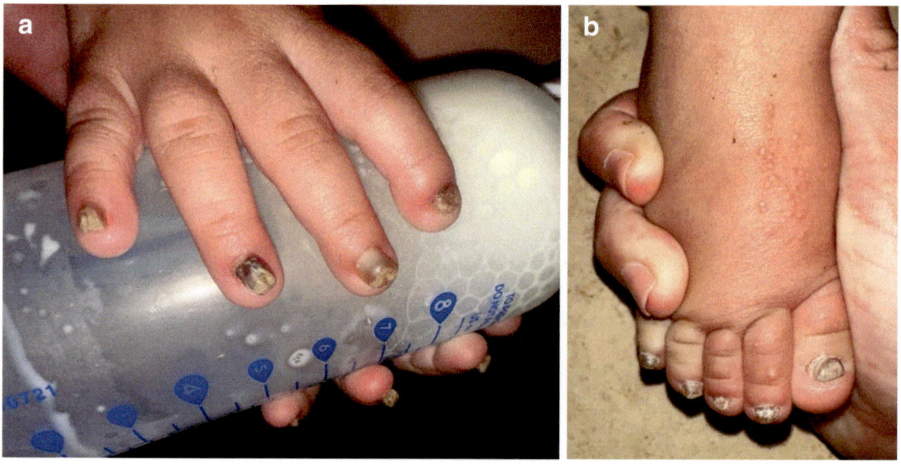

Fig. 51.9 (**a**) 1-Year-old male, Fitzpatrick type IV, pachyonychia congenita secondary to *KRT6A* mutation, with thickening and brown discoloration of the fingernails. (**b**) 1-Year-old male, Fitzpatrick type IV, pachyonychia congenita secondary to *KRT6A* mutation, with thickening and brown discoloration of the toenails. There are flat-topped flesh-colored papules on the dorsal foot (*courtesy of* the Pachyonychia Congenita Project)

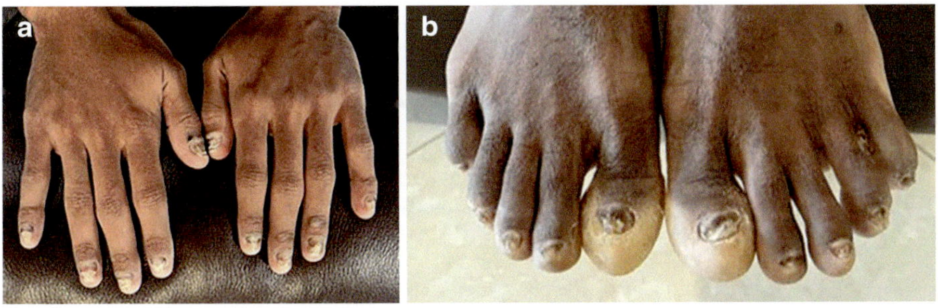

Fig. 51.10 (**a**) 36-Year-old male, Fitzpatrick type V, pachyonychia congenita secondary to *KRT6A* mutation, with thickening and brown discoloration of the fingernails. (**b**) 36-Year-old male, Fitzpatrick type V, pachyonychia congenita secondary to *KRT6A* mutation, with thickening and brown discoloration of the toenails. There is premature nail plate termination of the bilateral great toenails exposing the distal region (*courtesy of* the Pachyonychia Congenita Project)

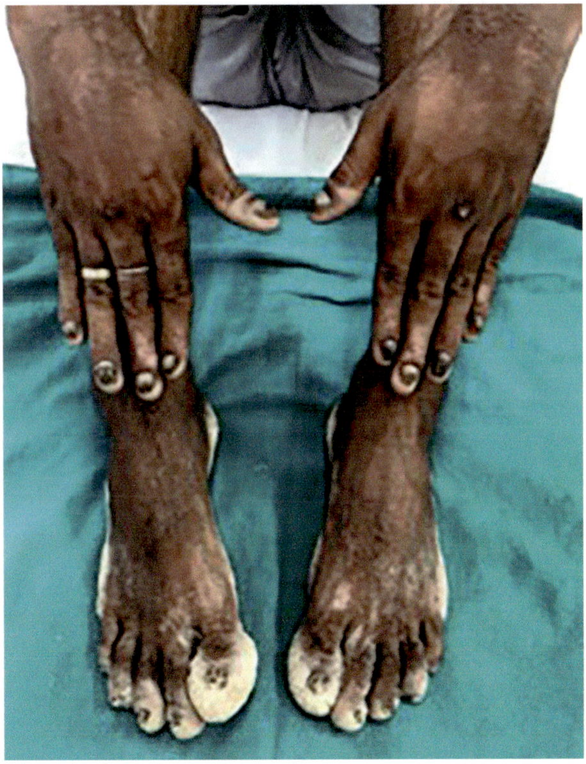

Fig. 51.11 Adult male, Fitzpatrick type VI, pachyonychia congenita secondary to *KRT6A* mutation, with thickening and brown discoloration of the fingernails and toenails. There is premature nail plate termination of the bilateral great toenails and hypopigmented patches of the dorsal hands and feet (*courtesy of* the Pachyonychia Congenita Project)

Acknowledgments We would like to thank the Pachyonychia Congenita Project for contribution of figures for this chapter.

References

1. Mccarthy RL, De Brito M, O'Toole E. Pachyonychia congenita: clinical features and future treatments. Keio J Med. 2023; https://doi.org/10.2302/kjm.2023-0012-IR.
2. Eliason MJ, Leachman SA, Feng B, Schwartz ME, Hansen CD. A review of the clinical phenotype of 254 patients with genetically confirmed pachyonychia congenita. J Am Acad Dermatol. 2012;67:680–6.
3. Kaspar RL. Challenges in developing therapies for rare diseases including pachyonychia congenita. J Investig Dermatol Symp Proc. 2005;10:62–6.
4. Shah S, Boen M, Kenner-Bell B, Schwartz M, Rademaker A, Paller AS. Pachyonychia congenita in pediatric patients: natural history, features, and impact. JAMA Dermatol. 2014;150(2):146–53.
5. Smith FJD, Hansen CD, Hull PR, et al. Pachyonychia congenita. 2006 Jan 27 [updated 2017 Nov 30]. In: Adam MP, Feldman J, Mirzaa GM, et al., editors. GeneReviews®. Seattle, WA: University of Washington; 1993–2024.
6. Bellet JS. Pediatric nail disorders. Dermatol Clin. 2021;39(2):231–43.
7. Wu TT, Eldirany SA, Bunick CG, Teng JMC. Genotype–structurotype–phenotype correlations in patients with pachyonychia congenita. J Invest Dermatol. 2021;141(12):2876–84.e4.
8. Stewart CL, Takeshita J, Hansen CD, Rubin AI. The histopathological features of the nail plate in pachyonychia congenita. J Cutan Pathol. 2020;47(4):357–62.

Epidermolysis Bullosa

52

Kaya L. Curtis and Shari R. Lipner

52.1 Description of Disease

Epidermolysis bullosa is a heterogeneous group of inherited blistering disorders characterized by mucocutaneous fragility [1]. The etiology is a mutation in cutaneous structural proteins. There are four types of epidermolysis bullosa classified by depth of blistering, including epidermolysis bullosa simplex (intraepidermal blistering), junctional epidermolysis bullosa (blistering in the lamina lucida of the basement membrane), dystrophic epidermolysis bullosa (blistering below the basement membrane), and Kindler epidermolysis bullosa (mixed skin cleavage pattern) [2, 3]. Classification is further divided into 34 subtypes (14 epidermolysis bullosa simplex, 9 junctional epidermolysis bullosa, and 11 dystrophic epidermolysis bullosa) [3, 4]. Each subtype of epidermolysis bullosa has different clinical manifestations and genetic mutations [2]. Classification may be challenging as there are multiple overlapping clinical signs between subtypes [3]. Nail matrix and bed abnormalities in epidermolysis bullosa are frequent and are caused by pathogenic alterations in the dermoepidermal junction [5]. Nail changes are included in the criteria for epidermolysis bullosa severity [6].

52.2 Epidemiology

Epidermolysis bullosa is a rare disease. In a prospective cross-sectional and longitudinal study [1] of 3271 patients in the National Epidermolysis Bullosa Registry 1986–2002, the estimated epidermolysis bullosa prevalence was 11 per million population and the estimated incidence was 20 per million live births. Male and female patients were equally affected with no difference in prevalence between racial or ethnic groups.

S. R. Lipner, *Atlas of Nail Disorders Across All Skin Colors*,
https://doi.org/10.1007/978-3-031-74272-9_52

52.3 Risk Factors

Epidermolysis bullosa is an inherited disorder, with at least 16 genes identified thus far [3]. There is variable expressivity between and within each subtype; therefore, there is a wide spectrum of presentations ranging from mild cutaneous features to severe cutaneous presentations and extracutaneous involvement [3, 7]. Trauma likely contributes to associated nail dystrophy, as is evidenced by more severe involvement of the great toenails [6].

52.4 Clinical Cutaneous Features

The characteristic sign of epidermolysis bullosa is cutaneous blister formation induced by minor mechanical trauma. In epidermolysis bullosa simplex, mechanical trauma causes superficial erosions, whereas mechanical trauma in junctional epidermolysis bullosa, dystrophic epidermolysis bullosa, and Kindler epidermolysis bullosa causes deeper ulcerations [3]. Oral, esophageal, tracheal, ocular, and genitourinary mucous membranes may also be affected. Patients with severe subtypes may have extramucocutaneous involvement, including osteoporosis, joint contractures, cardiomyopathy, renal amyloidosis, and growth delay [1, 4]. Patients with severe subtypes may have complications, including chronic infection, chronic pain, limb mutilation, squamous cell carcinoma, and early death [3, 8]. Squamous cell carcinoma is the leading cause of death. Cumulative risk of death from metastatic squamous cell carcinoma is 38.7% and 78.8% by 35 years and 55 years, respectively [1].

52.5 Clinical Nail Features

Nail changes in epidermolysis bullosa result from nail bed and nail matrix scarring, but there are no pathognomonic findings [6]. Nail findings may range from minor nail dystrophy to anonychia (absence of nail) [7]. Nail changes may be the first or only sign of epidermolysis bullosa, as observed in nail-only dominant dystrophic epidermolysis bullosa [6, 9–11]. In a systematic literature review [5] assessing nail changes in 74 epidermolysis bullosa patients, fingernail and toenail involvement occurred in 45.9% of patients, with an average of 13.8 nails affected per patient. The most common nail findings were nail dystrophy (48.6%), anonychia (43.2%), and pachyonychia (40.5%). Other nail findings include onychorrhexis, onycholysis, thickening, xanthonychia, onychomadesis, onychogryphosis, subungual hematoma, and nail matrix scarring resulting in micronychia [6].

52.5.1 Clinical Nail Features of Epidermolysis Bullosa Simplex

The nails are typically spared in localized epidermolysis bullosa simplex [6]. Onycholysis, onychomadesis, toenail thickening, and onychogryphosis may be observed in more severe epidermolysis bullosa simplex subtypes [6]. In a phenotype review of 130 epidermolysis bullosa simplex patients, nail changes included periodic shedding of fingernails and toenails in infants and great toenail thickening in adults [12]. Subungual hematomas may result from blister-associated bleeding underneath the nails.

52.5.2 Clinical Nail Features of Epidermolysis Junctional Epidermolysis Bullosa

Severe nail abnormalities are observed with most subtypes of junctional epidermolysis bullosa [6]. Subungual blistering may result in nail bed erosions leading to anonychia [6]. Other nail findings include paronychia, onycholysis, and periungual/subungual granulation tissue [6].

52.5.3 Clinical Nail Features of Dystrophic Epidermolysis Bullosa

Severity of nail abnormalities differs among various subtypes of dystrophic epidermolysis bullosa. Patients with nail involvement early in life are more likely to develop nail loss, as recurrent episodes of blistering result in nail bed and matrix scarring with eventual permanent anonychia [6]. Dystrophic epidermolysis bullosa, nails only (DEB-na) is a rare subtype of dystrophic epidermolysis bullosa in which nail changes are the predominant sign of disease [13]. In a case series [13] of two DEB-na patients, a 5-year-old boy presented with 20-nail dystrophy, specifically roughness, thickening, and xanthonychia of all 20 nail plates since birth, without associated skin findings. The other patient was a 27-year-old man who presented with recurrent blisters of the extremities associated with mild trauma. The patient had lost almost all toenails and the fingernails were short, rough, and embedded in the skin.

52.5.4 Clinical Nail Features of Kindler Epidermolysis Bullosa

Long and thick cuticles extending over half of the nail plate have been reported in patients with Kindler epidermolysis bullosa [14, 15].

52.6 Clinical Features in Skin of Color

Distinct clinical presentations of nail involvement in skin of color have not been characterized. Recurrent subungual blistering trauma may result in longitudinal melanonychia due to melanocytic activation in darker skin tones.

52.7 Requirements for Diagnosis

Diagnosis of the specific subtype of epidermolysis bullosa is important, as it allows for precision medicine, genetic counseling, and prognosis counseling [4]. Definitive diagnosis requires skin biopsy with immunofluorescence mapping, transmission electron microscopy, or genetic analysis [4, 16]. Skin biopsy with immunofluorescence mapping alone is diagnostic when the level of cleavage and subtype is identified. In cases in which immunofluorescence mapping does not identify the level of cleavage or subtype, diagnostic confirmation may be achieved with additional transmission electron microscopy or genetic analysis. Nail biopsy is not necessary for diagnosis. A family history of epidermolysis bullosa is a supportive feature, though a negative family history does not rule out the disease given variable expressivity.

52.8 Cases

Figures 52.1, 52.2, 52.3, 52.4, 52.5, 52.6, 52.7, 52.8, 52.9, and 52.10 demonstrate the presentation of epidermolysis bullosa in a clinical setting.

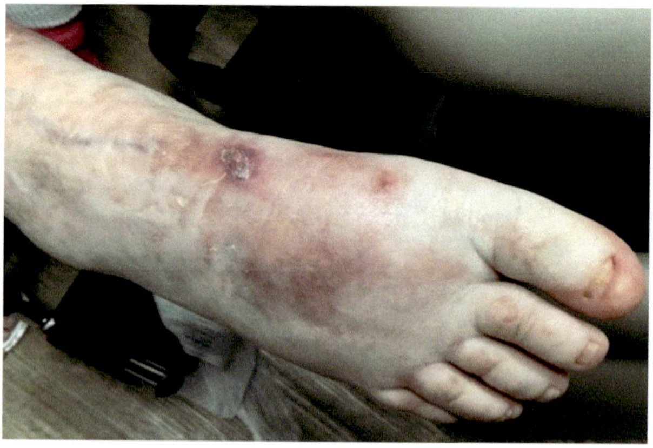

Fig. 52.1 A 24-year-old female, Fitzpatrick type I, syndromic epidermolysis bullosa simplex with nephropathy and epilepsy, with the dorsum of the right foot with a single bulla as well as dystrophic nail of first digit (*from* Dunn et al. [17]; *with permission*)

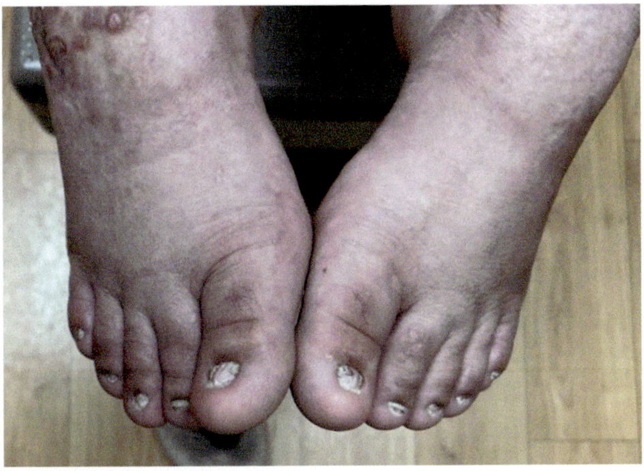

Fig. 52.2 A 35-year-old female, Fitzpatrick type II, epidermolysis bullosa pruriginosa, with dystrophic nail abnormalities. Onychorrhexis with signs of nail matrix scarring resulting in micronychia (*from* LaMonica et al. [18]; *with permission*)

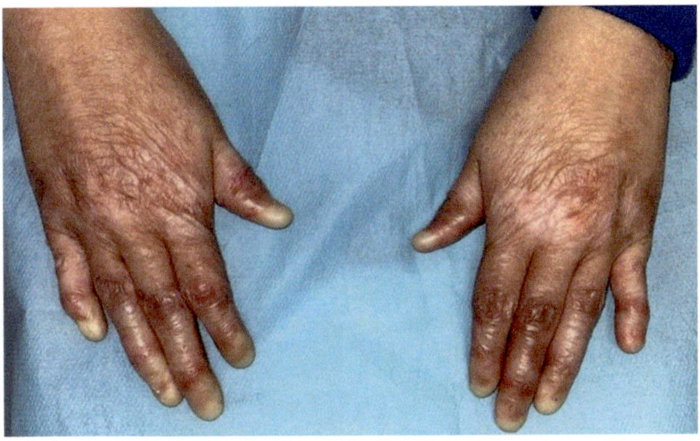

Fig. 52.3 A 27-year-old female, Fitzpatrick type III, recessive dystrophic epidermolysis bullosa, with view of the hands showing absence of nails, scarring, and deformity (*from* El Yacoubi et al. [19]; *with permission*)

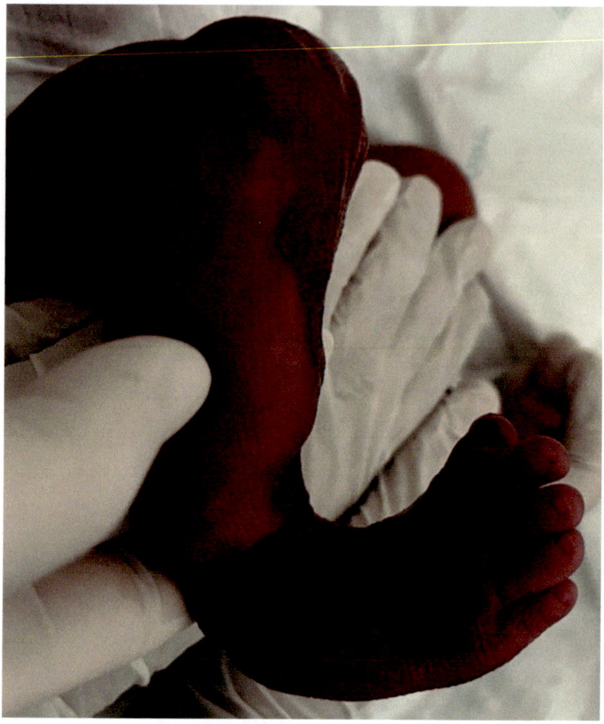

Fig. 52.4 A 10-day-old male, Fitzpatrick type IV, dominant dystrophic epidermolysis bullosa, with an S-shaped area of localized absence of skin accompanied by first toenail dystrophy and small erosions in both feet (*from* Ramos et al. [20]; *with permission*)

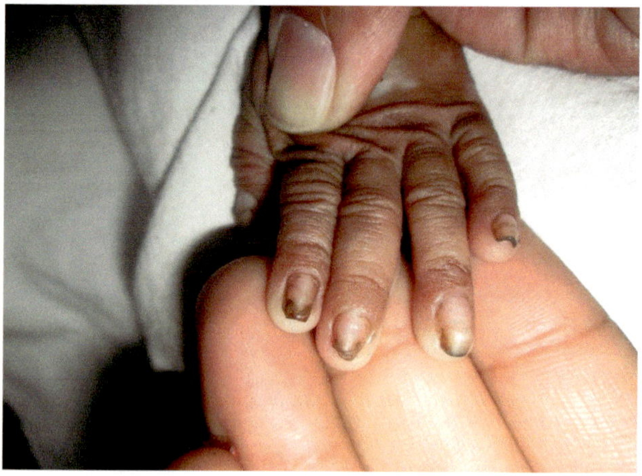

Fig. 52.5 A 4-month-old male child, Fitzpatrick skin type IV, with epidermolysis bullosa junctionalis, with multiple Beau's lines, partial nail shedding, and distal yellow-brown discoloration. The patient had recurrent blistering since birth (*courtesy of* Dr. Chander Grover, MD, DNB)

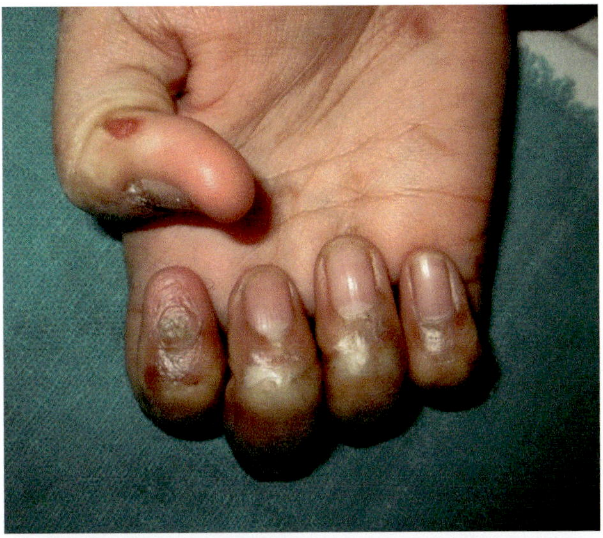

Fig. 52.6 An 18-year-old female, Fitzpatrick skin type IV, dystrophic epidermolysis bullosa, with scarring and acquired anonychia of multiple fingernails. There was a history of blistering followed by scarring since birth (*courtesy of* Dr. Chander Grover, MD, DNB)

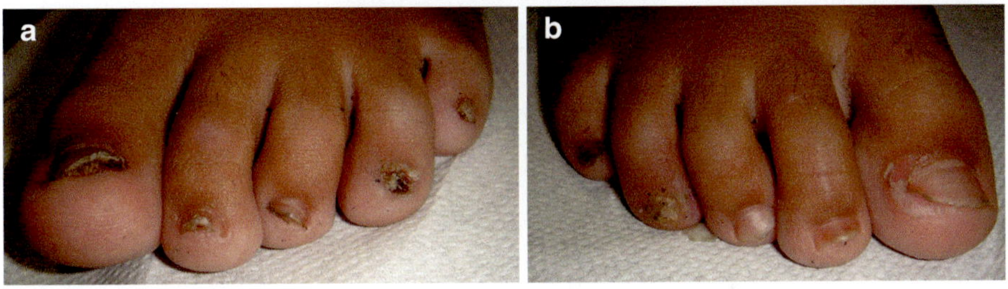

Fig. 52.7 (**a**) A 9-year-old female, Fitzpatrick type IV, epidermolysis bullosa, with brown discoloration and micronychia of the left toenails. (**b**) A 9-year-old female, Fitzpatrick type IV, epidermolysis bullosa, with partial nail shedding of the right fourth toenail and erosion of the right great toe (*courtesy of* Dr. Bertrand Richert, MD, PhD)

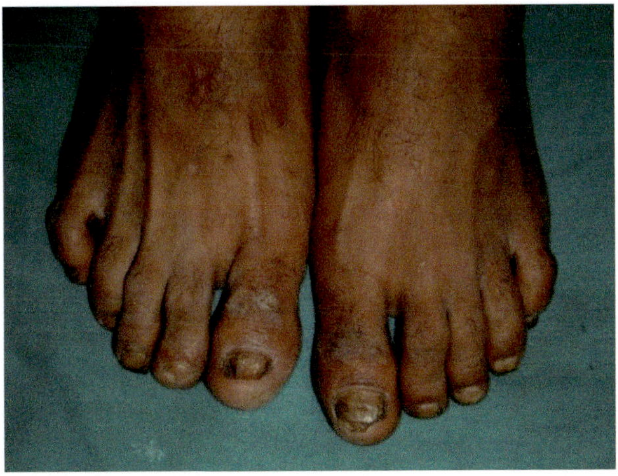

Fig. 52.8 A 28-year-old male, Fitzpatrick type IV, with epidermolysis bullosa pruriginosa, with thickening, discoloration, and dystrophy of multiple toenails. The patient presented with multiple pruritic lesions involving bilateral shins, followed by involvement of the extensor aspects of the arms (*courtesy of* Dr. Chander Grover, MD, DNB)

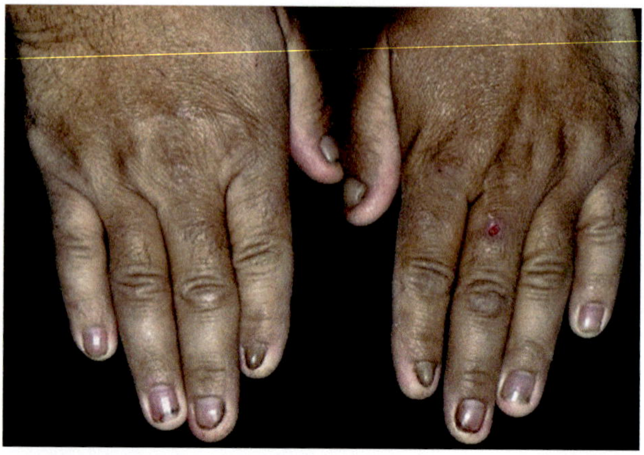

Fig. 52.9 A 45-year-old male, Fitzpatrick type V, syndromic epidermolysis bullosa without pulmonary involvement, with dystrophic nails (*from* Kinyó et al. [21]; *with permission*)

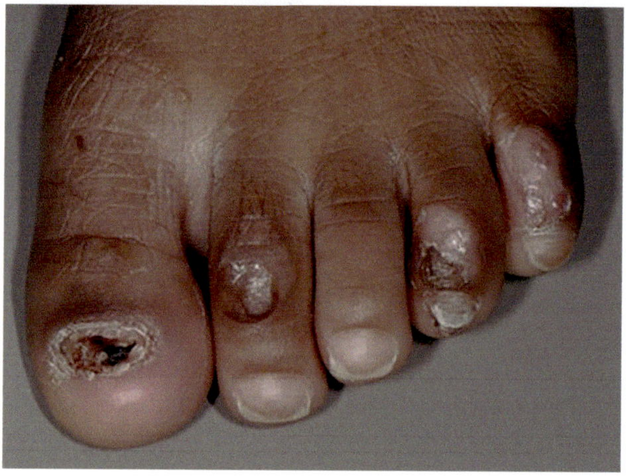

Fig. 52.10 A 3-year-old patient, Fitzpatrick type V, dominant dystrophic epidermolysis bullosa, with nail dystrophy, milia, and scarring (*from* Bellet [22]; *with permission*)

References

1. Fine JD, Eady RA, Bauer EA, Bauer JW, Bruckner-Tuderman L, Heagerty A, Hintner H, Hovnanian A, Jonkman MF, Leigh I, McGrath JA, Mellerio JE, Murrell DF, Shimizu H, Uitto J, Vahlquist A, Woodley D, Zambruno G. The classification of inherited epidermolysis bullosa (EB): report of the Third International Consensus Meeting on Diagnosis and Classification of EB. J Am Acad Dermatol. 2008;58(6):931–50.
2. Intong LR, Murrell DF. Inherited epidermolysis bullosa: new diagnostic criteria and classification. Clin Dermatol. 2012;30(1):70–7.
3. Mariath LM, Santin JT, Schuler-Faccini L, Kiszewski AE. Inherited epidermolysis bullosa: update on the clinical and genetic aspects. An Bras Dermatol. 2020;95(5):551–69.
4. Has C, Bauer JW, Bodemer C, Bolling MC, Bruckner-Tuderman L, Diem A, Fine JD, Heagerty A, Hovnanian A, Marinkovich MP, Martinez AE, McGrath JA, Moss C, Murrell DF, Palisson F, Schwieger-Briel A, Sprecher E, Tamai K, Uitto J, Woodley DT, Zambruno G, Mellerio JE. Consensus reclassification of inherited epidermolysis bullosa and other disorders with skin fragility. Br J Dermatol. 2020;183(4):614–27.

5. Pastrana-Arellano E, Morales-Olvera D, García-Romero MT. Nail involvement in patients with epidermolysis bullosa: a systematic review. Skin Health Dis. 2022;3(1):e183.
6. Tosti A, de Farias DC, Murrell DF. Nail involvement in epidermolysis bullosa. Dermatol Clin. 2010;28(1):153–7.
7. Bruckner-Tuderman L, Has C. Molecular heterogeneity of blistering disorders: the paradigm of epidermolysis bullosa. J Invest Dermatol. 2012;132(E1):E2–5.
8. Bardhan A, Bruckner-Tuderman L, Chapple ILC, Fine JD, Harper N, Has C, Magin TM, Marinkovich MP, Marshall JF, McGrath JA, Mellerio JE, Polson R, Heagerty AH. Epidermolysis bullosa. Nat Rev Dis Primers. 2020;6(1):78.
9. Dharma B, Moss C, McGrath JA, Mellerio JE, Ilchyshyn A. Dominant dystrophic epidermolysis bullosa presenting as familial nail dystrophy. Clin Exp Dermatol. 2001;26(1):93–6.
10. González-Cantero A, Sánchez-Moya AI, Pérez-Hortet C, Martinez-Lorenzo E, Gomez-Dorado B, Schoendorff-Ortega C. "Nails only" phenotype and partial dominance of p.Glu170Lys mutation in a family with epidermolysis bullosa simplex. Pediatr Dermatol. 2017;34(4):e205–6.
11. Tosti A, Piraccini BM, Scher RK. Isolated nail dystrophy suggestive of dominant dystrophic epidermolysis bullosa. Pediatr Dermatol. 2003;20(5):456–7.
12. Horn HM, Tidman MJ. The clinical spectrum of epidermolysis bullosa simplex. Br J Dermatol. 2000;142(3):468–72.
13. Yang R, Duan Y, Kong Q, Li W, Xu J, Xia X, Sang H. What do we learn from dystrophic epidermolysis bullosa, nails only? Idiopathic nail dystrophy may harbor a COL7A1 mutation as the underlying cause. J Dermatol. 2020;47(7):782–6.
14. Gupta V, Dogra D, Gupta N, Parveen S. Kindler's syndrome with long thick cuticles and mottled hyperpigmentation. Indian J Dermatol Venereol Leprol. 2011;77(1):66–8.
15. Nath AK, Chougule A, Thappa DM. Long cuticle of the nail in Kindler's syndrome: is it more than an incidental finding? Indian J Dermatol Venereol Leprol. 2009;75(3):314–5.
16. Has C, Fischer J. Inherited epidermolysis bullosa: new diagnostics and new clinical phenotypes. Exp Dermatol. 2019;28:1146–52.
17. Dunn C, Ambur A, Foss M, Nathoo R. Expanding the spectrum of epidermolysis bullosa simplex: syndromic epidermolysis bullosa simplex with nephropathy and epilepsy secondary to CD151 tetraspanin defect-a case report and review of the literature. JAAD Case Rep. 2022;23:136–40.
18. LaMonica LC, Lang-Houser M, Bresler SC, Mervak JE. Low-dose naltrexone as treatment for epidermolysis bullosa pruriginosa-associated refractory pruritus. JAAD Case Rep. 2023;38:82–5.
19. El Yacoubi O, Chbicheb S. Recessive dystrophic epidermolysis bullosa (RDEB): oral manifestation and management rules in oral surgery: a case report. Int J Surg Case Rep. 2023;102:107848.
20. Ramos FJM, Corpas TD, Corrales AE, Puchades AM. Congenital localized absence of skin (Bart syndrome) in a patient with dominant dystrophic epidermolysis bullosa. An Pediatr (Engl Ed). 2023;99(6):447–8.
21. Kinyó Á, Kovács AL, Degrell P, Kálmán E, Nagy N, Kárpáti S, Gyulai R, Saeidian AH, Youssefian L, Vahidnezhad H, Uitto J. Homozygous ITGA3 missense mutation in adults in a family with syndromic epidermolysis bullosa (ILNEB) without pulmonary involvement. J Invest Dermatol. 2021;141(11):2752–6.
22. Bellet JS. Pediatric nail disorders and selected genodermatoses with nail findings. In: Rubin AI, Jellinek NJ, Daniel CR, Scher RK, editors. Scher and Daniel's nails. 4th ed. Cham: Springer; 2018. https://doi.org/10.1007/978-3-319-65649-6_20.

Brachyonychia

53

Kaya L. Curtis and Shari R. Lipner

53.1 Description of Disease

Brachyonychia is characterized by a short, broad nail(s) with nail plate width exceeding length [1]. There is frequently associated bone and soft tissue deformity [2–4]. Brachyonychia may be hereditary or acquired.

53.2 Epidemiology

The epidemiology of brachyonychia is unknown. Hereditary brachyonychia affects patients of all ages. Acquired brachyonychia due to hyperparathyroidism (e.g., in chronic kidney disease) typically affects older patients. A female-to-male ratio of 3:1 has been previously reported [5].

53.3 Risk Factors

Hereditary brachyonychia is inherited in an autosomal dominant manner [6]. Pathogenesis in the hereditary form has been hypothesized to be due to premature closure of the cartilaginous line of the distal phalanx [7]. Acquired brachyonychia is primarily associated with acro-osteolysis (lytic destruction of the distal phalanges due to bone resorption) [2, 4, 8, 9]. In a cross-sectional study [10] of 235 atopic dermatitis pediatric patients, 10.2% of patients had nail abnormalities, of which brachyonychia was present in 8.3%. In a literature review of nail changes in acro-osteolysis, brachyonychia was the most commonly reported nail finding [11]. Acro-osteolysis may result from hyperparathyroidism (e.g., in chronic kidney disease, malabsorption, osteomalacia, and rickets) [1, 12, 13], onychophagia, leprosy [14, 15], frostbite or severe cold exposure [16], trauma, inflammatory diseases (such as scleroderma, Raynaud disease, and psoriatic arthritis), drugs (such as phenytoin),

S. R. Lipner, *Atlas of Nail Disorders Across All Skin Colors*,
https://doi.org/10.1007/978-3-031-74272-9_53

and tumors (such as epidermal inclusion cyst or glomus tumor) [12]. A case of acquired brachyonychia secondary to Erasmus syndrome (systemic sclerosis resulting from silica exposure) has also been reported [17]. In a retrospective cohort study [12] of eight chronic kidney disease patients on dialysis who presented with brachyonychia, X-ray demonstrated acro-osteolysis of the phalanges in all patients.

53.4 Clinical Features

On physical examination, brachyonychia is characterized by a short nail plate that is greater in width than length, with a "racquet" appearance. Lateral nail folds may be absent or very narrow [18, 19]. Hereditary brachyonychia is typically an isolated disorder; however, rarely may be associated with other syndromic congenital abnormalities [1], including cartilage-hair hypoplasia, Rubinstein–Taybi syndrome, Larsen syndrome, Brooke–Spiegler syndrome, Bardet–Biedl syndrome, and Stüve–Wiedemann syndrome [6, 20]. Hereditary brachyonychia primarily involves the thumbnails [1, 6], whereas acquired brachyonychia may involve additional digits [12].

53.5 Clinical Features in Skin of Color

Distinct clinical presentations of brachyonychia in skin of color have not been characterized. Patients with darker skin tones may have concurrent longitudinal melanonychia.

53.6 Requirements for Diagnosis

Brachyonychia is a clinical diagnosis. A family history of brachyonychia and nail involvement since birth is supportive of hereditary brachyonychia. It is important to elicit a history of onychophagia as it may be a potential etiology. A thorough medical history is conducted to assess for potential medical comorbidities resulting in acro-osteolysis. Exposures to cold or medications (e.g., phenytoin) that may result in acro-osteolysis may be elicited. X-ray may aid in diagnosis and may demonstrate lytic lesions of the distal phalanges. Baran et al. recommend measuring parathyroid hormone and serum 25 hydroxy-D3 in all patients with acquired brachyonychia to assess for hyperparathyroidism [1].

53.7 Cases

Figures 53.1, 53.2, 53.3, 53.4, 53.5, 53.6, and 53.7 demonstrate the presentation of brachyonychia in a clinical setting.

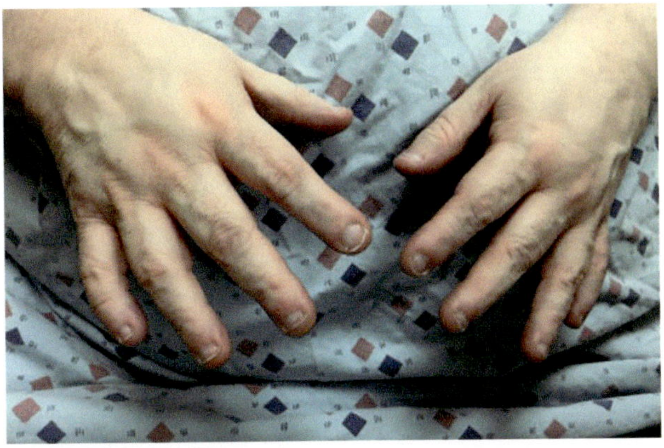

Fig. 53.1 44-Year-old male, Fitzpatrick type II, brachyonychia, with clinical brachyonychia of the fingernails. Etiology: Bardet-Biedl syndrome (*from* Detty et al. [6]; *with permission*)

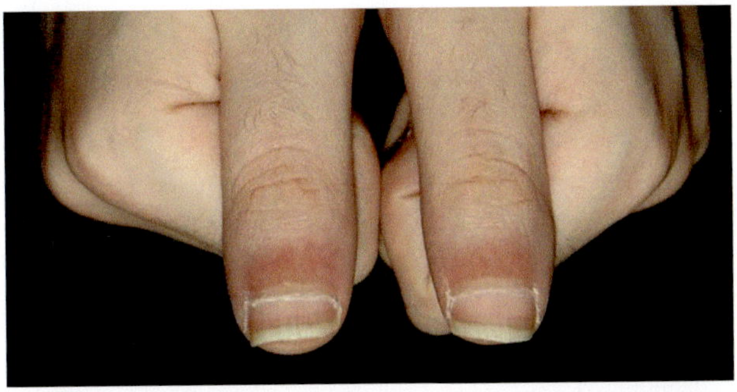

Fig. 53.2 20-Year-old male, Fitzpatrick type II, brachyonychia, with acquired racquet nail of the thumbs. Etiology: hyperparathyroidism (*from* Baran et al. [1]; *with permission*)

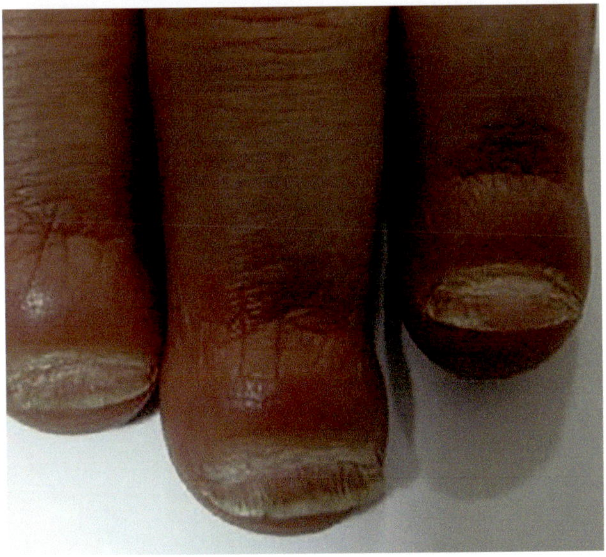

Fig. 53.3 16-Year-old female, Fitzpatrick type III, brachyonychia, with proximal onychoschizia and swelling of proximal nail folds. Etiology: acro-osteolysis from cold exposure (*from* El-Komy et al. [16]; *with permission*)

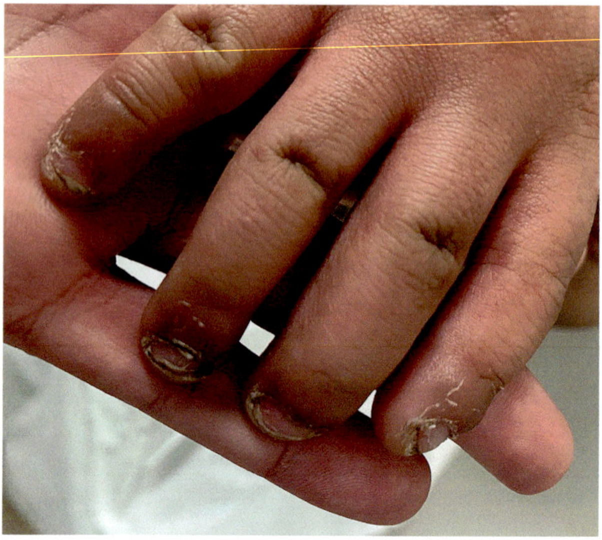

Fig. 53.4 Patient, Fitzpatrick type IV, brachyonychia, with dystrophic nails, with onycholysis, brachyonychia, and ragged cuticles. Etiology: Stüve-Wiedemann syndrome (*from* Almuhanna et al. [20]; *with permission*)

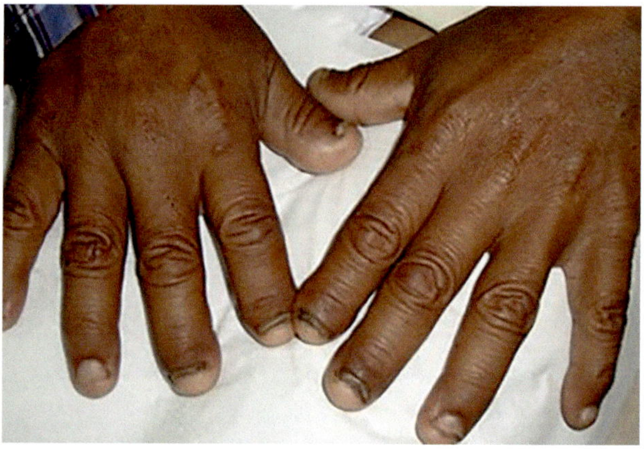

Fig. 53.5 Adult patient, Fitzpatrick type IV, brachyonychia, brachyonychia in a patient with 16 years of chronic kidney disease and 3 years of hemodialysis (*from* Rosales Figueroa et al. [12]; *with permission*)

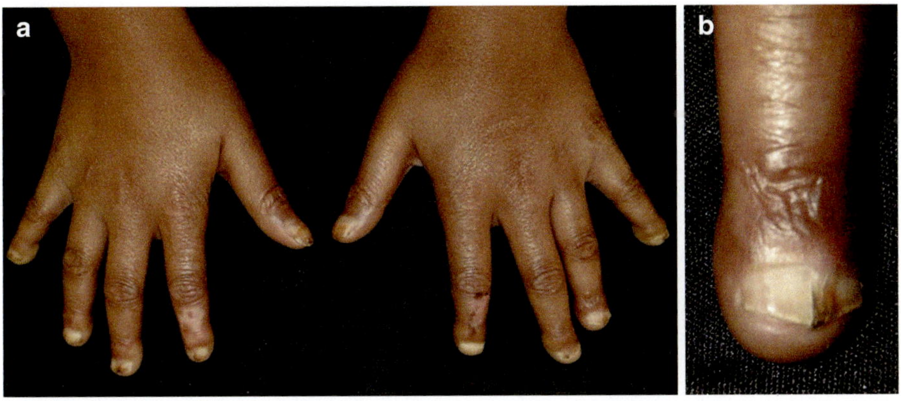

Fig. 53.6 (**a**) 10-Year-old female, Fitzpatrick type V, brachyonychia, with symmetric involvement with shortening of digits, brachyonychia, longitudinal ridging, and pterygium formation. Note the dyspigmentation of the skin of the second digits bilaterally. Etiology: idiopathic acro-osteolysis. (**b**) 10-Year-old female, Fitzpatrick type V, brachyonychia, with prominent pterygium. Etiology: idiopathic acro-osteolysis (*from* Gray et al. [11]; *with permission*)

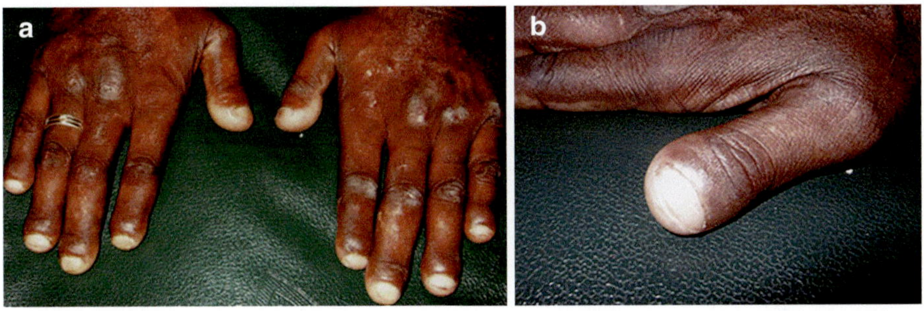

Fig. 53.7 (**a**) 35-Year-old male, Fitzpatrick type V, brachyonychia, with dorsal view of the hands showing racquet nails. Etiology: Erasmus syndrome. (**b**) 35-Year-old male, Fitzpatrick type V, brachyonychia, with racquet nail of the thumb. Etiology: Erasmus syndrome (*from* Vetrichevvel et al. [17]; *with permission*)

References

1. Baran R, Turkmani MG, Mubki T. Acquired racquet nails: a useful sign of hyperparathyroidism. J Eur Acad Dermatol Venereol. 2014;28(2):257–9.
2. Datta PK, Ghosh S, De A. Idiopathic non-familial acro-osteolysis: a rare case report. Indian J Dermatol. 2012;57(6):486–8.
3. Fairris GM, Rowell NR. Acquired racket nails. Clin Exp Dermatol. 1984;9(3):267–9.
4. Scher RK. Acro-osteolysis and the nail unit. Br J Dermatol. 1986;115(5):638–9.
5. Ronchese F. The racket thumb-nail. Dermatologica. 1973;146(3):199–202.
6. Detty SQ, Hinshaw MA, Tuite MJ, Means AD. Brachyonychia in a patient with Bardet-Biedl syndrome: case report and review of this rare syndrome. JAAD Case Rep. 2019;5(8):672–4.

7. Burrows H. Developmental abbreviation of terminal phalanges. Br J Radiol. 1938;11:165–76.
8. Harzy T, Benbouazza K, Lazrak N, Amine B, Hassouni NH. Idiopathic phalangeal acroosteolysis: a case report. Joint Bone Spine. 2003;70:146–8.
9. Todd G, Saxe N. Idiopathic phalangeal osteolysis. Arch Dermatol. 1994;130(6):759–62.
10. Chung BY, Choi YW, Kim HO, Park CW. Nail dystrophy in patients with atopic dermatitis and its association with disease severity. Ann Dermatol. 2019;31(2):121–6.
11. Gray NA, Scott C, Ngwanya RM, Pillay K, Isaacs T. Nail changes in acro-osteolysis: a case report and review of the literature. JAAD Case Rep. 2019;5(12):1033–6.
12. Rosales Figueroa JD, Chang P. Brachyonychia associated with acroosteolysis in chronic kidney disease: how phalange shape influences nail morphology. Skin Appendage Disord. 2018;4(4):264–7.
13. Rasi A, Soltani-Arabshahi R, Naraghi Z. Circumscribed juvenile-onset pityriasis rubra pilaris with hypoparathyroidism and brachyonychia. Cutis. 2006;77:218–22.
14. Belinchón Romero I, Ramos Rincón JM, Reyes Rabell F. Las uñas en la lepra [Nail involvement in leprosy]. Actas Dermosifiliogr. 2012;103(4):276–84. Spanish.
15. Rajput CD, Nikam BP, Gore SB, Malani SS. Nail changes in leprosy: an observational study of 125 patients. Indian Dermatol Online J. 2020;11(2):195–201.
16. El-Komy MH, Baran R. Acroosteolysis presenting with brachyonychia following exposure to cold. J Eur Acad Dermatol Venereol. 2015;29(11):2252–4.
17. Vetrichevvel TP, Renita L, Shobana S, Anandan S. Acquired racquet nails in Erasmus syndrome. Int J Dermatol. 2010;49(8):932–3.
18. Richert B, Choffray A, de la Brassinne M. Cosmetic surgery for congenital nail deformities. J Cosmet Dermatol. 2008;7(4):304–8.
19. Baran R. Nail contour variations. In: Pediatric nail disorders. CRC Press; 2016. p. 22–35.
20. Almuhanna N, Alogayell L, Alkhezzi S, Al-Malki S, Alhamazani R, Altassan F, Alsuhibani A, Alowairdhi Y, Alekrish K, Alhomida FA. A rare presentation of multiple eruptive vellus hair cysts and dystrophic nails in a pediatric patient with Stüve-Wiedemann syndrome. JAAD Case Rep. 2023;38:89–91.

Index

S. R. Lipner, *Atlas of Nail Disorders Across All Skin Colors*,
https://doi.org/10.1007/978-3-031-74272-9

V

W

X

Y

GPSR Compliance

The European Union's (EU) General Product Safety Regulation (GPSR) is a set of rules that requires consumer products to be safe and our obligations to ensure this.

If you have any concerns about our products, you can contact us on ProductSafety@springernature.com

In case Publisher is established outside the EU, the EU authorized representative is:

Springer Nature Customer Service Center GmbH
Europaplatz 3
69115 Heidelberg, Germany

Batch number: 10317666

Printed by Printforce, the Netherlands